Gynecologic Ultrasound

Guest Editors

SANDRA J. ALLISON, MD
DARCY J. WOLFMAN, MD

ULTRASOUND CLINICS

www.ultrasound.theclinics.com

April 2010 • Volume 5 • Number 2

SAUNDERS an imprint of ELSEVIER, Inc.

W.B. SAUNDERS COMPANY
A Division of Elsevier Inc.

1600 John F. Kennedy Boulevard • Suite 1800 • Philadelphia, Pennsylvania 19103-2899

http://www.theclinics.com

ULTRASOUND CLINICS Volume 5, Number 2
April 2010 ISSN 1556-858X, ISBN-13: 978-1-4377-2337-3

Editor: Barton Dudlick

Ultrasound Clinics (ISSN 1556-858X) is published quarterly by W.B. Saunders, 360 Park Avenue South, New York, NY 10010-1710. Months of publication are January, April, July, and October. Business and editorial offices: 1600 John F. Kennedy Boulevard, Suite 1800, Philadelphia, Pennsylvania 19103-2899. Accounting and circulation offices: 6277 Sea Harbor Drive, Orlando, FL 32887-4800. Periodicals postage paid at New York, NY, and additional mailing offices. Subscription prices are $204 per year for (US individuals), $279 per year for (US institutions), $102 per year for (US students and residents), $232 per year for (Canadian individuals), $312 per year for (Canadian institutions), $247 per year for (international individuals), $312 per year for (international institutions), and $123 per year for (Canadian and foreign students/residents). To receive student/resident rate, orders must be accompanied by name of affiliated institution, date of term, and the signature of program/residency coordinator on institution letterhead. Orders will be billed at individual rate until proof of status is received. Foreign air speed delivery is included in all Clinics subscription prices. All prices are subject to change without notice. **POSTMASTER:** Send address changes to *Ultrasound Clinics,* Elsevier Health Sciences Division, Subscription Customer Service, 3251 Riverport Lane, Maryland Heights, MO 63043. **Customer Service (orders, claims, online, change of address): Telephone: 1-800-654-2452 (U.S. and Canada); 314-447-8871 (outside U.S. and Canada). Fax: 314-447-8029. E-mail: journalscustomerservice-usa@elsevier.com (for print support); journalsonlinesupport-usa@elsevier.com (for online support).**

Reprints: For copies of 100 or more, of articles in this publication, please contact the Commercial Reprints Department, Elsevier Inc., 360 Park Avenue South, New York, NY 10010-1710. Tel.: (+1) 212-633-3812; Fax: (+1) 212-462-1935; E-mail: reprints@elsevier.com.

Contributors

GUEST EDITORS

SANDRA J. ALLISON, MD
Associate Professor of Radiology, Director, Division of Ultrasound, Georgetown University Hospital, Washington, DC

DARCY J. WOLFMAN, MD
Assistant Professor of Radiology, Georgetown University Hospital, Washington, DC

AUTHORS

SUSAN J. ACKERMAN, MD
Professor, Department of Radiology, Medical University of South Carolina, Charleston, South Carolina

SANDRA J. ALLISON, MD
Associate Professor of Radiology, Director, Division of Ultrasound, Georgetown University Hospital, Washington, DC

TERESITA L. ANGTUACO, MD
Professor of Radiology and Obstetrics, and Gynecology, Department of Radiology, University of Arkansas for Medical Sciences, Little Rock, Arkansas

MUNAZZA ANIS, MD
Assistant Professor, Department of Radiology, Medical University of South Carolina, Charleston, South Carolina

OKSANA H. BALTAROWICH, MD
Associate Professor of Radiology, Division of Diagnostic Ultrasound, Department of Radiology, Thomas Jefferson University, Philadelphia, Pennsylvania

ASHLEY CORBETT BRAGG, MD
Radiology Resident, Department of Radiology, University of Arkansas for Medical Sciences, Little Rock, Arkansas

NATASHA BRASIC, MD
Clinical Instructor, Ultrasound and Breast Imaging, Department of Radiology and Biomedical Imaging, University of California San Francisco, San Francisco, California

MARION BRODY, MD
Fellow, Abdominal Imaging, Department of Radiology, Hospital of the University of Pennsylvania, Philadelphia, Pennsylvania

LAWRENCE A. CICCHIELLO, MD
Department of Diagnostic Radiology, Yale University School of Medicine, New Haven, Connecticut

BEVERLY COLEMAN, MD, FACR
Professor and Associate Chairman of Radiology, Department of Radiology, Hospital of the University of Pennsylvania, Philadelphia, Pennsylvania

VICKIE A. FELDSTEIN, MD
Professor of Clinical Radiology and Obstetrics, Gynecology and Reproductive Sciences, Department of Radiology and Biomedical Imaging, University of California San Francisco, San Francisco, California

ULRIKE M. HAMPER, MD, MBA
Professor of Radiology and Urology Director, Division of Ultrasound, Department of Diagnostic Radiology, The Johns Hopkins Medical Institutes, Baltimore, Maryland

MINDY M. HORROW, MD, FACR
Director of Body Imaging, Department of Radiology, Albert Einstein Medical Center; Associate Professor of Radiology, School of Medicine, Thomas Jefferson University, Philadelphia, Pennsylvania

ABID IRSHAD, MD
Associate Professor, Department of Radiology, Medical University of South Carolina, Charleston, South Carolina

ANNA S. LEV-TOAFF, MD, FACR
Professor of Radiology, Department of Radiology, Hospital of the University of Pennsylvania, Philadelphia, Pennsylvania

DOLORES H. PRETORIUS, MD
Professor of Radiology, Department of Radiology, University of California San Diego, San Diego, California

LESLIE M. SCOUTT, MD
Professor of Radiology and Chief, Ultrasound Service, Department of Diagnostic Radiology, Yale University School of Medicine, New Haven, Connecticut

CECILE A. UNGER, MD
Resident, Department of Vincent Obstetrics and Gynecology, Massachusetts General Hospital, Boston, Massachusetts

MILENA M. WEINSTEIN, MD
Assistant, Division of Urogynecology and Reconstructive Pelvic Medicine, Department of Vincent Obstetrics and Gynecology, Massachusetts General Hospital, Boston, Massachusetts

DARCY J. WOLFMAN, MD
Assistant Professor of Radiology, Georgetown University Hospital, Washington, DC

Contents

Preface **xi**

Sandra J. Allison and Darcy J. Wolfman

Technical Approach

Avoiding Pitfalls in Transvaginal Sonography of the Female Pelvis **177**

Oksana H. Baltarowich and Leslie M. Scoutt

Transvaginal sonography (TVS) is currently the preferred method for sonographic evaluation of the female pelvis. Although TVS allows for more accurate diagnosis of female pelvic conditions, one must be aware of potential pitfalls in technique, protocols and interpretation of images.These may all lead to errors in diagnosis and possibly to inappropriate treatment of the patient. This article discusses the potential areas where pitfalls may occur as it takes the reader through the components of a transvaginal sonographic examination of the pelvis in a step-wise fashion.

Pearls and Pitfalls in Sonohysterography **195**

Sandra J. Allison, Mindy M. Horrow, and Anna S. Lev-Toaff

Sonohysterography is a useful adjunct to transvaginal sonography, especially for evaluation of the endometrium and adjacent lesions. The examination is well tolerated, with few complications. Knowledge of potential technical and interpretive pitfalls is essential to minimize patient discomfort, prevent nondiagnostic procedures, and ensure accurate interpretation. Proper technique will increase the efficiency and success rate of the procedure by allowing the practitioner to obtain diagnostic information for the patient and her referring physician.

Clinical Approach

Ultrasound Evaluation of Gynecologic Causes of Pelvic Pain **209**

Lawrence A. Cicchiello, Ulrike M. Hamper, and Leslie M. Scoutt

Ultrasound should be considered the first-line imaging modality of choice in women presenting with acute or chronic pelvic pain of suspected gynecologic or obstetric origin because many, if not most, gynecologic/obstetric causes of pelvic pain are easily diagnosed on ultrasound examination. Since the clinical presentation of gynecologic causes of pelvic pain overlaps with gastrointestinal and genitourinary pathology, referral to CT or MRI, especially in pregnant patients, should be considered if the US examination is nondiagnostic.

Ultrasound for Pelvic Pain: Nongynecologic Causes **233**

Susan J. Ackerman, Abid Irshad, and Munazza Anis

Acute pelvic pain in women is a common presenting complaint that can result from various conditions. Because these conditions can be of gynecologic or nongynecologic origin, they may pose a challenge to the diagnostic acumen of physicians, including radiologists. A thorough workup should include clinical

history, physical examination, laboratory data, and appropriate imaging studies, all of which should be available to the radiologist for evaluation. Ultrasound is the primary imaging modality in women with acute pelvic pain because of its high sensitivity, low cost, wide availability, and lack of ionizing radiation, particularly when a gynecologic disorder is suspected as the underlying cause. However, other modalities such as computed tomography (CT) and magnetic resonance imaging (MRI) may be very helpful, especially when a nongynecologic condition is suspected.

Dysfunctional Uterine Bleeding: Diagnostic Approach and Therapeutic Options **245**

Natasha Brasic and Vickie A. Feldstein

Abnormal uterine bleeding is a common symptom in pre- and postmenopausal women and appropriate triage of patients may be made with transvaginal sonography (TVUS) and, in some cases, subsequent saline-infused sonohysterography (SIS). Techniques, pitfalls, possible findings at TVUS and SIS are discussed, including focal and diffuse findings such as endometrial polyps, submucosal leiomyomas, and endometrial hyperplasia. Management recommendations based on disease process are discussed. Endometrial findings on TVUS and management of these findings in patients taking tamoxifen are addressed. A general algorithm is proposed in the workup of abnormal uterine bleeding.

The Ultrasound Workup of Adnexal Masses **257**

Marion Brody and Beverly Coleman

Adnexal masses, both painful and asymptomatic, are commonly encountered entities in clinical practice. Ultrasound is generally the initial imaging evaluation, because it is readily available, inexpensive, and has a high negative predictive value. The goal is to identify distinguishing features of the adnexal mass and to assess its malignant potential. In some cases, follow-up ultrasound or MRI may be necessary. In this article, adnexal masses are classified as cystic, complex, or solid based on pattern recognition.

Sonographic Evaluation of Patients Treated with Uterine Artery Embolization **277**

Sandra J. Allison and Darcy J. Wolfman

Uterine artery embolization (UAE) is one of the treatment options for patients with symptomatic fibroids. Ultrasound can be used in the preprocedural work-up of patients considering UAE. It can also be used to follow-up patients after the procedure and to assess for complications in patients who present with pain after UAE.

Applications of Ultrasound in Gynecologic Oncology **289**

Darcy J. Wolfman and Sandra J. Allison

In patients with gynecologic malignancy, ultrasound (US) has many established applications, including the diagnosis and staging of ovarian cancer, endometrial cancer, and gestational trophoblastic disease (GTD); detection of recurrent and/or metastatic disease, including ovarian and cervical cancer and GTD; and diagnosis and guidance for treatment of postoperative complications.

Future

Three-Dimensional Gynecologic Ultrasound 299

Ashley Corbett Bragg and Teresita L. Angtuaco

Three-dimensional (3D) ultrasound has introduced added value to pelvic sonography. It has allowed the display of coronal images not previously possible with 2D ultrasound, enhancing the accuracy of ultrasound in the diagnosis of uterine anomalies due to its capability of outlining both external uterine contour and endometrial abnormalities. The ability of 3D ultrasound ability to define endometrial pathology is superior to that of 2D ultrasound and complementary to that of saline infusion sonohysterography (SIS). The volumetric data it provides improve work flow efficiency and allow off-line data analysis. Consultation with referring clinicians and other specialists is made possible through storage of data sets that can be manipulated without the need for repeat studies.

Pelvic Floor Imaging 313

Cecile A. Unger, Milena M. Weinstein, and Dolores H. Pretorius

Pelvic floor ultrasound is a valuable adjunct in elucidation of cause, diagnosis, and treatment of pelvic floor disorders. Three-dimensional ultrasound specifically has been shown to have many advantages over conventional imaging modalities. Proper evaluation of pelvic floor muscle function, strength, and integrity is an important component of diagnosis and treatment of pelvic floor disorders. The pelvic floor muscle training used to change the structural support and strength of muscle contraction requires clinicians to be able to conduct high-quality measurements of pelvic floor muscle function and strength. Ultrasound is a useful modality to assess the pelvic floor and its function. As practitioners become more familiar with the advantages and capabilities of ultrasound, this tool should become part of routine clinical practice in evaluation and management of pelvic floor disorders.

Index 331

Ultrasound Clinics

FORTHCOMING ISSUES

July 2010

Genitourinary Ultrasound
Mukund Joshi, MD, and Paul Sidhu, MD, *Guest Editors*

October 2010

Vascular Ultrasound
Beatrice L. Madrazo, MD, *Guest Editor*

January 2011

Advanced Obstetric Ultrasound
Theodore Dubinsky, MD, and Manjiri Dighe, MD, *Guest Editors*

RECENT ISSUES

January 2010

Pediatric Ultrasound, Part 2
Brian D. Coley, MD, *Guest Editor*

October 2009

Pediatric Ultrasound Part 1
Brian D. Coley, MD, *Guest Editor*

July 2009

Advances in Ultrasound
Vikram Dogra, MD, *Guest Editor*

GOAL STATEMENT

The goal of the *Ultrasound Clinics* is to keep practicing radiologists and radiology residents up to date with current clinical practice in ultrasound by providing timely articles reviewing the state of the art in patient care.

ACCREDITATION

The *Ultrasound Clinics* is planned and implemented in accordance with the Essential Areas and Policies of the Accreditation Council for Continuing Medical Education (ACCME) through the joint sponsorship of the University of Virginia School of Medicine and Elsevier. The University of Virginia School of Medicine is accredited by the ACCME to provide continuing medical education for physicians.

The University of Virginia School of Medicine designates this educational activity for a maximum of 15 *AMA PRA Category 1 Credits*™ for each issue, 60 credits per year. Physicians should only claim credit commensurate with the extent of their participation in the activity.

The American Medical Association has determined that physicians not licensed in the US who participate in this CME activity are eligible for a maximum of 15 *AMA PRA Category 1 Credits*™ for each issue, 60 credits per year.

Credit can be earned by reading the text material, taking the CME examination online at http://www.theclinics.com/home/cme, and completing the evaluation. After taking the test, you will be required to review any and all incorrect answers. Following completion of the test and evaluation, your credit will be awarded and you may print your certificate.

FACULTY DISCLOSURE/CONFLICT OF INTEREST

The University of Virginia School of Medicine, as an ACCME accredited provider, endorses and strives to comply with the Accreditation Council for Continuing Medical Education (ACCME) Standards of Commercial Support, Commonwealth of Virginia statutes, University of Virginia policies and procedures, and associated federal and private regulations and guidelines on the need for disclosure and monitoring of proprietary and financial interests that may affect the scientific integrity and balance of content delivered in continuing medical education activities under our auspices.

The University of Virginia School of Medicine requires that all CME activities accredited through this institution be developed independently and be scientifically rigorous, balanced and objective in the presentation/discussion of its content, theories and practices.

All authors/editors participating in an accredited CME activity are expected to disclose to the readers relevant financial relationships with commercial entities occurring within the past 12 months (such as grants or research support, employee, consultant, stock holder, member of speakers bureau, etc.). The University of Virginia School of Medicine will employ appropriate mechanisms to resolve potential conflicts of interest to maintain the standards of fair and balanced education to the reader. Questions about specific strategies can be directed to the Office of Continuing Medical Education, University of Virginia School of Medicine, Charlottesville, Virginia.

The faculty and staff of the University of Virginia Office of Continuing Medical Education have no financial affiliations to disclose.

The authors/editors listed below have identified no professional or financial affiliations for themselves or their spouse/partner:

Susan J. Ackerman, MD; Sandra J. Allison, MD (Guest Editor); Teresita L. Angtuaco, MD; Munazza Anis, MD; Oksana H. Baltarowich, MD; Matthew J. Bassignani, MD (Test Author); Ashley Corbett Bragg, MD; Marion Brody, MD; Lawrence A. Cicchiello, MD; Beverly Coleman, MD; Vikram S. Dogra, MD (Consulting Editor); Barton Dudlick (Acquisitions Editor); Vickie A. Feldstein, MD; Ulrike M. Hamper, MD, MBA; Mindy M. Horrow, MD; Abid Irshad, MD; Anna S. Lev-Toaff, MD; Cecile A. Unger, MD; Milena M. Weinstein, MD; Darcy J. Wolfman, MD (Guest Editor).

The authors/editors listed below have identified the following professional or financial affiliations for themselves or their spouse/partner:

Natasha Brasic, MD is employed by and owns stock in Gilead Sciences.

Dolores H. Pretorius, MD has an equipment loan from General Electric, and has an equipment loan from and is a consultant for Phillips Medical Systems.

Leslie M. Scoutt, MD is an educational consultant for Philips.

Disclosure of Discussion of Non-FDA Approved Uses for Pharmaceutical Products and/or Medical Devices.

The University of Virginia School of Medicine, as an ACCME provider, requires that all faculty presenters identify and disclose any off-label uses for pharmaceutical and medical device products. The University of Virginia School of Medicine recommends that each physician fully review all the available data on new products or procedures prior to clinical use.

TO ENROLL

To enroll in the *Ultrasound Clinics* Continuing Medical Education program, call customer service at 1-800-654-2452 or visit us online at www.theclinics.com/home/cme. The CME program is available to subscribers for an additional fee of $205.00.

Preface

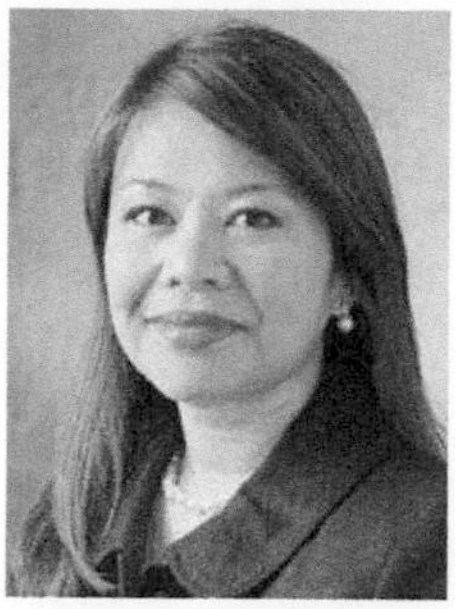 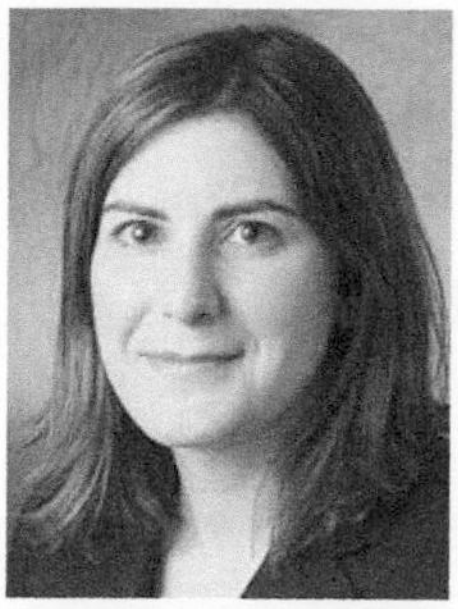

Sandra J. Allison, MD   Darcy J. Wolfman, MD
Guest Editors

During the planning stages of this edition of *Ultrasound Clinics*, we bounced around many ideas on how to make this issue of gynecologic ultrasound appealing and useful to practicing radiologists. It is not infrequent during resident and fellow readout that one of our trainees comments on how the pearls we are dispatching are not easily found in books. This is usually said when we are sharing scanning tricks or discussing how to approach certain patients. These observations were the seed for the organization of this issue.

The first part includes practical tips and tricks for performing transvaginal sonography and sonohysterography. The second part addresses work-up of patients based on their presentation: bleeding, pain, or adnexal mass. This is followed by articles on sonographic work-up or follow-up of patients commonly encounter in practices: those who have undergone uterine artery embolization and those who are treated for gynecologic malignancy. Finally, the issue ends with articles about more recent advances in ultrasound. There are practical tips for 3-D imaging and applications for its use in assessing the pelvic floor.

Much like an apprenticeship, ultrasound is an art that is passed down from teacher to pupil. Ultrasound is unique in radiology in that obtaining the images is oftentimes more difficult than the interpretation and this skill is not easily learned. We were both fortunate to have learned the art of ultrasound from some of the best in the field. The contributing authors are well-known masters and teachers of ultrasound and people from whom we have personally learned.

The authors all took our mission to heart and have written wonderful articles that address practical and up-to-date topics in ultrasound. We hope that with this issue, their tricks of the trade and systematic approach to working up patients are passed down to the readers and that you, the readers, will learn from our teachers and this issue as much as we did.

ACKNOWLEDGMENTS

We were warned that editing a volume could be a painful experience but we have to thank all the authors for proving that to be completely untrue. It could not have been an easier or a more enjoyable experience given the talent and professionalism that ooze from this group. Anna Lev-Toaff deserves a special thank you for being involved from the beginning; we owe the learning and experience we gained with this project to her. Leslie Scoutt got us through the very early stages by providing us with invaluable insight and solicited advice. In the 11th hour, Larry Needleman saved us by digging up that last needed image. Michael McCullough provided professional photography. Ashley

Ultrasound Clin 5 (2010) xi–xii
doi:10.1016/j.cult.2010.05.001

Stowell was a word processing whiz. And finally, our families have been unwavering in their support and encouragement.

Sandra J. Allison, MD
Department of Radiology
Georgetown University Medical Center
3800 Reservoir Road, NW
Washington, DC 20007, USA

Darcy J. Wolfman, MD
Department of Radiology
Georgetown University Hospital
3800 Reservoir Road, NW
Washington, DC 20007, USA

E-mail addresses:
sa263@gunet.georgetown.edu (S.J. Allison)
DJW106@gunet.georgetown.edu (D.J. Wolfman)

Avoiding Pitfalls in Transvaginal Sonography of the Female Pelvis

Oksana H. Baltarowich, MD[a,*], Leslie M. Scoutt, MD[b]

KEYWORDS

- Transvaginal sonography • Transvaginal pelvic scanning
- Pitfalls • Pelvic ultrasonography
- Ultrasonographic scanning techniques

At present, transvaginal sonography (TVS) is the preferred method for sonographic evaluation of the female pelvis. Although the transvaginal technique has numerous advantages in comparison with transabdominal imaging of the pelvis and allows for more accurate diagnosis as a result of increased spatial and soft tissue resolution, one must be aware of potential pitfalls in technique, protocols, and interpretation of images that may lead to errors in diagnosis and inappropriate treatment of the patient. This article examines the places where pitfalls may occur while analyzing the components of a TVS examination of the pelvis in a stepwise method.

KNOW THE OB-GYN HISTORY

Several pitfalls can be avoided even before the probe is placed into the vagina. Knowledge of the patient's clinical history is more important in imaging the female pelvis than in most other ultrasonogaphic examinations because the appearance of the normal anatomy and the type of potential pathologic conditions vary depending on the hormonal status of the patient. Before performing any pelvic sonogram the sonographer should, at a minimum, know the patient's age, parity, last menstrual period, and hormonal status, particularly infertility treatment, hormone replacement therapy, and use of SERMs—selective estrogen receptor modulators (tamoxifen used in the past, raloxifene used most commonly at present). For example, the list of differential diagnoses for a small round cystic mass within a thickened endometrium is very different for a woman of reproductive age than for a postmenopausal woman on raloxifene therapy (**Fig. 1**). Similarly, a personal history of certain types of malignancies makes a pelvic mass more suspicious for recurrence or metastasis. Use of assisted reproductive techniques alerts one to the increased risk of heterotopic pregnancies, which have become increasingly popular over the years. At present, 1% to 3% of pregnancies achieved following assisted reproduction technology are heterotopic pregnancies.[1]

One should also be aware of special clinical circumstances that might influence the sonographic technique or protocol. Transvaginal evaluation of cervical length is routinely conducted in patients with preterm labor. However, in the case of preterm rupture of the membranes, transperineal sonography may be the preferred method for cervical evaluation[2] because this approach carries a lower potential risk of infection. If transperineal sonography proves to be inadequate, then TVS of the cervix may be required.

[a] Division of Diagnostic Ultrasound, Department of Radiology, Thomas Jefferson University, 132 South 10th Street, Suite 796B Main Building, Philadelphia, PA 19107-5244, USA
[b] Ultrasound Service, Department of Radiology, Yale University School of Medicine, 333 Cedar Street, PO Box 208042, New Haven, CT 06520-8042, USA
* Corresponding author.
E-mail address: oksana.baltarowich@jefferson.edu

Ultrasound Clin 5 (2010) 177–193
doi:10.1016/j.cult.2010.03.009
1556-858X/10/$ – see front matter

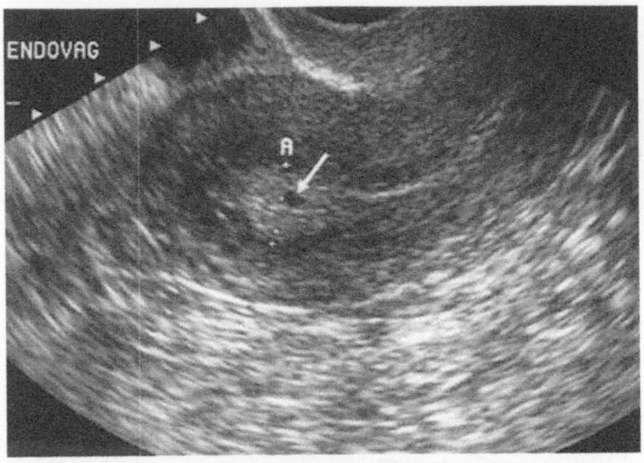

Fig. 1. Transvaginal sagittal sonogram demonstrates a thick endometrium measured as A, containing a small cystic area (*arrow*). Without knowledge of the patient's age and gynecologic history, the list of differential diagnoses is long and varied. If the patient is in child-bearing years, such an appearance of endometrium could represent an early intrauterine pregnancy. But in this 65-year-old patient on SERM, it represented cystic change in a surgically proven endometrial polyp.

Listening to the patient and scanning over the area where the patient experiences pain help to avoid missing a diagnosis or performing an inappropriate or incomplete study. For example, a patient who presents for pelvic sonography with pain may actually be experiencing abdominal wall pain from causes such as abdominal wall endometriosis (**Fig. 2**), malignant lymph node metastasis, hernia, rectus sheath hematoma, or abscess. Examination of the anterior abdominal wall requires a high-frequency linear array transducer. The curved array probe typically used for transabdominal scanning does not have adequate near-field resolution to evaluate the anterior abdominal wall, and the transvaginal probe does not have adequate depth or a large enough field of view to image the more distant anterior subcutaneous tissues. In another example, a patient presenting with right-sided pelvic pain, on closer questioning, may explain that her pain started in the flank and settled in the right pelvis. Using this information, transabdominal sonography (TAS) of the kidneys and TVS with attention to the right ureterovesical junction (UVJ) becomes important to assess for hydronephrosis and a right UVJ calculus (**Fig. 3**).[3]

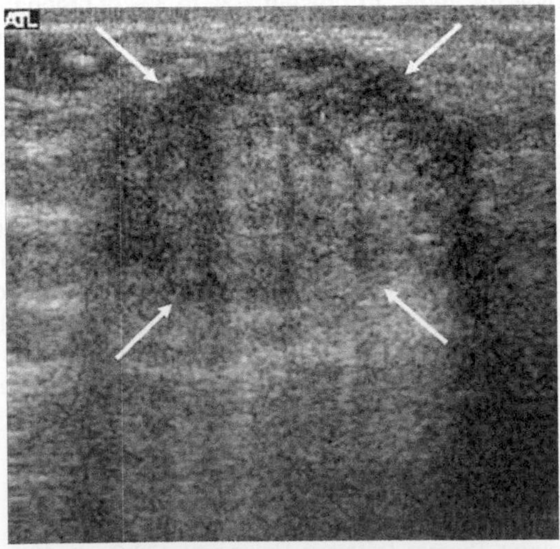

Fig. 2. A 30-year-old woman was scanned transvaginally for indication of "pelvic pain." However, on further questioning she pointed to her abdominal wall as the source of pain. An image obtained using a high-frequency 10-MHz linear array transducer shows a solid abdominal wall mass (*arrows*) that was proven by biopsy to be endometriosis.

One should always attempt to answer the clinician's question. If a good clinician feels a mass on pelvic examination and it is not identified on the initial sonogram, then one should be persistent and continue searching the sonogram. Dermoid cysts of the ovary and pedunculated subserosal myomas, especially when they are solitary, are notorious for having high miss rates when evaluating the female pelvis with ultrasonography.

PRESCAN TRANSABDOMINALLY

TAS offers a general pelvic overview, whereas transvaginal scanning provides a focused or targeted higher-resolution evaluation of pelvic structures. To avoid tunnel vision, one should first look at the big picture. Although TVS has replaced TAS as the primary method for evaluation of the female pelvis because of the improved resolution afforded by the use of higher frequency transvaginal transducers, TAS is still considered as a complementary imaging technique and is particularly important for evaluation of the upper pelvis. However, a painful and uncomfortably full bladder is no longer considered necessary for transabdominal evaluation of the female pelvis, and although a partially full bladder provides a more limited view of the pelvis, in most cases it will be adequate to avoid diagnostic errors.[4,5]

At the authors' institutions, investigation of the female pelvis begins by a quick transabdominal prescan, which is performed irrespective of how full the bladder is at the time of presentation. Most women have a partially full bladder when this limited transabdominal scan is performed.

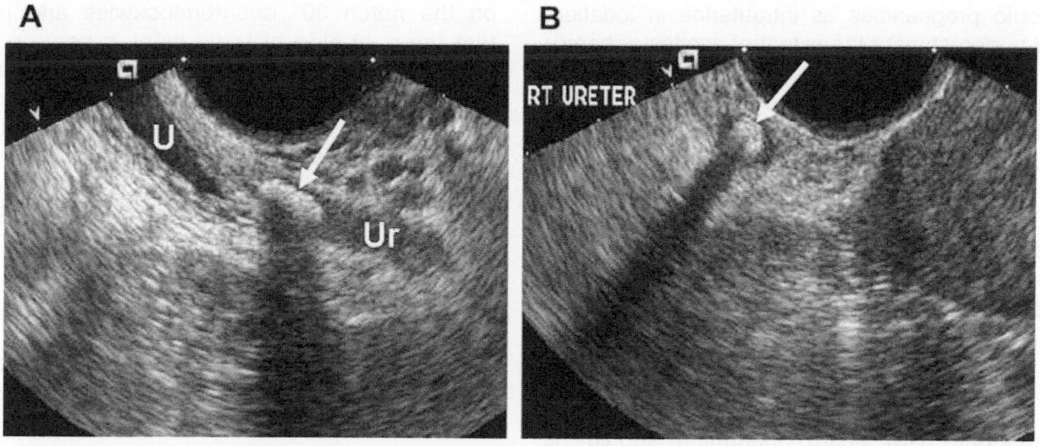

Fig. 3. (*A*) Transvaginal longitudinal sonogram along the course of the distal right ureter (Ur) shows a shadowing calculus (*arrow*) at the ureterovesical junction near the empty urinary bladder (U). (*B*) Transaxial transvaginal sonogram through the distal right ureter also demonstrates the shadowing calculus (*arrow*).

The patient is then asked to void completely and the pelvis is subsequently scanned transvaginally. In a study of 206 patients reported by Benacerraf and coworkers,[5] TVS alone was thought to be sufficient to visualize all the findings in 83.5% of patients. An additional 15% of patients required TAS without a full bladder with only 1.5% of patients requiring TAS examination with a completely full bladder to identify all the clinically important findings.

The transabdominal prescan with an empty or partially full bladder does not offer an optimal evaluation of pelvic structures, but is important because it actually directs the transvaginal ultrasound (which way the uterus is pointing), provides an estimation of the uterine size (best way to measure the uterus), and is the best way to search for masses above the fundus of the uterus such as a pedunculated myoma (**Fig. 4**) or a large ovarian mass, and to evaluate for intra-abdominal fluid.[6–11] Some ectopic pregnancies are seen only on TAS examination. In addition, the transverse transabdominal scan of an anteverted uterus may show a true coronal section of the uterus providing the best visualization of the fundal contour, which is important when there is a question of a congenital anomaly.

If patients are scanned only transvaginally, then one is likely to miss, incompletely visualize, or misinterpret a large pelvic mass, incompletely scan a large uterus, miss a pedunculated subserosal myoma, miss an ectopic or intrauterine pregnancy in a high pelvic location, misinterpret some

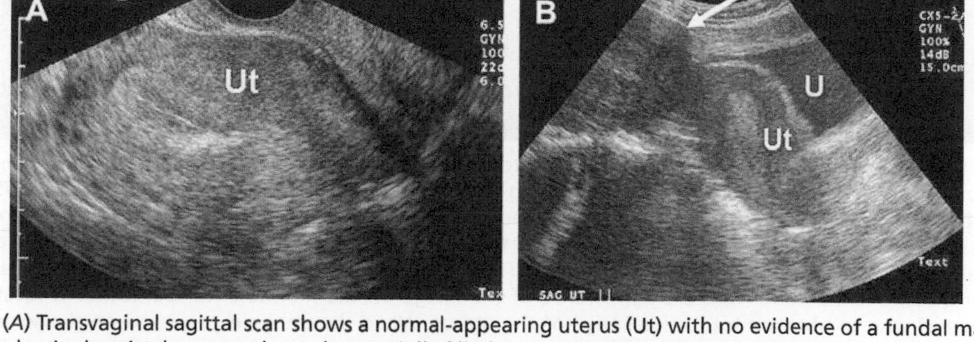

Fig. 4. (*A*) Transvaginal sagittal scan shows a normal-appearing uterus (Ut) with no evidence of a fundal mass. (*B*) Transabdominal sagittal prescan through a partially filled urinary bladder (U) shows a large pedunculated myoma (*arrow*) attached to the fundus of the uterus (Ut) that would have been missed by TVS alone.

ectopic pregnancies as intrauterine in location, and underestimate the extent of ascites or hemoperitoneum, which is easily detected on a quick scan through the right upper quadrant. Because high-resolution transvaginal probes have decreased beam penetration, uteri longer than 8 to 10 cm cannot be completely evaluated by TVS. An intrauterine or extrauterine gestational sac in or above an enlarged uterus may not be imaged transvaginally and may be missed altogether.

CHECK BEAM ORIENTATION

Ultrasound (US) beam orientation should be checked either by touching the surface of the probe before insertion or by checking after the transducer is placed into the vagina. Usually the handle of a transvaginal probe is marked with a notch, groove, or a flat surface to mark the "up side" of the US beam. The examiner should keep his or her thumb on the notch while scanning. On a sagittal image of the pelvis, the urinary bladder should appear in the upper left-hand corner of the image on the monitor (see **Fig. 3**A). This action ensures that the image is not reversed and helps one recognize whether the uterus is anteverted or retroverted. When coronal/axial scans are performed, the operator should rotate the probe with the thumb on the notch 90° counterclockwise and note that the right side of the patient is now on the left side of the monitor. This procedure ensures that the image is not reversed and correctly places a mass in the right or left side of the pelvis. In summary, there are 3 ways to check for correct beam orientation on the image: (1) touch the surface of the probe; (2) the urinary bladder should be imaged in the left upper corner of the sagittal image; (3) on the coronal image, the right side of the patient should be projected on the left side of the monitor. Therefore, the left side of the image on the monitor should move when the right side of patient's pelvis is probed.

UNDERSTAND IMAGE PROJECTION

By convention, most manufacturers display the narrowest part of the beam, which is always closest to the transducer face as it exits the transducer, at the top of the image. Therefore for TVS, the image has to be rotated 90° from the way the beam enters the body (**Fig. 5**). This technique becomes important for understanding how fluid-fluid levels project on an image, and anterior-posterior or cranial-caudal locations of masses in the uterus or adnexa (**Fig. 6**).

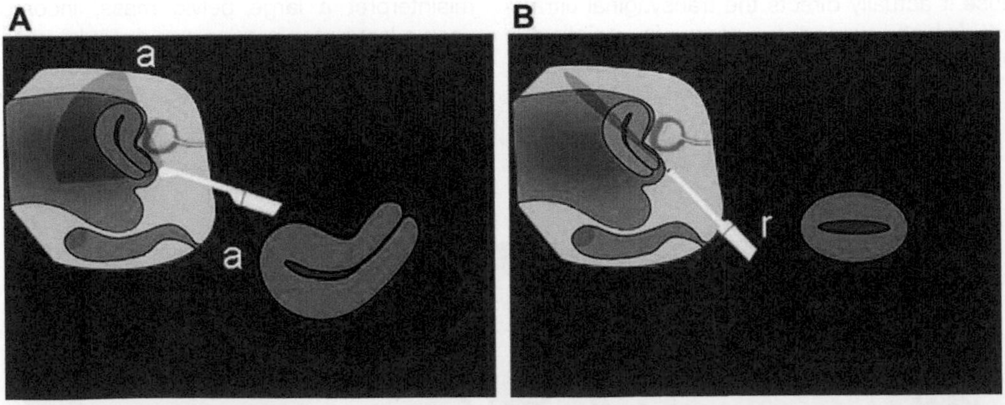

Fig. 5. (*A*) A transvaginal sagittal scan of an anteverted/anteflexed uterus and the appearance of the image on the monitor. US images are projected on the viewing monitor at 90° angles to the orientation of the US beam in the body. The apex (narrowest portion) of the beam is located at the face of the transducer, but is projected on the monitor at a 90° rotation so that it appears at the top of the image. The location of the anterior abdominal wall (a) is shown on both the transabdominal and transvaginal scans. (*B*) A transvaginal transverse scan of an anteverted/anteflexed uterus and the appearance of the image on the monitor. The transducer is rotated 90° counterclockwise to obtain a transverse image of the uterus. When the image is projected on the screen, it is also turned 90° so that the apex of the beam is at the top of the image on the monitor. The right side (r) of the uterus is on the left side of the image.

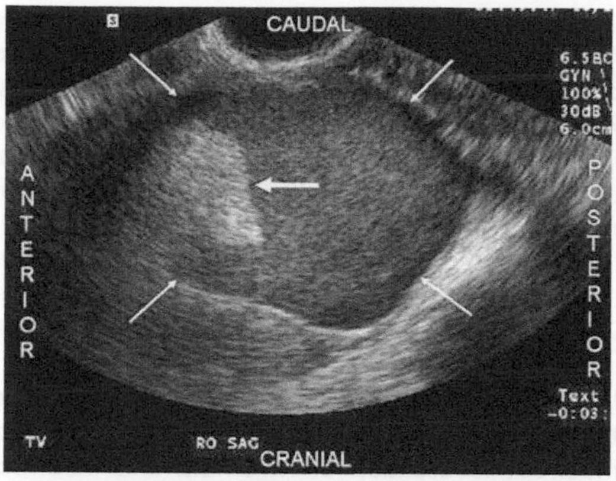

Fig. 6. Transvaginal sagittal scan of the right adnexa shows a cystic mass (*thin arrows*) filled with internal echoes and layering of hyperechoic material (*thick arrow*) in the nondependent portion of the mass (note anterior direction). Findings are virtually diagnostic of a fat-fluid level in a benign dermoid cyst of the ovary with hyperechoic fat floating on top of serous fluid with low-level echoes. Cranial, caudal, anterior, and posterior labels refer to orientation in the patient's body. The apex of the beam is at the top of the image.

DOCUMENT THE URINARY BLADDER

Another pitfall is forgetting to look at the urinary bladder before scanning the reproductive organs. Because the patient is asked to void before the transvaginal scan, the bladder is typically collapsed and small, and therefore may be hard to see. To find the empty bladder, one must deliberately angle the probe anteriorly without exerting pressure. Too much pressure on the bladder and urethra is uncomfortable for the patient and may also completely appose the bladder walls, thus making the bladder unrecognizable.

Identification of the urinary bladder aids in recognition of pelvic masses that are located anterior to the uterus. Occasionally a cystic mass anterior to the uterus is misinterpreted as the urinary bladder. This pitfall can be avoided by an initial careful search for the bladder (**Fig. 7**). This preliminary step may also help find the occasional unsuspected bladder tumor and identify lower urinary tract conditions not conventionally imaged by TVS (**Fig. 8**).

DOCUMENT THE CERVIX

After the probe is placed into the vagina and the position of the urinary bladder is documented, the next step is to examine the uterine cervix. The entire cervix should be imaged separately from the uterus with the beam directed as perpendicular to the cervix as possible to show the entire cervical length and to include a clearance of 2 to 3 cm beyond its borders. This simple step is often bypassed, which may lead to several pitfalls. Documentation of the cervix helps to avoid missing a mass within the

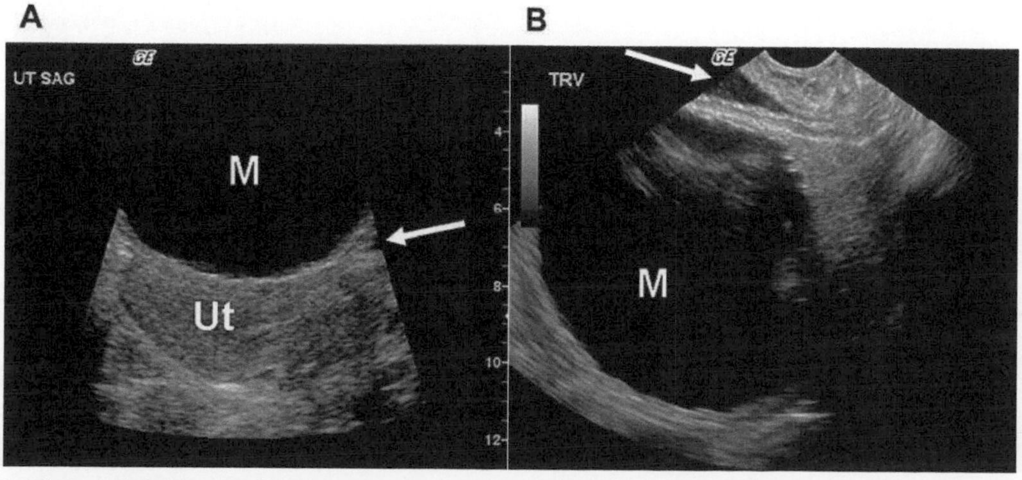

Fig. 7. (*A*) Transabdominal midline sagittal sonogram demonstrates the uterus (Ut) behind a large cystic structure (M) that was thought initially to be a distended urinary bladder. However, the bladder (*arrow*) was actually compressed by the mass (M) and was collapsed and small. (*B*) Transvaginal sagittal scan of the pelvis shows the collapsed urinary bladder (*arrow*) and the large cystic mass (M), which was mistaken for the urinary bladder on the transabdominal scan.

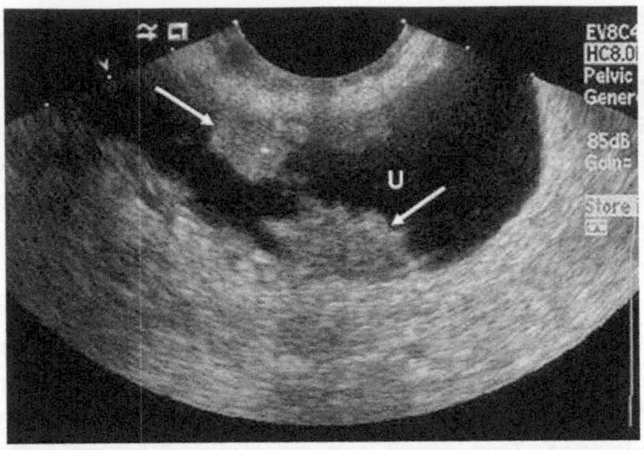

Fig. 8. Transvaginal sonogram of the urinary bladder (U) in an 80-year-old patient with postmenopausal bleeding shows 2 incidental irregularly outlined bladder wall masses (*arrows*) that proved to be transitional cell carcinomas. The pelvic organs were normal. The bleeding was a result of hematuria, not vaginal bleeding.

cervix, such as a polyp, a prolapsing myoma (**Fig. 9**), or a potentially life-threatening cervical ectopic pregnancy (**Fig. 10**). Documentation reminds one to look at the deep cul-de-sac, which may be the only place where echogenic free fluid, representing hemoperitoneum or pus, or masses such as peritoneal implants may be visualized.

In addition, the linear echo of the endocervical canal serves as a guide to the endometrial cavity, helping to align the beam with the linear echo of the endometrium and identifying the true longitudinal midline plane of the uterus. Accurate measurement of the endometrium must be made on a true midline longitudinal image of the uterus. Finding the endometrial cavity helps to locate intrauterine pregnancies and avoid the rare, but dangerous misinterpretation of an ectopic pregnancy as an intrauterine pregnancy (**Fig. 11**).

DETERMINE UTERINE POSITION

Identification of variations of uterus position during the transvaginal scan helps to avoid pitfalls of incorrect localization of myomata and incorrect endometrial measurement, which may lead to the erroneous conclusion of a falsely thickened endometrium and thus result in unnecessary invasive procedures. This mistake may occur when the endometrium is measured in an oblique or coronal plane (**Fig. 12**) rather than in the true midline longitudinal plane of the uterus. Usually the longitudinal axis of the uterus corresponds to the sagittal plane of the body (**Fig. 13**). One must find the longitudinal midline of the uterus by taking into account any obliquity of the uterus from the midline sagittal plane of the body (**Fig. 14**), tilting of the uterus anteriorly or posteriorly in the pelvis, or rotation of the uterus around its longitudinal axis (**Figs. 15** and **16**).

One should have a clear understanding of the sonographic appearances of uteri in various anatomic positions, including anteverted/anteflexed, retroverted/retroflexed, and mid-position (**Figs. 17–19**). The 90° view is just that—whatever is the resultant imaging plane of the uterus after

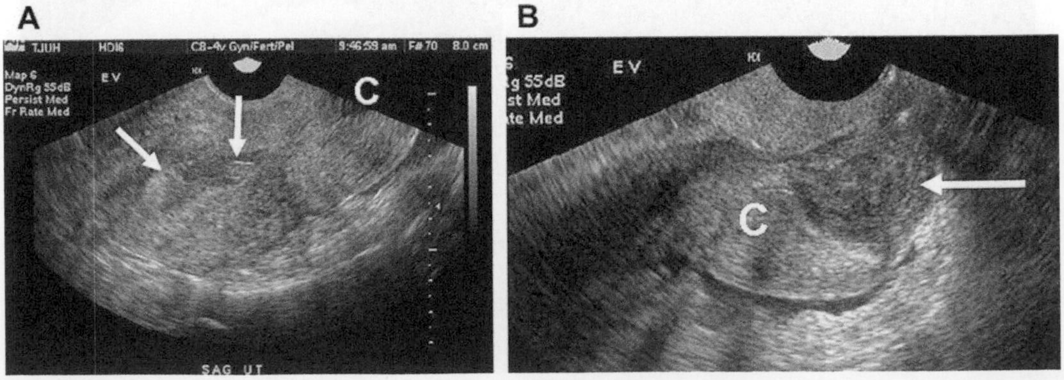

Fig. 9. (*A*) Midline transvaginal sonogram of the uterus demonstrates heterogeneous echoes (*arrows*) that were due to blood within the distended endometrial cavity, but the entire cervix (C) is not included in the image. (*B*) Transvaginal sagittal sonogram directed squarely at the cervix (C) shows that there is an endocervical mass (*arrow*), proven to be a polypoid myoma, protruding through the external cervical os. This mass was beyond image *A* and would have been missed. There is a small amount of free fluid in the cul-de-sac.

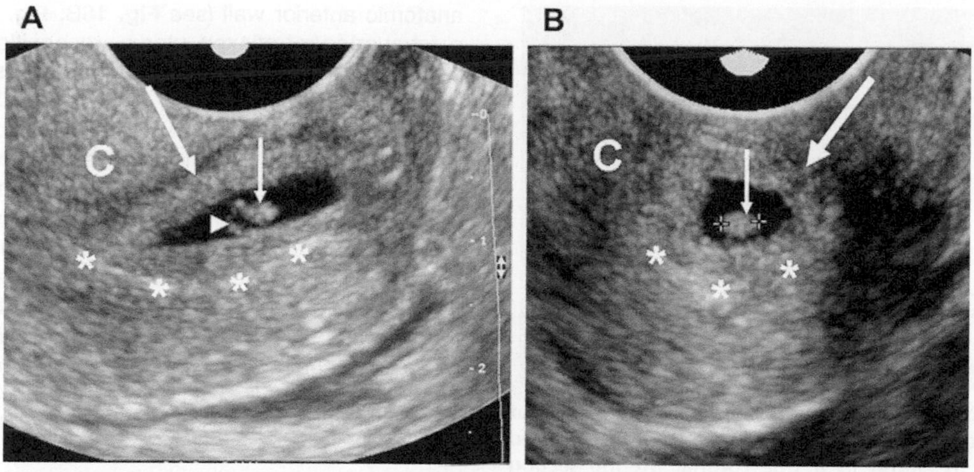

Fig. 10. (*A*) Transvaginal midline sagittal sonogram of the cervix (C) demonstrates a gestational sac (*thick arrow*) with an embryo (*thin arrow*) and yolk sac (*arrowhead*) representing a cervical ectopic pregnancy implanted under the endocervical lining (*asterisk*). (*Adapted from* Bryan-Rest R, Scoutt LM. Ectopic pregnancy. In: Fielding J, Brown D, Thurmon A, editors. Gynecologic imaging. Elsevier (estimated publishing date: June 2011); with permission.) (*B*) Transvaginal 90° transaxial sonogram of the cervix (C) demonstrates the gestational sac (*thick arrow*) and the embryo (*thin arrow*) representing a cervical ectopic pregnancy implanted under the endocervical lining (*asterisk*).

one rotates the transducer 90° counterclockwise from the midline longitudinal plane of the given uterus. Depending on the anatomic position of the uterus in the pelvis, the 90° view may be a true transverse/transaxial, oval-shaped section (see **Figs. 17** and **18**), a coronal/frontal cut (see **Fig. 19**), or a nonstandard oblique section that includes parts of the uterine corpus and cervix. The true transaxial sections or 90° views of anteverted/anteflexed and retroverted/retroflexed uteri have an oval shape, but the location of the anterior wall is different (see **Figs. 17** and **18**).

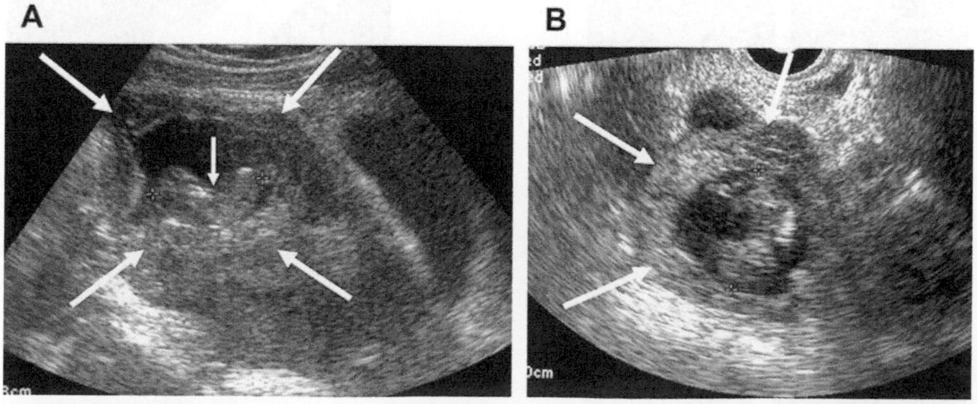

Fig. 11. (*A*) Transabdominal sagittal sonogram shows a gestational sac (*large arrows*) containing an embryo (*small arrow*) that was thought to be an intrauterine pregnancy, but was actually an extrauterine gestational sac. The intrauterine location of the pregnancy was never established on the transabdominal examination, because the normal linear echo of the endocervical canal was never connected with the endometrial "stripe." (*B*) An inaccurate transvaginal US scan also concluded that the pregnancy was intrauterine. Blood and trophoblastic tissue surrounding the gestational sac (*arrows*) looked like myometrium while the caudal end of the sac was obscured by shadowing from bowel gas. If the linear echo of the endocervical canal was properly connected to the endometrial "stripe," then the empty endometrial cavity and the ectopic location of the pregnancy would have been identified.

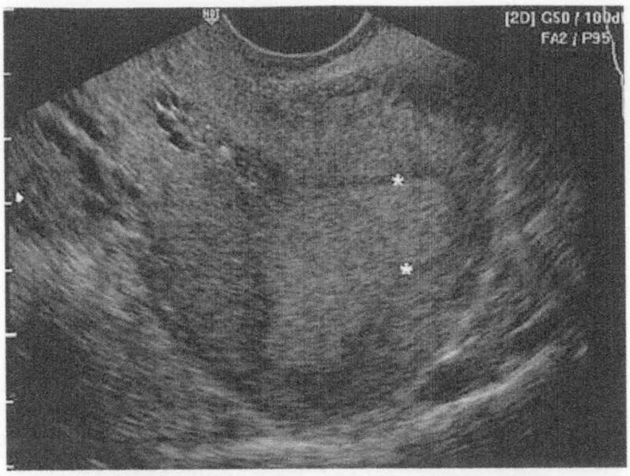

Fig. 12. Transvaginal scan in the sagittal plane of a patient's pelvis shows a retroverted and rotated uterus, resulting in a true coronal uterine section that shows the width of the endometrial cavity instead of the expected linear endometrial "stripe." As this was not understood at the time of scanning, endometrial thickness (*asterisks*) was incorrectly measured. A true midline longitudinal image of such a uterus is found by rotating the transducer 90°. Only then can the endometrium be measured correctly, as shown in the uterus in Fig. 1A.

The anterior wall of an anteverted/anteflexed uterus is located closer to the transducer on the 90° transaxial scan (see **Fig. 17**B), but in a retroverted/retroflexed uterus it is deeper and is further from the transducer, although it is still the anatomic anterior wall (see **Fig. 18**B; **Fig. 20**). In a retroverted/retroflexed uterus, recognition that the deepest appearing myoma in the pelvis originates from the anterior wall of the uterus, rather than from the posterior wall, avoids incorrect localization of the myoma for the surgeon (see **Fig. 20**). Recognition that the uterus is suspended in the middle of the pelvis (**Fig. 21**) helps to anticipate that transvaginal images will probably be suboptimal, because the uterus lies parallel to the US beam, which is the least optimal angle for B-mode scanning. The more optimal technique for scanning such a uterus may be transabdominal imaging, where it is perpendicular to the US beam, thus optimizing the angle for B-mode scanning.

CHECK TECHNIQUE

Attention to sonographic technique, especially with regard to transducer frequency, angle of insonation, and depth, gain, and focus settings, is also important to avoid missed diagnoses. Decreased penetration of the beam is a disadvantage of TVS because of the use of higher frequency transducers. Therefore, the scan

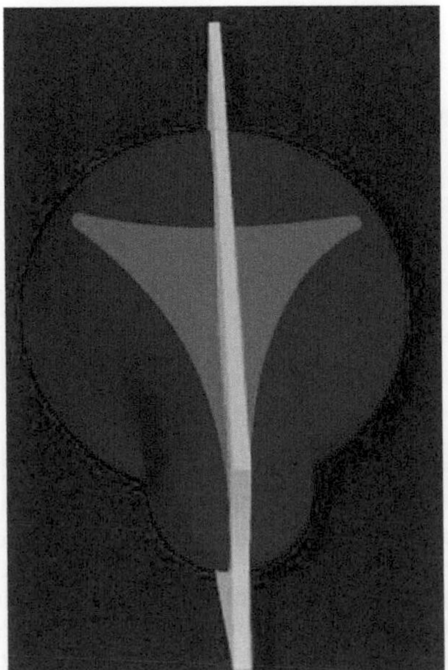

Fig. 13. The midline sagittal plane of a normal uterus in standard position in the midline of the pelvis without tilt or rotation.

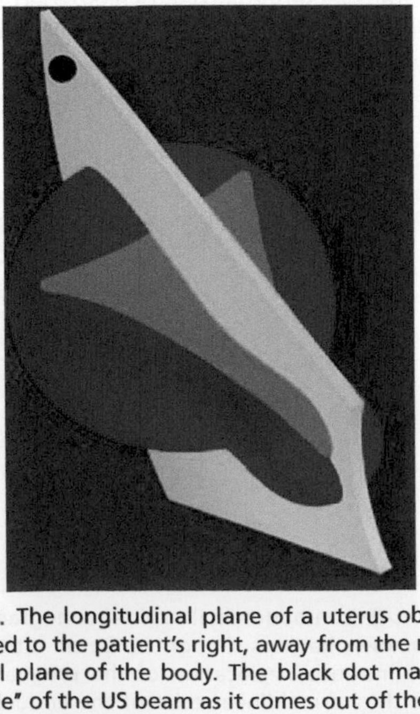

Fig. 14. The longitudinal plane of a uterus obliquely oriented to the patient's right, away from the midline sagittal plane of the body. The black dot marks the "up side" of the US beam as it comes out of the transducer, and is parallel to the position of the thumb of the scanning hand on the notched surface on the transducer. To obtain the true midline longitudinal plane of the uterus itself, the transducer must be angled to the right.

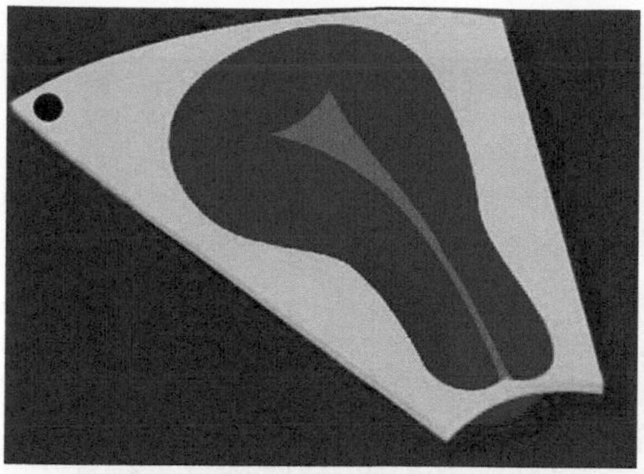

Fig. 15. An obliquely positioned uterus that is also rotated 90° counterclockwise in the pelvis. The transducer must be angled to the right and rotated 90° counterclockwise to obtain the midline longitudinal plane of the uterus. The black dot marks the "up side" of the US beam as it comes out of the transducer, and is parallel to the position of the thumb of the scanning hand on the notched surface on the transducer.

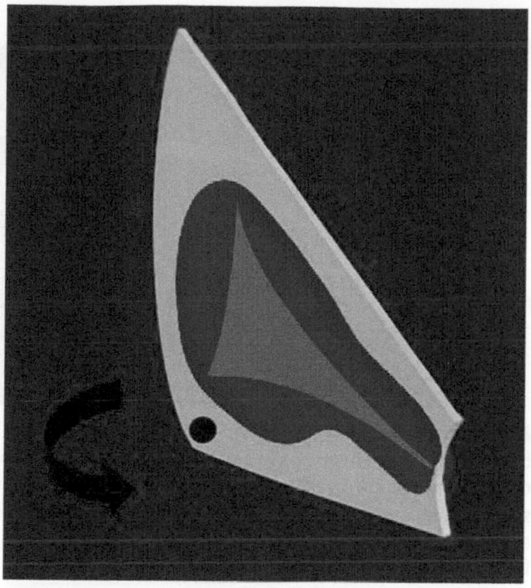

Fig. 16. To obtain the 90° coronal view of the uterus shown in **Fig. 15** the transducer must be rotated another 90° counterclockwise. The black dot marks the "up side" of the US beam as it comes out of the transducer, and is parallel to the position of the thumb of the scanning hand on the notched surface on the transducer. Essentially the transducer is rotated 180° counterclockwise from the midline longitudinal plane of a uterus obliquely positioned in the pelvis, as shown in **Fig. 14**, and the thumb of the scanning hand ends up facing the floor.

should be started at the maximal depth setting so as to see as deep into the pelvis as possible. After one is assured that the uterus is identified and unsuspected masses are not cut off at the edge of the image, the depth setting is decreased so that the image is larger and can be scrutinized for finer details (**Fig. 22**). It is always good practice to keep a clear margin of visibility for 2 to 3 cm beyond the margin of the uterus, ovary, or area of interest (**Fig. 23**). Scanning with maximal depth and using limited transabdominal scans to prescan the pelvis are the 2 best ways to avoid incomplete evaluation of an enlarged uterus or nonvisualization of a high pelvic mass or fluid collection.

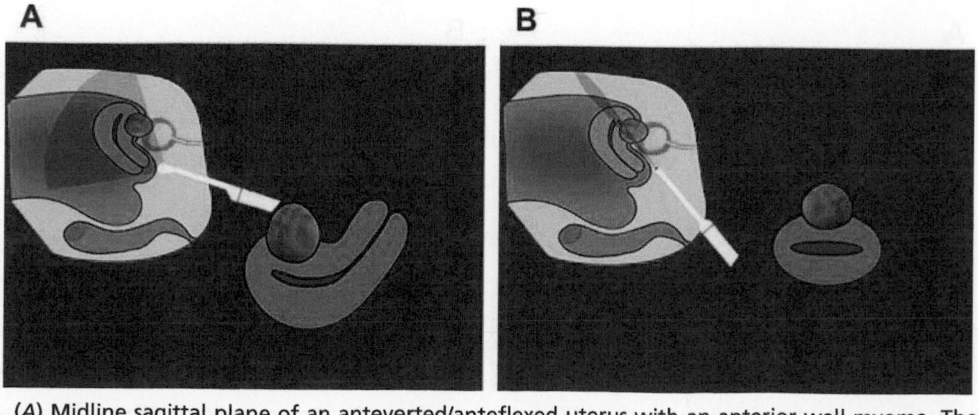

Fig. 17. (*A*) Midline sagittal plane of an anteverted/anteflexed uterus with an anterior wall myoma. The corresponding TVS image, as it is projected on the monitor, is also shown. (*B*) TVS image of an anteverted/anteflexed uterus with an anterior wall myoma showing the corresponding 90° view. Note the oval shape of the uterus and the location of the myoma on the anterior uterine wall, where it is closest to the transducer face.

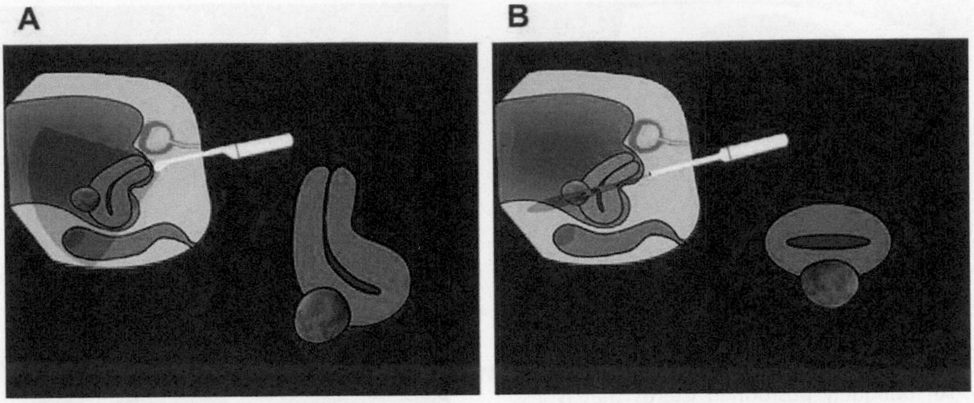

Fig. 18. (*A*) TVS image showing the midline sagittal plane of a typical retroverted/retroflexed uterus. Note the location of the anterior wall myoma on the image as it is projected on the monitor. (*B*) Illustration and US image of a retroverted/retroflexed uterus with an anterior wall myoma showing the corresponding 90° view. Note the similar oval shape of the uterus, but the different location of the anterior wall myoma, as compared with the anteverted uterus in **Fig. 14**. The myoma on the anterior wall of a retroverted/retroflexed uterus is located farther from transducer face and deeper on the image.

Gain settings, including the time-gain-compensation (TGC) curve and overall gain, should be adjusted so that false echoes are not created in fluid. The best way to decide if the echoes in a mass or fluid collection are real or artifactual is to compare the echogenicity with a known fluid structure, ideally the urinary bladder or ovarian follicle, at a similar depth. If the urinary bladder is anechoic and the pelvic mass or fluid contains echoes, then the echoes are real (**Fig. 24**). To test this hypothesis, start by lowering the gain until the bladder and the mass or pelvic fluid are free of echoes. Now slowly increase the gain. If the mass fills in with echoes before the urinary bladder, then the echoes are real. If they fill in at the same time, then the echoes are artifactual. This test becomes very important in analysis of pelvic fluid that may represent hemoperitoneum or in analysis of complex ovarian cystic masses.

BLIND SPOTS IN THE PELVIS

One must be aware of the blind spots in the pelvis on transvaginal scanning. These blind spots

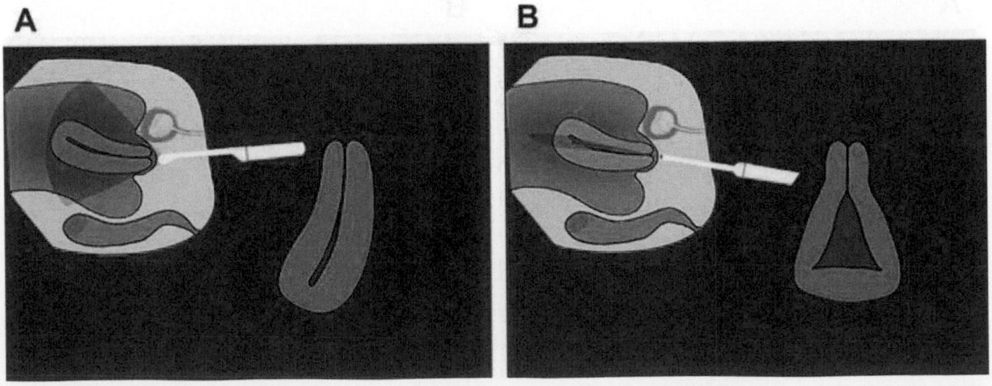

Fig. 19. (*A*) Transvaginal image showing the midline sagittal plane of a uterus in mid-position in the pelvis. Such a uterus has no or minimal flexion and lies parallel to the US beam. (*B*) The corresponding 90° view of the uterus in mid-position in the pelvis is a true coronal or frontal section of the uterus, and has a very different appearance from the 90° views of anteverted and retroverted uteri in **Figs. 17** and **18**, respectively.

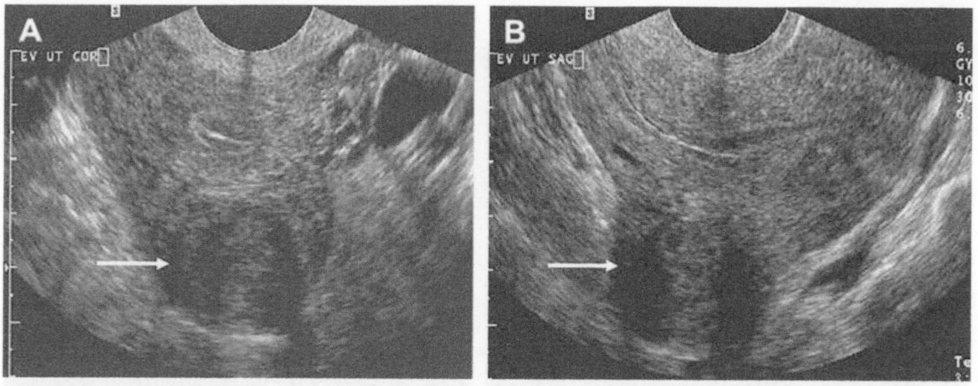

Fig. 20. (*A*) Transvaginal 90° ("coronal" or "transverse") scan of a uterus shows a myoma on the deep wall (*arrow*). One cannot be certain whether the myoma is located on the anterior or posterior wall of the uterus without knowledge of the uterine position on the longitudinal scan. (*B*) Transvaginal sagittal scan of the uterus shows that the uterus is retroverted/retroflexed, therefore the myoma (*arrow*) is on the anterior wall of the uterus.

include areas in the upper pelvis above the fundus of the uterus, laterally along the pelvic side walls, deep in the cul-de-sac, and markedly anterior to the uterus. Evaluation of these areas is especially important when searching for ovaries or ectopic pregnancies. Transabdominal imaging is helpful in such cases.

MANEUVER THE PROBE

Maneuvers with the transvaginal probe may help to solve diagnostic dilemmas in the pelvis. Exerting pressure on masses with the probe helps to check for mobility, separate masses in close proximity, separate a mass from the ovary, or

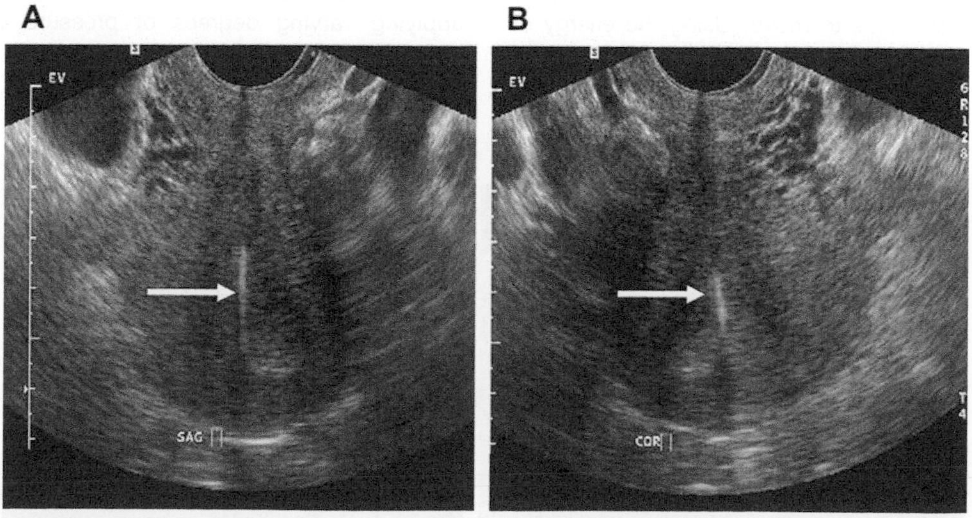

Fig. 21. (*A*) Transvaginal sagittal scan of the pelvis shows a longitudinal section of a uterus in mid-position in the pelvis with a barely visible intrauterine device (*arrow*) within the endometrial cavity. Resolution is poor because the uterus is parallel to the US beam. (*B*) Transvaginal 90° scan of the same uterus shows a true coronal section of the uterus with an intrauterine device (*arrow*). Resolution remains poor because the uterus is still parallel to the US beam.

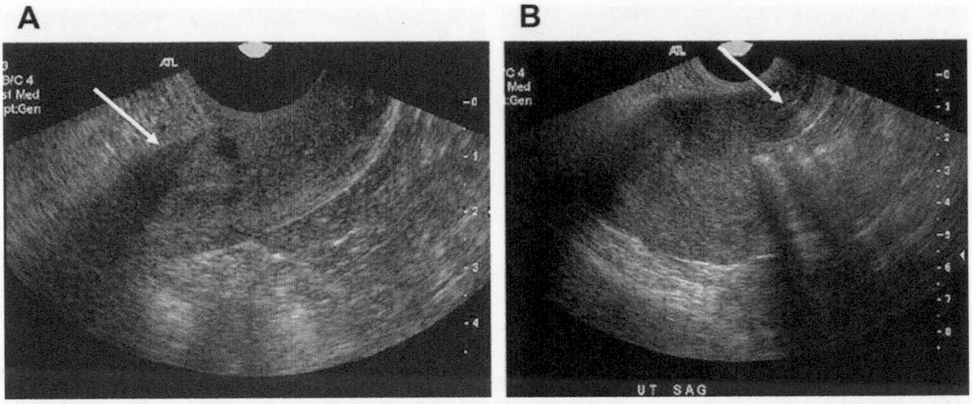

Fig. 22. (*A*) Initial transvaginal sagittal scan set at shallow depth shows a structure that was mistaken for a small uterus. This structure is actually the cervix (*arrow*) and the rest of the uterus is not imaged. (*B*) Subsequent transvaginal sagittal image obtained using maximal depth setting shows the extent of the entire retroflexed uterus with the cervix (*arrow*) near the top of the image. This sequence of events while scanning should be reversed: begin scanning with maximal depth and an open field to obtain an idea about uterine size and position, then change to more shallow depth to focus on details of the organ.

elicit pain that helps to localize and identify pathology. Using the nonscanning hand for pressing and simultaneously pulling down on the anterior abdominal wall with the intention of displacing an ovary in a high location into the pelvis is a helpful technique, and one should be persistent about identifying both ovaries to ensure a complete examination. Either the scanning hand with the probe or the palpating hand on the abdominal wall may be used to cause movement of the internal contents of a complex cystic mass or to prove that echoes are real by causing particles to move. Using the energy of color or spectral Doppler to move particles in fluid, called acoustic streaming, may also be helpful.[12,13] Whenever there appears to be a septated cystic mass, especially if it is elongated, the probe should be maneuvered by twisting and turning movements of the hand to try to unravel a potentially folded dilated tubular mass (**Fig. 25**) because a hydrosalpinx has much different clinical consequences for the patient than a septated ovarian mass. Another useful maneuver is to change location of the transducer tip from the anterior to the posterior fornix while applying varying degrees of pressure on the

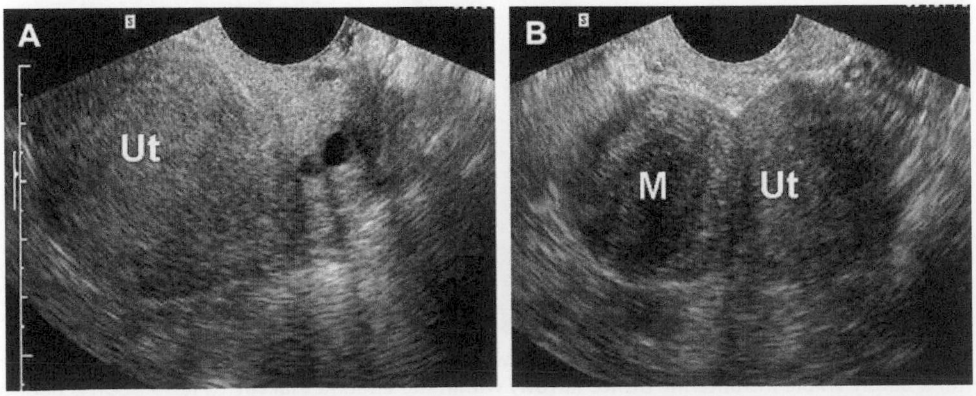

Fig. 23. (*A*) Transvaginal sagittal scan of the uterus (Ut) cuts off part of the fundus and anterior wall of the uterus. (*B*) Maneuvering and angling of the transducer to include the entire anterior wall of the uterus (Ut) reveals an exophytic myoma (M) that was cut off from the image in *A*.

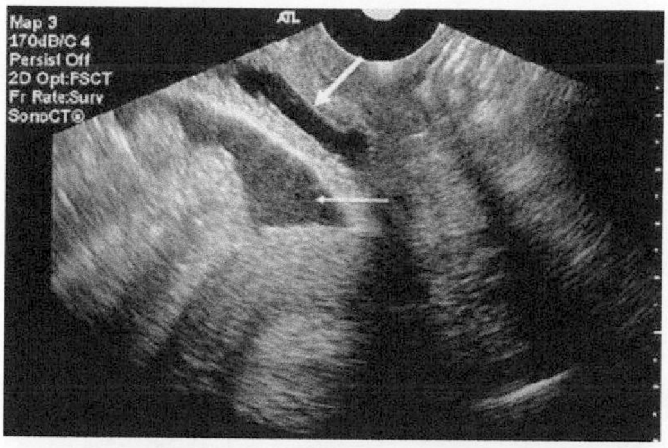

Fig. 24. Transvaginal sonogram of the pelvis shows an empty urinary bladder containing anechoic urine (*thick arrow*) and echogenic free fluid, and hemoperitoneum (*thin arrow*) in the cul-de-sac. Comparison of the echoes in the pelvic fluid with anechoic fluid in the bladder confirms that the echoes in the pelvic fluid are real and not artifactual.

cervix to change the position of the uterus in the pelvis to a more favorable scan plane (**Figs. 26** and **27**).

DOPPLER EVALUATION

Doppler investigation is helpful in evaluating many types of pelvic pathology. Color or spectral Doppler US helps to differentiate a pelvic vessel from a hydrosalpinx (**Fig. 28**). One can avoid misinterpretation of axially imaged uterine vessels for ovaries, so-called pseudo-ovaries, simply by using color Doppler US or scanning at 90° to elongate the vessels.

Using Doppler to help evaluate unusual cystic pelvic masses may help to avoid misdiagnosis of a vascular mass, such as an iliac artery aneurysm for an ovarian cyst, which could lead to unnecessary surgery in a postmenopausal woman. Doppler evaluation should also be considered for any unusual area of myometrial echogenicity that includes myometrial inhomogeneity, irregular cystic changes, or an area of tortuous tubular cystic structures. Such an area may be caused by a uterine arterial venous malformation, which is a congenital or acquired vascular plexus of arteries and veins within the uterine myometrium or endometrium. Proper diagnosis would help to avoid dilation and curettage or surgery, which may cause massive hemorrhage or on occasion might lead to hysterectomy.

Although Doppler US investigation is often helpful in the evaluation of pelvic masses, one should exercise caution concerning the role of Doppler US in the diagnosis of ovarian torsion. The US diagnosis of ovarian torsion is not as certain as testicular torsion. The spectrum of Doppler US findings in ovarian torsion ranges from complete lack of arterial and venous flow through variations in arterial and venous flow to completely normal blood flow in the ovary.[14,15] Because it is possible to demonstrate normal blood flow in an ovary undergoing torsion (**Fig. 29**), one must first look for signs of torsion on the gray-scale image. These

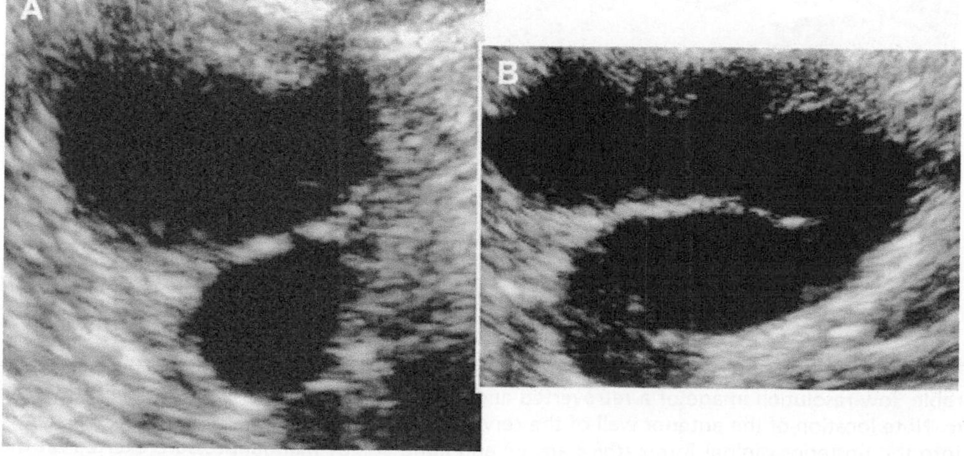

Fig. 25. (*A*) Transvaginal sonogram of the adnexa shows a septated cytic mass, which could be mistaken for a septated ovarian mass. (*B*) After manipulation by twisting and turning of the transducer, a fluid-filled tubular structure, representing a hydrosalpinx, is unfolded.

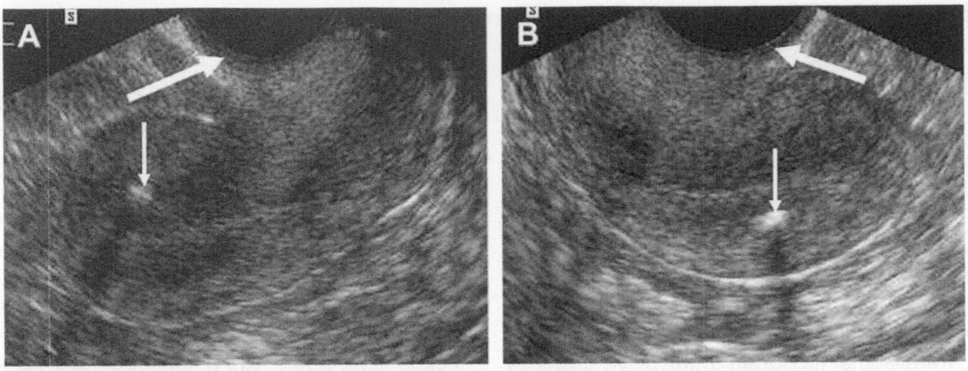

Fig. 26. (*A*) Transvaginal sagittal scan with the transducer in the anterior vaginal fornix (*thick arrow*) shows an anteverted uterus with a calcification in the anterior wall (*thin arrow*). (*B*) Moments later the transducer is gently manipulated into the posterior vaginal fornix (*thick arrow*) and light manual pressure exerted on the uterus. The uterus becomes retroverted/retroflexed. Note the position of the calcification (*thin arrow*), which marks the location of the anterior wall.

signs include an enlarged edematous ovary with peripherally displaced follicles or an ovarian mass that serves as the lead for the twist around a fulcrum. The twisted vascular pedicle sign, which is a round mass composed of several concentric stripes of alternating echogenicity creating a target appearance adjacent to the twisted ovary, is another reliable sign of ovarian or adnexal torsion.[16] Any one of these findings in the presence of significant pelvic pain should lead to the proper diagnosis, despite the presence of blood flow in an adnexal mass. Waiting for complete absence of arterial and venous blood flow to make a diagnosis of ovarian torsion usually leads to a diagnosis of ovarian necrosis, which is not reversible. It is far more important to make the diagnosis of ovarian torsion in a salvageable ovary before infarction has occurred. A potential pitfall in the demonstration of blood flow by color Doppler US is flash artifact that can mimic blood flow. Any evidence of blood flow seen on color Doppler US scan must be confirmed with a spectral tracing, which will confirm real flow by demonstrating a venous or arterial waveform.

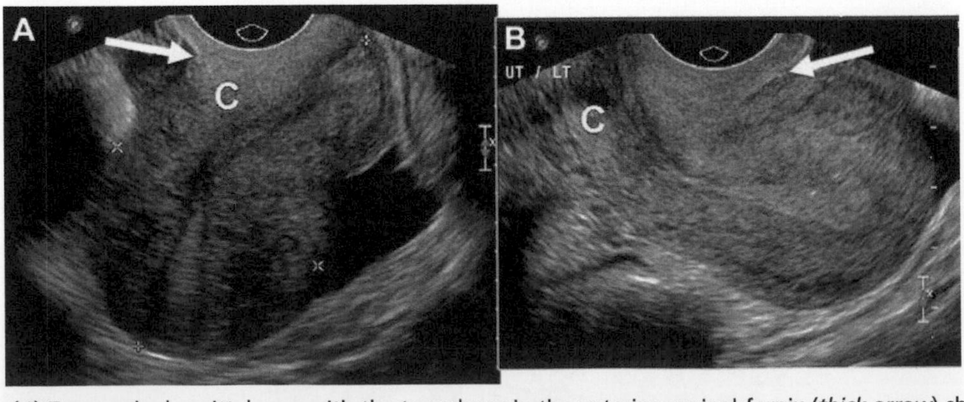

Fig. 27. (*A*) Transvaginal sagittal scan with the transducer in the anterior vaginal fornix (*thick arrow*) shows an unfavorable, low-resolution image of a retroverted and mildly retroflexed uterus that is almost parallel to the US beam. Note location of the anterior wall of the cervix (C). (*B*) Moments later the transducer is gently manipulated into the posterior vaginal fornix (*thick arrow*) and light, steady manual pressure exerted on the uterus. The uterus changes into a more retroverted/retroflexed position and the body, fundus, and endometrium become more perpendicular to the sound beam, thus creating an image with better resolution. Note location of the anterior wall of the cervix (C).

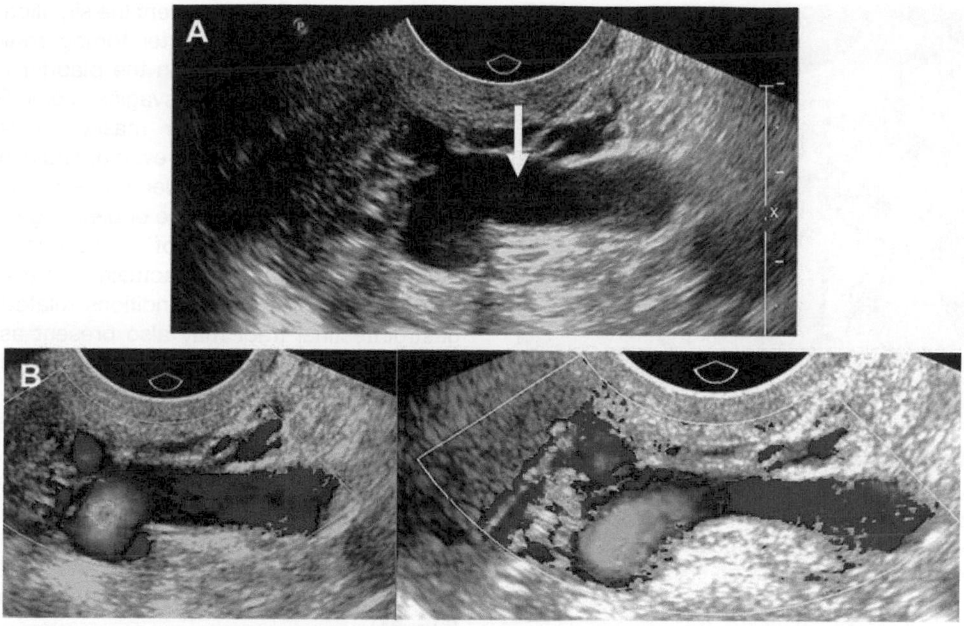

Fig. 28. (*A*) Transvaginal scan shows a dilated, fluid-filled tubular structure that resembles a hydrosalpinx (*arrow*). (*B*) Transvaginal color Doppler scan shows blood flow in the structure, which is a pelvic varix.

Another word of caution concerns the "ring of fire," which refers to concentric enhancement of vessels on color or power Doppler interrogation around the perimeter of a mass, originally described in ectopic pregnancy.[17] Unfortunately, the "ring of fire" is not a reliable sign of ectopic pregnancy. The "ring of fire" is also caused by circumferential increased vascularity in the wall of the corpus luteum, which is a much more common event than ectopic pregnancy. A cystic mass with a thick echogenic rim and a "ring of fire" within the ovary is much more likely to be

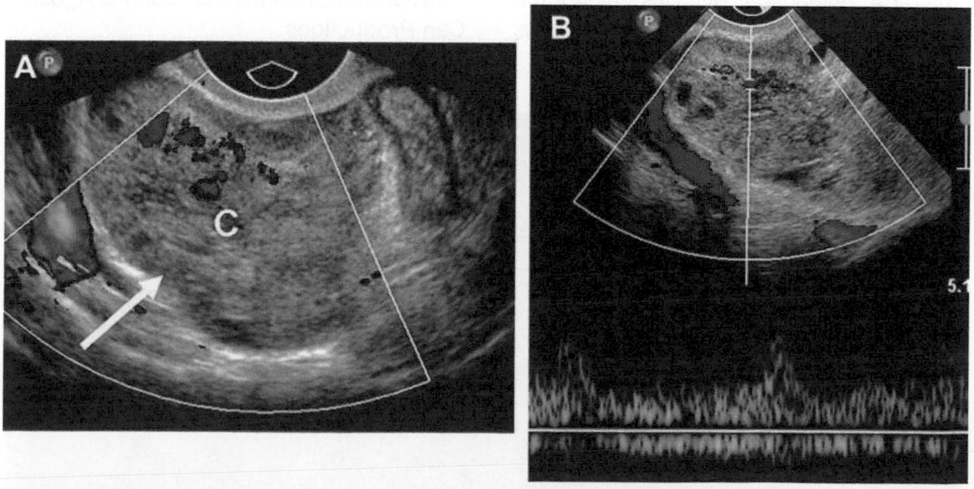

Fig. 29. (*A*) Transvaginal color Doppler scan shows an enlarged painful ovary (*arrow*) with a heterogeneous center (C) and blood flow that was proven to be an ovarian torsion at laparoscopy. (*B*) Spectral Doppler tracing confirms presence of arterial blood flow seen on color Doppler US scan of the ovary. Laparoscopy showed that the ovary was twisted and anemic, but not infarcted. The ovary was untwisted, normal blood flow returned, and the ovary was salvaged.

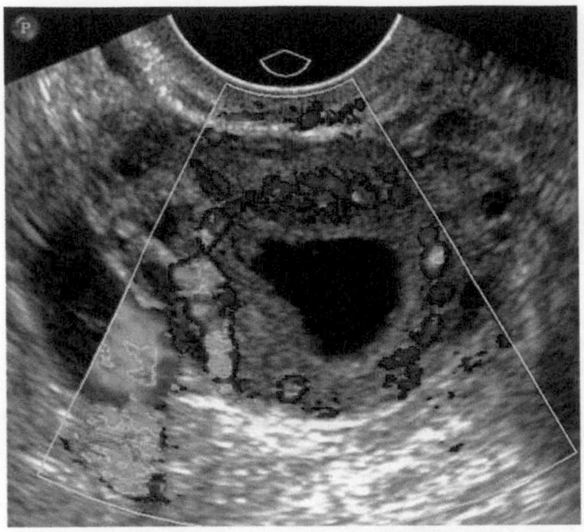

Fig. 30. Color Doppler image of a corpus luteum demonstrates a "ring of fire" as a result of normal blood vessels within the periphery of this common physiologic entity. There was no ectopic pregnancy.

a corpus luteum (**Fig. 30**) than the rare (<0.5% of all ectopic pregnancies) ovarian ectopic pregnancy.

THINK BEYOND GYNECOLOGIC CONDITIONS FOR PELVIC PAIN

Considering nongynecologic sources of pain in the pelvis expands the differential diagnosis and may lead to correct diagnosis, for which a good clinical history is also critical. Lower urinary tract abnormalities often present as pelvic pain. Distal ureteral calculi may be diagnosed by TVS, when the calculus is at the ureterovesical junction, thus sparing a young female patient the significant radiation dose from a computer tomographic scan (see **Fig. 3**). Ureteric jets in the bladder may be easier to detect with transvaginal color Doppler US. Unsuspected bladder masses have been observed in young women, even during evaluation of early pregnancy. Bladder masses have also been found to be the source of bleeding in elderly women complaining of "postmenopausal bleeding," which was actually unrecognized hematuria (see **Fig. 8**). Conditions related to the gastrointestinal tract may also present as pelvic pain. Abnormally thickened large or small bowel loops may be observed in inflammatory bowel diseases. Pericolonic abscesses, such as those associated with diverticulitis, may be well visualized. Occasionally pelvic pain from a low appendix with acute inflammation mimics ovarian pain. This situation may occur when the inflamed tip of a pelvic appendix touches the ovary or surrounding tissues and incites inflammation (**Fig. 31**).

TVS has become the preferred method for sonographic evaluation of the pelvis because of its higher resolution, better detail, and more confidence in diagnosis of pelvic pathology. Unfortunately, there are numerous opportunities for missed diagnosis or incorrect interpretation with TVS. Knowledge of the pitfalls and a systematic, orderly approach for examination of every patient helps to minimize the potential for errors.

ACKNOWLEDGMENTS

Artwork was created by John D'Agostino of Tin Can Productions.

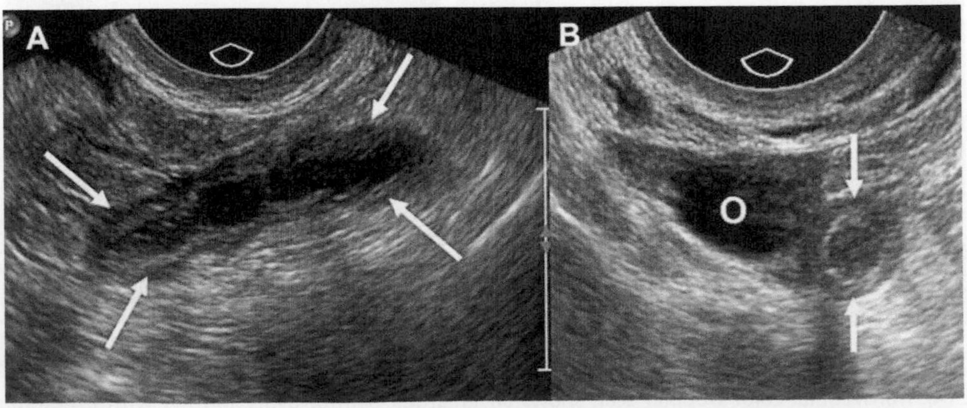

Fig. 31. (*A*) Transvaginal sonogram shows the longitudinal section of a blind-ending, fluid-filled, thick-walled, noncompressible, tubular structure (*arrows*) in the right pelvis that represents an acutely inflamed pelvic appendix. (*B*) Transvaginal sonogram shows the transaxial section of the acutely inflamed pelvic appendix (*arrows*) adjacent to the right ovary (O).

REFERENCES

1. Fernandez H, Gervaise A. Ectopic pregnancies after infertility treatment: modern diagnosis and therapeutic strategy. Hum Reprod Update 2004; 10:503–13.
2. Hertzberg BS, Livingston E, DeLong DM, et al. Ultrasonographic evaluation of the cervix: transperineal versus endovaginal imaging. J Ultrasound Med 2001;20:1071–8.
3. Laing FC, Benson CB, DiSalvo DN, et al. Distal ureteral calculi: detection with vaginal US. Radiology 1994;192:545–8.
4. Benacerraf BR. Filling of the bladder for pelvic sonograms: an ancient form of torture. J Ultrasound Med 2003;22:239–41.
5. Benacerraf BR, Shipp TD, Bromley B. Is the full bladder still necessary for pelvic sonography? J Ultrasound Med 2000;19:237–41.
6. Tessler FN, Schiller VL, Perrella RR, et al. Transabdominal versus endovaginal pelvic sonography: prospective study. Radiology 1989;170:553–6.
7. Mendelson EB, Bohm-Velez M, Joseph N, et al. Gynecologic imaging: comparison of transabdominal and transvaginal sonography. Radiology 1988; 166:321–4.
8. Leibman AJ, Kruse B, McSweeney MB. Transvaginal sonography: comparison with transabdominal sonography in the diagnosis of pelvic masses. AJR Am J Roentgenol 1988;151(1):89–92.
9. Coleman BG, Arger PH, Grumbach K, et al. Transvaginal and transabdominal ultrasound: prospective comparison. Radiology 1988;168:639–43.
10. Andolf E, Jorgensen C. A prospective comparison of transabdominal and transvaginal ultrasound with surgical findings in gynecologic disease. J Ultrasound Med 1990;9:71–5.
11. Hill LM, Breckle R. Value of a postvoid scan during adnexal sonography. Am J Obstet Gynecol 1985; 152:23–5.
12. Edwards A, Clarke L, Piessens S, et al. Acoustic streaming: a new technique for assessing adnexal cysts. Ultrasound Obstet Gynecol 2003; 22:74–8.
13. Clarke L, Edwards A, Pollard K. Acoustic streaming in ovarian cysts. J Ultrasound Med 2005;24:617–21.
14. Albayram F, Hamper UM. Ovarian and adnexal torsion: spectrum of sonographic findings with pathologic correlation. J Ultrasound Med 2001;20: 1083–9.
15. Pena JE, Ufberg D, Cooney N, et al. Usefulness of Doppler sonography in the diagnosis of ovarian torsion. Fertil Steril 2000;73:1047–50.
16. Lee EJ, Kwon HC, Joo HJ, et al. Diagnosis of ovarian torsion with color Doppler sonography: depiction of twisted vascular pedicle. J Ultrasound Med 1998; 17:83–9.
17. Pellerito JS, Taylor KJ, Quedens-Case C, et al. Ectopic pregnancy: evaluation with endovaginal color flow imaging. Radiology 1992;183:407–11.

Pearls and Pitfalls in Sonohysterography

Sandra J. Allison, MD[a,*], Mindy M. Horrow, MD[b,c], Anna S. Lev-Toaff, MD[d]

KEYWORDS

- Ultrasound • Pelvic • Sohohysterography
- Saline infused sonohysterography
- Hysterosonography • Pitfalls • Technique

Sonohysterography (SHG) is a technique involving instillation of fluid into the endometrial cavity while imaging with transvaginal sonography (TVS) to improve visualization of the endometrium, endometrial cavity, and endometrial-myometrial interface. SHG can also be used to assess tubal patency. The most common indication in premenopausal and postmenopausal patients is abnormal uterine bleeding. Infertility, recurrent abortion, and suspected congenital or acquired uterine abnormalities are among the additional indications for the procedure.[1] It is more accurate than TVS alone and less invasive than hysteroscopy for the detection of endometrial pathology.[2,3]

Although hysteroscopy permits histologic sampling, SHG is less invasive, less costly, requires no sedation, and is rarely associated with complications. It can decrease the rate of negative hysteroscopy and may redirect therapy for those in whom hysteroscopy is not appropriate.[3] SHG can determine whether endometrial pathology is focal or diffuse, determine the appropriate technique for histologic sampling, document and provide information to direct the method of resection (or other treatment) of submucosal or intracavitary fibroids, and define intramural abnormalities such as fibroids or adenomyosis for which hysteroscopy/biopsy are not useful. SHG is often of practical use to the clinician by determining any structural cause of abnormal bleeding (vs dysfunctional uterine bleeding) and to guide appropriate sampling and therapeutic or other management options.

Many of the aspects of planning and performing SHG involve techniques in pelvic examination that may not be widely known. Some are infrequently required but can rescue an otherwise unsuccessful examination. The first half of this article discusses the technique of the procedure, including practical tips for a successful, comfortable examination. The second half of the article covers issues related to interpretation, with emphasis on avoiding pitfalls.

PREPROCEDURAL CONSIDERATIONS

Scheduling

In premenopausal women the procedure is optimally performed when the endometrium is at its thinnest but before ovulation to avoid inadvertently flushing out a fertilized ovum. This time frame spans days 4 and 10 of the menstrual cycle. If performed too early, blood may obscure pathology or be confused with polyps. If performed later in the secretory phase, physiologic thickening of the endometrium may result in false positives and false negatives.[4,5] In a patient with intermenstrual bleeding, intracavitary blood may be unavoidable, in which case extra-brisk injections of fluid may be needed to flush out blood or the catheter may be

[a] Division of Ultrasound, Georgetown University Hospital, 3800 Reservoir Road, Northwest, Washington, DC 20007-2113, USA
[b] Department of Radiology, Albert Einstein Medical Center, 5501 Old York Road, Philadelphia, PA 19141-3098, USA
[c] School of Medicine, Thomas Jefferson University, 1025 Walnut Street, Philadelphia, PA 19107, USA
[d] Department of Radiology, Hospital of the University of Pennsylvania, Ground Dulles, 3400 Spruce Street, Philadelphia, PA 19104, USA
* Corresponding author.
E-mail address: sa263@gunet.georgetown.edu

Ultrasound Clin 5 (2010) 195–207
doi:10.1016/j.cult.2010.03.008
1556-858X/10/$ – see front matter

manipulated to break up clots. On occasion, color Doppler can be useful to distinguish between an adherent blood clot and an intracavitary mass or to detect a clot adherent to a mass. In patients with irregular cycles, the procedure should be performed after obtaining a negative pregnancy test.

In postmenopausal patients, the procedure can be performed at any time. Patients on cyclical hormone treatment should be scheduled at the conclusion of the progesterone treatment phase, as for premenopausal patients. Active bleeding is not a contraindication, however the procedure should be performed with the understanding that blood clots may simulate or obscure pathology.

Contraindications to scheduling patients include pregnancy and active pelvic inflammatory disease (PID) for fear of exacerbating the latter. An intrauterine device (IUD) is a relative contraindication. The authors have occasionally encountered a patient with an IUD in whom SHG is required; in these cases prophylactic antibiotics were used and no complications were encountered.

Risks and Concerns

There are a few reports of pelvic infection related to SHG.[6,7] Tubal occlusion and peritubal adhesions are associated with increased risk for stasis of saline within the pelvis. Patients with this condition may benefit from antibiotic prophylaxis.[6] For this reason, preliminary transvaginal ultrasonography (TVUS) is strongly recommended to detect uterine/adnexal tenderness or hydrosalpinx that would mandate deferring the procedure or antibiotic prophylaxis. If the patient's history and physical examination, as well as preliminary TVUS findings, are consistent with active PID, the examination can be delayed until after a course of antibiotics to minimize risk of exacerbating the condition.

Other reasons to perform preliminary TVUS include screening for ovarian pathology and assessing the size and position of the uterus (ie, retroflexion), the latter providing a guide to the likely position of the cervix. In a retrodisplaced uterus the cervix will be located more anteriorly. If the uterus is enlarged, the outer plastic cannula may need to be cut short to permit a greater length of catheter to be advanced into the uterine cavity. Infrequently, in the presence of large myomas, imaging of the displaced/elongated uterine cavity may require transabdominal imaging.

There is a theoretical risk of seeding the peritoneal cavity in performing SHG in patients with ovarian, fallopian, or uterine malignancy. Devore and colleagues[8] performed a study addressing this concern in patients with endometrial carcinoma undergoing conventional x-ray hysterosalpingogram (HSG). They found no difference in survival between patients with and without tubal occlusion who had endometrial carcinoma and underwent HSG. The preliminary TVUS should ideally be performed under the supervision of, or by, the same person who is performing the SHG. The authors have occasionally noted that, whereas preview of preliminary images obtained by the technologist may be unremarkable, speculum placement reveals that the cervix is not easily visualized or atypically oriented.

Reducing Anxiety

There are several reasons for patients to present to the ultrasound suite with anxiety, including embarrassment related to pelvic examination, previous painful experience with gynecologic procedures, fear of the unknown, or concern about the results. It may be helpful to instruct patients to take a nonsteroidal antiinflammatory drug (NSAID) 30 to 60 minutes before the procedure, typically one they normally take for menstrual cramping.[9] An extra few minutes to explain to the patient what is to be expected in terms of discomfort related to speculum, catheter placement, and saline injection will help allay patient anxiety. It is helpful to explain why distention of the endometrial cavity aids in diagnosis. All personnel present for the procedure should be introduced to the patient.

Although some patients prefer a more interactive position (ie, semisupine with maximized operator-patient eye contact), others prefer to be more supine, thereby avoiding seeing any instruments and focusing attention elsewhere until the procedure has been completed. Slight elevation of the head is preferred to pool fluid in the pelvis, especially when tubal evaluation is required. Because the patient will be in a vulnerable position for an extended period of time, careful attention to lighting, draping, patient orientation with respect to the door, and minimizing personnel in the room is important. The patient should not be placed in the lithotomy position until the last possible minute after the procedure is explained and the procedure tray and catheters are fully prepped. Minimizing interruptions and intrusions into the room will help considerably in reducing anxiety.

TECHNICAL ISSUES

Patient Positioning

It is preferable to perform the examination with the patient in a semiupright lithotomy position. Place the patient with thighs flexed and abducted, and feet in stirrups. Positioning the buttocks extending slightly over the edge of the examination table will allow more room to manipulate the probe. If a stretcher with stirrups is unavailable, the patient can be placed in a frogleg position and an angled pad can be placed under the pelvis, preferably with cutout to allow probe maneuvering.

For patients who have hip or knee problems, it may be necessary to manually support the affected limb in an unflexed position. For obese patients (or other rare circumstances) in whom the cervix cannot be visualized in the lithotomy position, asking the patient to flex her hips and hold her knees as much toward the chest as possible has helped to bring the cervix into view.

Speculum Choice

Specula come in 2 basic shapes (Pederson and Graves) and are made of metal and plastic; both shapes are available in small, medium, and large sizes.[10] Several sizes should be available so that the appropriate sized speculum may be selected to minimize discomfort and ensure visualization of the cervix. A Pederson speculum is narrow with straight blades; the medium size is usually the most comfortable for sexually active women. A small Pederson is available for patients with a small introitus (virgins and elderly women). The Graves speculum is slightly wider than the Pederson. The end of the blades has a biconcave, duckbill shape. This speculum is a good choice for obese women or those who have undergone vaginal delivery. A large Graves can be used for very obese women or those with multiple vaginal births or vaginal prolapse. For those with redundant vaginal folds (often seen in very obese women), it may be helpful to cut off the thumb of a glove and place it over a large Graves speculum to compress the redundant vaginal folds outward.[11] The Miller speculum has a single-hinge design, allowing the catheter to pass through the open side during speculum withdrawal.

Preprocedural knowledge of uterine flexion and version and cervical orientation can be useful in directing speculum and catheter placement. Scarring from a cesarean section may cause tethering of the cervix and lower uterine segment. Warming the speculum and using adequate lubricating gel will prevent the patient from tensing her muscles, which can hinder speculum and catheter placement. In tense patients, having them bear down or Valsalva, or gently pressing on the perineal body may also ease speculum insertion.

A preliminary TVUS can be useful to assess the position and orientation of the cervix. The speculum can then be oriented accordingly toward cervix. In cases of severe retroversion, placement of the speculum upside down may make cervical access easier. If the cervix is posteriorly positioned, having the patient push down on the uterus just above the pubic symphysis will aid in elevating the cervix into view. A Valsalva maneuver may bring the uterus into view. This technique may be especially helpful in patients with redundant vaginal folds or those with rectoceles or cystoceles. If a tenaculum is needed to straighten the uterus to allow catheter placement or to allow cervical dilatation, it should be placed at the 12 or 6 o'clock position on the exocervix. Sufficient tissue must be grasped so that traction on the tenaculum does not tear the cervix. Closing the tenaculum during a cough decreases discomfort. Infiltration of the exocervix at the 12 or 6 o'clock position with 1% lidocaine using a 22- or 25-gauge needle provides local anesthesia and is our preferred technique to minimize discomfort in the few cases in which a tenaculum is required during SHG.

In our anecdotal experience, the authors rarely resort to using a tenaculum. The cervix can be displaced to straighten the endocervical canal using any long instrument such as a forceps with cotton ball or long speculum. In the setting of a mobile cervix, steady forward pressure on the os with the catheter stiffener is usually sufficient to pin down the cervix and gain access with the catheter.

Catheter Choice

Catheters designed specifically for SHG are available.[12] Balloon-tip catheters are popular options because the inflated balloon can prevent leakage of saline and catheter displacement. They are less likely to become dislodged during ultrasound probe insertion and removal of the speculum. Typically, they do not require a tenaculum for cervical traction. Balloon catheters ensure a better seal, requiring less fluid instillation.[13] A balloon may also be useful in patients with patulous or incompetent cervix or enlarged uterus.

Thin pediatric feeding catheters can be used, although these are not equipped with a balloon. Foley catheters have a balloon but are generally too flexible, limiting the ability to cannulate the cervix. Goldstein and ZUI 2.0 catheters are equipped with stoppers for the external cervical os, but the seal is not as effective as that of the balloon catheter. In general, soft-tip catheters are favored because they prevent endometrial shearing, which can mimic other pathology.

Cervical Stenosis

On occasion, cervical stenosis will prevent catheter placement. Cervical stenosis is the most common cause of SHG failure.[14] Risk factors for stenosis include nulliparity, history of cone biopsy or loop electrosurgical excision procedure, or peri/postmenopausal status. Screening for these factors before the procedure may prompt the physician to have alternatives available in case access cannot be achieved. If access cannot be gained with a 5 Fr catheter, there are a few options to consider. The Seldinger technique involves using a 0.038 glide wire to initially gain access, then advancing a 5 Fr tapered dilator over the wire and performing the study through the dilator.[6] Other alternatives include inserting a metal stylet through the catheter to stiffen it, or using a coaxial catheter.[15]

In patients with acute anteflexion, retroflexion or cervical stenosis, the catheter may be difficult to pass without traction on cervix by applying a tenaculum. Cervical dilators may assist in gentle dilatation of a stenotic cervix.

In rare cases, when the cervix is very fibrotic, the authors have managed to instill fluid via a 22-gauge spinal needle placed into the cervical canal following local anesthesia and traction on cervix with a tenaculum to straighten the uterocervical canal. Even a minimal amount of fluid can yield diagnostic results, especially in a postmenopausal woman. In patients with cervical stenosis, a balloon is usually not needed to prevent leakage.

Inability to place the catheter beyond the internal os should be documented in the report and the possibility of mass or adhesions should be raised; this may be relevant in patients undergoing assisted reproduction or patients with history of failed office endometrial biopsy.

Catheter Placement

Before catheter placement, it is important to flush air from the catheter, fill the balloon with saline, and aspirate as much air as possible from the balloon. This process may require several attempts. Air introduced into the endometrial cavity can limit visualization (**Fig. 1**). Because the initial catheter placement is not performed under ultrasound visualization, the catheter should be advanced as far as possible. After the speculum is removed and replaced with the vaginal probe, the catheter may be optimally positioned and the balloon inflated.

It is best to inflate the balloon within the endometrial cavity. A fully inflated balloon in the endocervical canal can obscure pathology and result in pain. In the authors' experience, patients report less pain with the balloon inflated in the endometrial canal than the endocervical canal. Some cervical canals cannot accommodate the balloon, whereas some are too patulous to maintain the balloon. In this situation, the balloon can easily be dislodged during saline injection or speculum withdrawal. When the balloon is placed in endocervical canal, it cannot be advanced to dislodge clots or break up thin adhesions. In this position, it is more difficult to optimize uterine distension to establish enough pressure to send fluid through fallopian tubes to evaluate for patency.

When placed at the internal os, balloon catheters ensure a better seal, requiring less fluid instillation. It can also prevent leakage of fluid through a patulous cervix and allow better distention of the uterus (**Fig. 2**). Initially inflating the balloon in the endometrial canal, and then retracting it to occlude the internal os, is recommended to provide an unobscured view of the endometrial cavity (see **Fig. 2**).

The distended balloon may obscure pathology. Once the uterine cavity is optimally evaluated, the balloon should be deflated and the catheter slowly withdrawn while instilling more fluid to ensure adequate visualization of the lower uterine segment and cervical canal (**Fig. 3**).

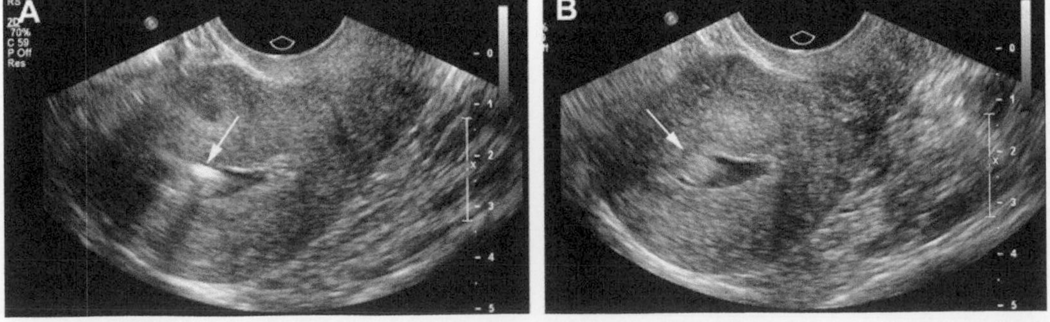

Fig. 1. Air obscuring pathology. (*A*) Sagittal TVUS obtained during SHG shows air (*arrow*) in the endometrial cavity. (*B*) After the air dissipated, a polyp (*arrow*) was revealed.

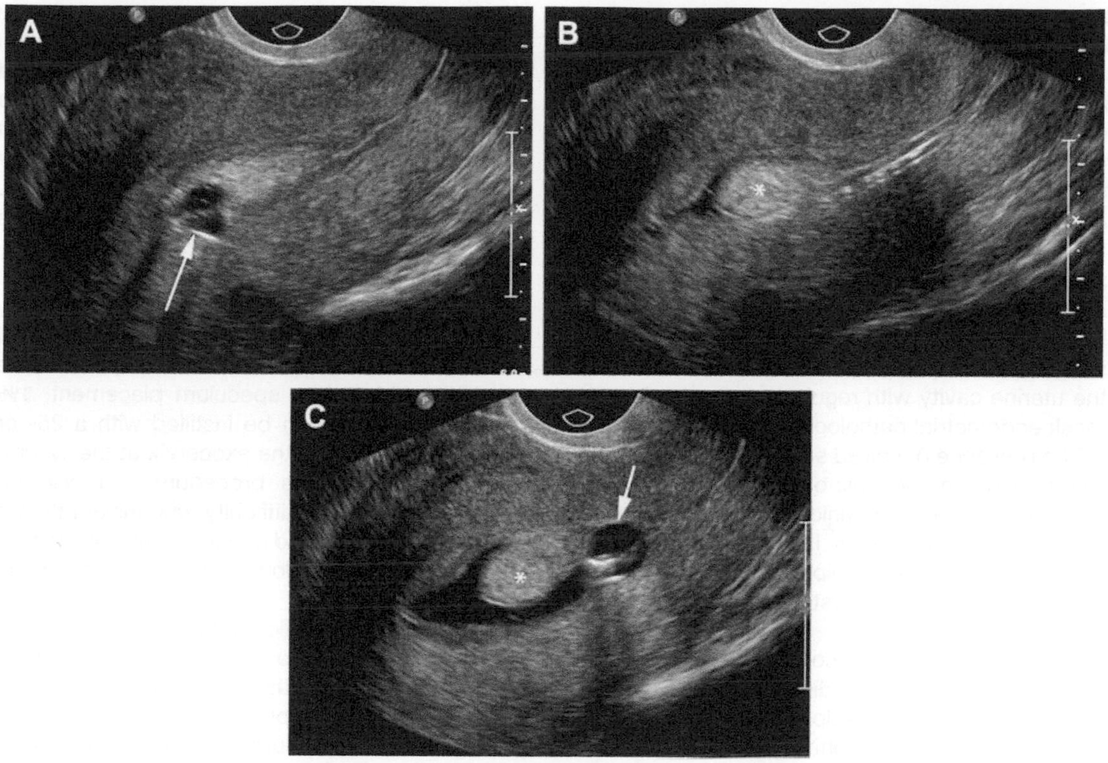

Fig. 2. Pull-back technique. (*A*) Sagittal TVUS shows catheter balloon (*arrow*) in the fundus. (*B*) With the balloon deflated and catheter retracted, instilled saline outlines a polyp (*asterisk*) that was originally obscured by the balloon. (*C*) The balloon (*arrow*) can be distended and pulled back to occlude the internal os and allow better distension of the endometrial cavity and show the attachment site of the polyp.

Contrast Choice and Instillation

In most cases, sterile saline is used for the procedure. When malignancy is suspected, it is theorized that sterile water or hypertonic saline may be preferred to induce cell lysis and potentially decrease or eliminate the risk of peritoneal spread; however, this theory remains unproven.

A steady, moderate rate of injection should produce optimal distention of the cavity. Warming the saline may prevent cramping. Overdistention of the endometrial cavity is painful and may result in underestimation of the size or extent of pathology.[16]

At the conclusion of the procedure, the pelvis should be rescanned. An increase in free fluid

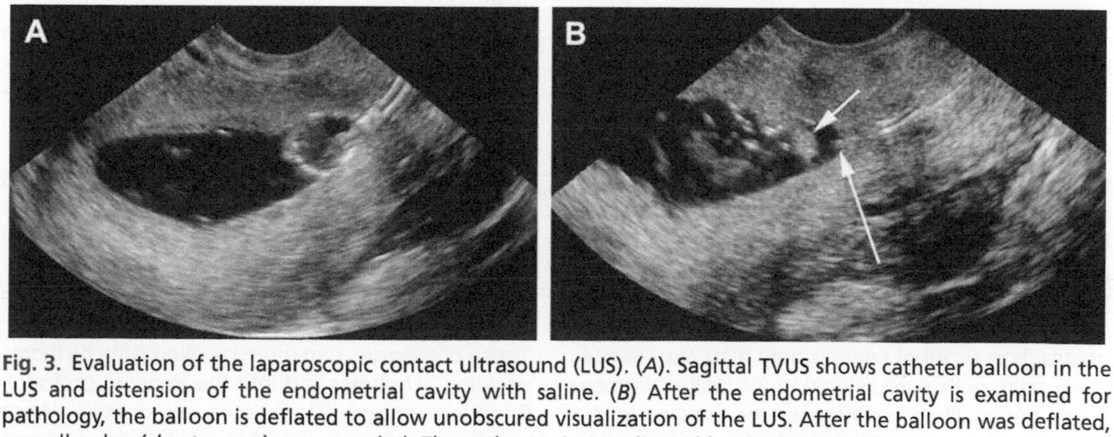

Fig. 3. Evaluation of the laparoscopic contact ultrasound (LUS). (*A*). Sagittal TVUS shows catheter balloon in the LUS and distension of the endometrial cavity with saline. (*B*) After the endometrial cavity is examined for pathology, the balloon is deflated to allow unobscured visualization of the LUS. After the balloon was deflated, a small polyp (*short arrow*) was revealed. The catheter tip is indicated by the long arrow.

implies tubal spill, and, therefore, patency of at least 1 fallopian tube. The absence of free fluid suggests bilateral tubal blockage but may also be to the result of corneal spasm or debris in the cornua or tubal isthmus.[17] For the workup of infertility, detection of tubal adhesions or tubal obstruction is essential because it may play a role in infertility in up to 35% of cases.[18]

The fallopian tubes can be evaluated with sonosalpingography using agitated saline after SHG.[19] Agitated saline contains multiple suspended gas bubbles, rendering it echogenic. If needed, this imaging should be performed after evaluation of the uterine cavity with regular saline so as not to mask endometrial pathology.

The presence of spilled saline in the adnexa will also provide an anechoic background in which to observe spill of echogenic agitated saline from the patent fallopian tubes. In a study by Campbell and colleagues,[20] sonosalpingography was found to be as accurate as hysterosalpingography for tubal patency.

Tubal patency can be confirmed if there is free flow of agitated saline distally for at least 10 seconds without hydrosalpinx formation. Lack of interstitial flow or peritoneal fluid accumulation implies proximal obstruction, whereas hydrosalpinx formation without spill implies distal segment tubal obstruction.[21]

Agitated saline can be prepared by filling a 30-mL syringe with 20 mL of saline and 10 mL of air. A suspension of microbubbles is produced by back-and-forth exchanges of saline and air via a 3-way stopcock with another syringe containing 1 mL of air. The agitated saline can then be injected through the same sonohysterogram catheter and each adnexa observed for spill. The authors anticipate that an ultrasound contrast medium may be available for use instead of agitated saline in the near future.

Pain Control

Pain is highly variable from patient to patient. Several factors may correlate with the occurrence and intensity of pain. Rapid distension of the postmenopausal uterus or any more than minimal inflation of the balloon in postmenopausal patients may produce significant discomfort. Adenomyosis tends to make the uterus sensitive, and affected patients may experience moderate to severe pain up to 1 hour after SHG. Premedication with ibuprofen may be helpful. Women with tubal obstruction or tubal ligation may also experience more pain, with overdistension (or lack of egress from uterus) likely serving as the cause. Intrauterine adhesions (which may or may not be visible) may cause diminished uterine distensibility and therefore pain. In addition, patients with chronic PID present with hydrosalpinx and decreased tolerance to additional distention. It is important to prescreen for signs of active PID and to consider premedication with antibiotics if hydrosalpinx is found on the preprocedural scan. One can also administer antibiotics after the scan and monitor the patient for signs of reactivation of PID.

If there is any indication that the patient may have a low threshold for pain, by her frame of mind at the time of presentation or by excessive initial discomfort with speculum placement, 1% buffered lidocaine can be instilled with a 25- or 22-gauge needle into the exocervix at the 12 or 6 o'clock position. This procedure can also be performed if there is difficulty with initial attempt to cannulate cervix, and makes the use of a tenaculum painless and allows for cervical dilatation without discomfort.

If the uterus is anteflexed or retroflexed, or the cervix is stenotic and a 5 French catheter cannot be passed, local anesthesia can also be administered, a tenaculum applied, and gentle traction placed on the tenaculum to straighten the canal and allow ready passage of the catheter or to offer some countertraction when cervical dilatation is required. Gentle dilatation can be safely performed with a graduated plastic dilator. The authors have had the occasional patient in whom cervical dilatation could not be achieved; in these few cases softening of the cervix with planaria was accomplished, followed by successful SHG.

Documentation

Images should be obtained in sagittal and axial planes, preferably with cine clips for capturing dynamic information or three-dimensional (3D) volumes that can be reconstructed for clarification.

If a balloon was positioned in the lower uterine segment, a second series of images should be obtained with the balloon deflated and saline being administered while the catheter is being withdrawn.

The planes of scanning are limited with TVUS because the vaginal probe has limited mobility within the confines of the vagina. Suboptimal endometrial visualization may also occur with angulated uteri, limiting the ability of the probe to image perpendicular to the long axis of the uterus. These challenges can often be overcome by incorporating 3D ultrasound into the imaging protocol. Because sonographic images are obtained from a volume rather than a slice of data, the images may be less dependent on the operator, and additional findings can be made after the patient has left the department by scrolling through the volume data.[22] There is greater freedom to manipulate or rotate the volume as necessary to clarify findings and obtain additional detail.

If the uterus is enlarged by fibroids, imaging can be performed transabdominally after transcervical instillation of saline. Even when the uterus is not enlarged beyond the field of view, shadowing from a fibroid may obscure visualization of the endometrial canal. The canal may also be better visualized with a lower-frequency transabdominal transducer in this situation.

DIAGNOSTIC PROBLEMS AND LIMITATIONS

Air

Inadvertently filling the balloon with air will obscure posterior structures. The catheter should be thoroughly flushed with sterile saline before insertion to remove as much air as possible. Air within the catheter that is introduced into the uterine cavity may obscure abnormalities (see **Fig. 1**).

Air may also make its way into the myometrium early after injection (**Fig. 4**). One should not assume that this is an indication of myometrial intravasation through a defect in the endometrium caused by catheterization as it may alternatively be related to air insinuating itself through myometrial cracks associated with adenomyosis.[23,24]

Endometrial Lesions

The normal, physiologically thickened endometrium of the secretory phase may mask or simulate a true endometrial lesion (**Fig. 5**). Endometrial hyperplasia, which generally presents as diffuse endometrial thickening, may be particularly difficult to distinguish from secretory endometrium. For this reason, the optimal time to perform SHG is during the proliferative phase. Blood clots may simulate focal endometrial lesions. Gentle catheter manipulation and saline flushing during real-time sonography will diminish the likelihood of mistaking an adherent blood clot for a true lesion. True endometrial lesions may be compressible but they cannot be flushed from their location. Menstrual debris may also be mistaken for adhesions, although debris should not limit uterine distensibility; filmy adhesions and linear debris can be dislodged with the catheter. Vascular polyps may be distinguished from blood clots using color Doppler (**Fig. 6**).[25]

Submucosal fibroids may present occasionally in an intracavitary location but can usually be differentiated from polyps by their echogenicity, which is similar to myometrium. Polyps are typically isoechoic to endometrium and are more echogenic than fibroids on ultrasound. In addition, the echogenic endometrium can often be seen covering the surface of the intracavitary fibroid, further supporting the diagnosis. Doppler imaging of fibroids usually shows circumferential flow rather than the single central feeding vessel typical of polyps (**Fig. 6C**). When palpated with the catheter, myomas are firm, whereas endometrial lesions are soft.

Tamoxifen-related changes are nonspecific and the diagnosis should be considered in the appropriate patient population. SHG can be useful in tamoxifen-treated women even in the setting of prior negative endometrial biopsy.[26,27] This is especially true for polyps, which are often missed during blind biopsies because of their focal nature. Because mucinous metaplasia may occur in tamoxifen-associated polyps, biopsy is important.

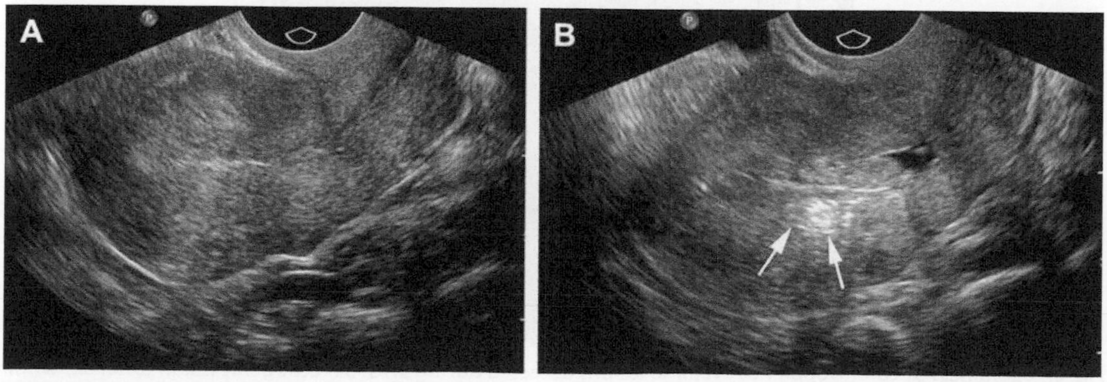

Fig. 4. Air in myometrium. (*A*) Preprocedure sagittal TVUS shows ill-defined echogenic nodules in the myometrium with blurring of the endometrial-myometrial interface. (*B*) After instillation of saline, echogenic foci (*arrows*) in the myometrium are considered to represent air within myometrial cracks associated with adenomyosis.

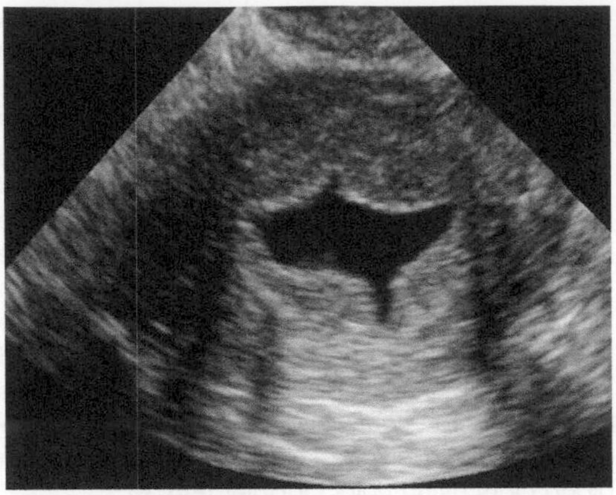

Fig. 5. Secretory endometrium. Transverse TVUS obtained during SHG shows physiologically thickened endometrium of the secretory phase, which can simulate endometrial lesions such as polyps.

Endometrial thickening with cystic spaces and submucosal cystic changes are also known tamoxifen effects.[28,29]

Cystic change in an endometrial abnormality is nonspecific and should not be used as a diagnostic feature. It may occur in polyps due to hemorrhage, infarction, inflammation, and dilated glands (**Fig. 7**).[4,30] Atypical polyps may also contain larger cystic spaces. Endometrial hyperplasia may also be focal and contain cysts in approximately 50% of cases, with concomitant polyps in approximately 25%.[31,32] Thus, TVUS cannot distinguish reliably between polyps and endometrial hyperplasia.

Endometrial cancer is typically diffuse, presenting with endometrial thickening, but may present in polypoid or focal form.[21,33] The appearance is nonspecific, making it difficult to distinguish from polyps and hyperplasia (**Fig. 8**A). With polyps, the endometrial-myometrial interface is preserved. If a clear distinction is not seen, invasion may be suggested (**Fig. 8**B). Heterogeneity, irregular margins, and lack of uterine distensibility are other suspicious sonographic features that warrant further evaluation. Color Doppler is not reliable in differentiating a benign from a malignant process.[16]

A few theoretical concerns exist regarding intraperitoneal seeding as a sequela of SHG. Although a handful of small prospective studies have found that this is of doubtful significance, until further

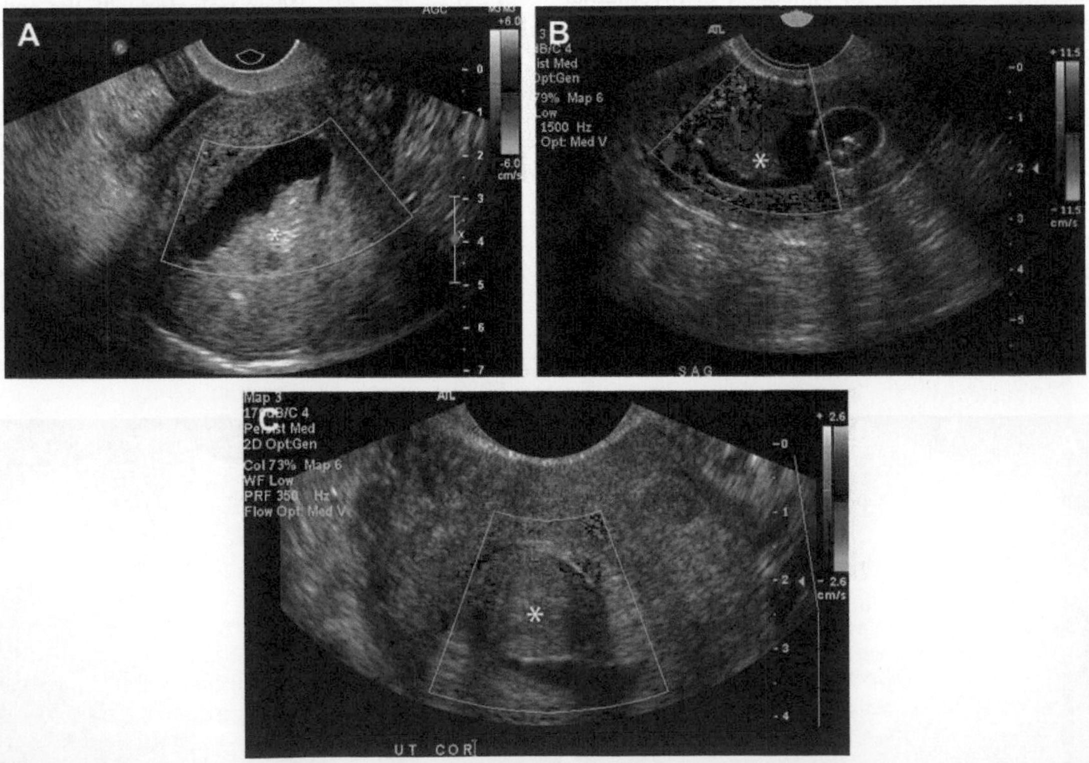

Fig. 6. Usefulness of color Doppler to evaluate lesions detected during SHG. (*A*) Echogenic lesion (*asterisk*) within the endometrial cavity without color Doppler flow is most compatible with a blood clot. This lesion could be displaced by the catheter to confirm diagnosis. (*B*) Lesion (*asterisk*) with a feeding vessel is most compatible with endometrial polyp. (*C*) Color Doppler shows vessels draping over this lesion (*asterisk*) with absence of detectable intralesional vascularity most compatible with a fibroid.

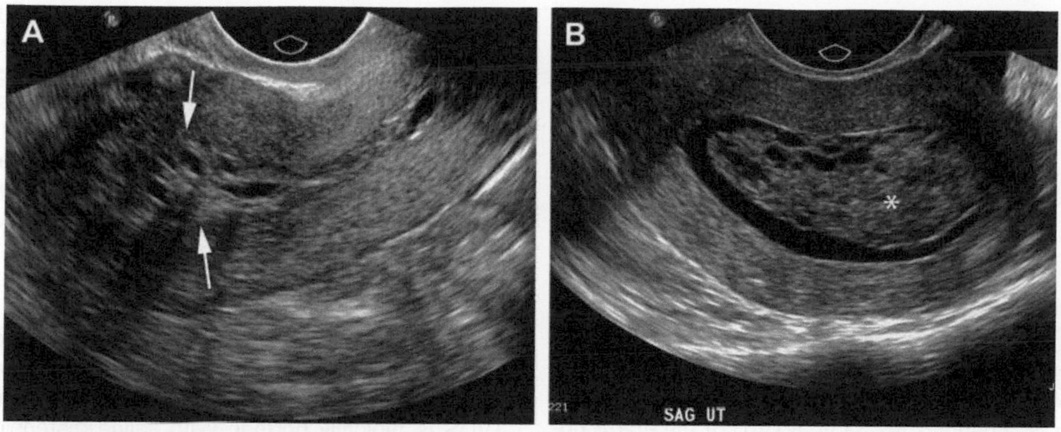

Fig. 7. Cystic change in an endometrial abnormality. (*A*) TVUS of a patient with abnormal uterine bleeding shows a thickened endometrial echo complex with associated cysts (*arrows*). This finding is nonspecific as polyps and hyperplasia may present with cysts. (*B*) Sagittal TVUS obtained during SHG showing fluid around a tamoxifen polyp (*asterisk*), distinguishing it from hyperplasia.

research is available, vigorous flushing and large volumes of saline should be avoided in these cases.[33,34] The use of sterile water rather than saline may be superior because it may cause lysis of any free neoplastic cells.[35]

Intramural Lesions

Of all fibroids, those in a submucosal location are most likely to cause bleeding. In the evaluation of abnormal uterine bleeding, SHG can be used to confirm the submucosal location of fibroids.[36] These fibroids are typically broad based, well defined, and hypo- to isoechoic to myometrium, in contrast to echogenic polyps, which are isoechoic to endometrium. Submucosal myomata are only considered intracavitary if they form acute margins with the endometrium. For treatment planning, it is important to note the number of fibroids, the amount of myometrial penetration or depth, and to describe the extent of any intracavitary component. The approach to treating a large broad-based fibroid is different from that of treating a small almost entirely pedunculated fibroid.[37] The remaining peripheral rim of myometrial tissue should be measured because it is a determining factor for hysteroscopic removal of fibroids. If the fibroid projects into the lumen by more than 50% of its surface, it can usually be hysteroscopically removed.[3]

Adenomyosis, including focal adenomyomas, are less well defined than fibroids and are

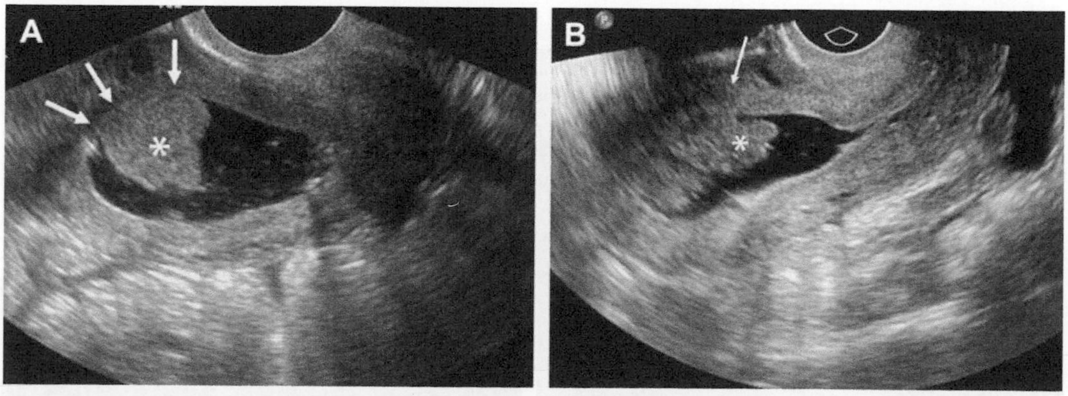

Fig. 8. Polyp versus cancer. (*A*). Sagittal TVUS shows a polyp (*asterisk*) projecting into uterine cavity. The endometrial-myometrial interface (*arrows*) is preserved, which suggests that this is likely a polyp. (*B*) Sagittal TVUS shows an echogenic lesion (*asterisk*) projecting into the uterine cavity. In this case a clear distinction between the lesion and the myometrium is not seen (*long arrow*) and myometrial invasion cannot be excluded. Pathology was consistent with endometrial cancer.

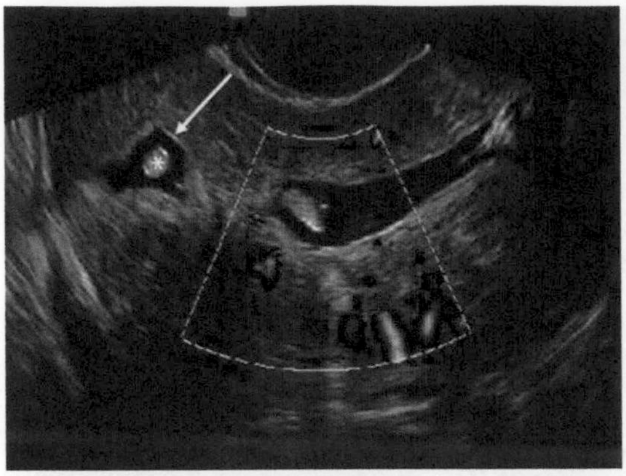

Fig. 9. Adenomyosis. Sagittal TVUS of the uterus obtained during SHG shows fluid distending a crack in the myometrium (*arrow*). These cracks are believed to relate to myometrial penetration of endometrial implants and to correlate with deep diverticula of contrast seen on hysterosalpingography of patients with adenomyosis. Within the crack is an adenomyotic nodule (*asterisk*).

characterized by myometrial heterogeneity and tiny cysts. Color Doppler imaging may show a penetrating vascular pattern. Unlike fibroids, they rarely present with mass effect and most commonly cause diffuse uterine enlargement. When focal, they may look masslike; distinguishing them from fibroids is important, because the treatment options are different. A feature that has recently been described and is not associated with fibroids is the presence of myometrial cracks that fill with fluid during SHG (**Fig. 9**).[24] The early appearance and persistence of echogenic foci in the myometrium has been postulated to be related to air bubbles entering these cracks.

Adenomyosis may present with pseudoendometrial thickening on TVUS because it obscures the endometrial margins. In postmenopausal patients this pitfall can lead to unnecessary biopsies that can be prevented by evaluating with SHG (**Fig. 10**). In addition, the heterogeneity of adenomyosis and blurring of the endometrial boundary can also mask other lesions (**Fig. 11**).

Manifestations of Uterine Scarring

Adhesions result from uterine trauma, most commonly curettage performed in a recent postpartum uterus. In the absence of trapped fluid, TVUS is typically normal. With saline distension, bridging echogenic bands may be found (**Fig. 12**). These bands can vary in length, thickness, and orientation and, when severe, may constrict or obliterate the uterine cavity as in Asherman syndrome.[13] On occasion, endometrial scarring manifests as focal or global decreased distensibility of the uterus. Lysis of adhesions can be performed for these patients. SHG is a useful tool to evaluate for adequacy of the procedure and recurrence.

In patients who have undergone a cesarean delivery, a triangular defect in the lower uterine segment anterior myometrium may be manifest on the sonohysterogram (**Fig. 13**). This cesarean section niche, with an average depth of 6 mm,[38] may be a cause of intermenstrual bleeding. With conventional TVUS the prominent overhanging tissue on the edge of the niche may simulate a fibroid or polyp. SHG can confirm the niche, ruling out focal lesions. In patients who have undergone myomectomy, other niches may be present or the uterine cavity may appear distorted. Again, care must be taken not to confuse the

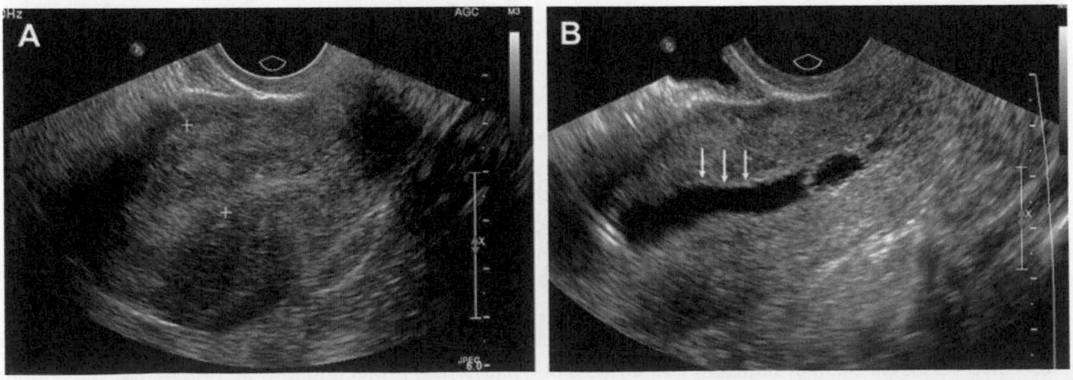

Fig. 10. Pseudoendometrial thickening. This 57-year-old woman presented with intermittent vaginal spotting for 3 months. (*A*) Sagittal TVUS shows apparent endometrial thickening. The apparent myometrial invasion was concerning for cancer. SHG was ordered along with magnetic resonance imaging (MRI). (*B*) Sagittal TVUS obtained during HSG shows an atrophic endometrium (*arrow*). MRI revealed endometrial atrophy and adenomyosis.

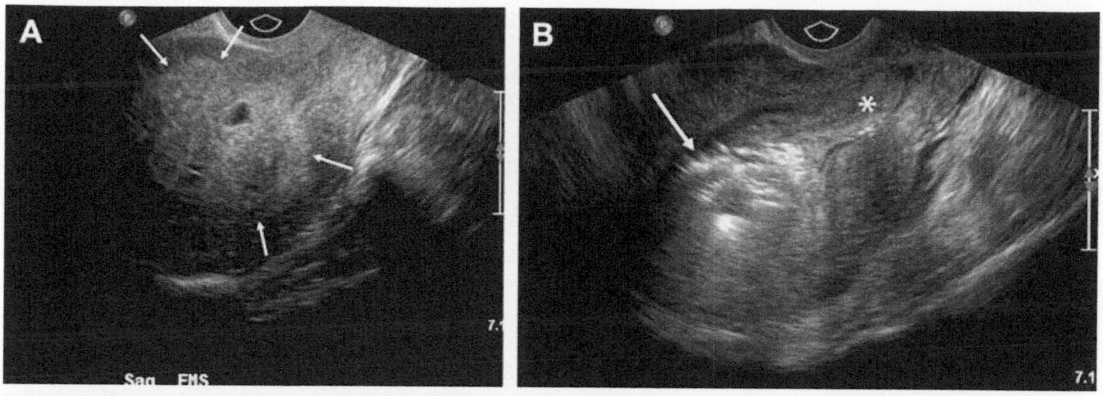

Fig. 11. Adenomyosis masking additional pathology. (*A*) Preprocedural sagittal TVUS shows echogenic lesion extending from endometrium into myometrium with myometrial cyst most compatible with adenomyosis. (*B*) During SHG, air entered myometrial cracks in area of adenomyosis. An incidental polyp (*asterisk*) that was obscured by the adenomyosis on the preliminary scan was revealed.

edges of each scar for pathology. In extreme cases, differentiation from congenital malformation may be difficult. Three-dimensional ultrasound, with its reformatting capabilities, may provide additional invaluable information in these patients.

Congenital Malformations

SHG is less invasive and less expensive than hysteroscopy as a screening examination for infertility patients.[39] It is safer, more informative, and better tolerated than hysteroscopy. SHG is faster and less expensive than MR for evaluating Mullerian duct anomalies with similar diagnostic accuracy.[40] The addition of 3D imaging to SHG results in sensitivities and specificities approaching 100% for diagnosis of an arcuate uterus and major uterine Mullerian duct anomalies.[41] An accurate description of the external fundal contour and internal cavity morphology is necessary to appropriately triage patients for interventional therapy.[42,43] This information is more easily provided by coronal reformatted images. In addition, the volume can be optimally rotated to ensure accuracy of measurements.

SUMMARY

SHG is a useful adjunct to TVS, especially for evaluation of the endometrium and adjacent lesions. The examination is well tolerated, with few complications. Knowledge of potential technical and interpretive pitfalls is essential to minimize patient discomfort, prevent nondiagnostic procedures, and ensure accurate interpretation. Proper technique will increase the efficiency and success rate of the procedure by allowing the practitioner

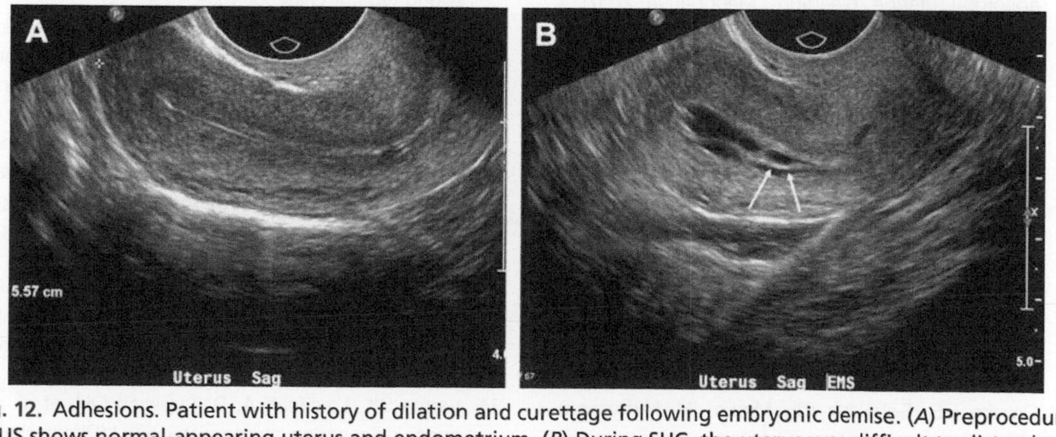

Fig. 12. Adhesions. Patient with history of dilation and curettage following embryonic demise. (*A*) Preprocedural TVUS shows normal-appearing uterus and endometrium. (*B*) During SHG, the uterus was difficult to distend and adhesions (*arrows*) were found.

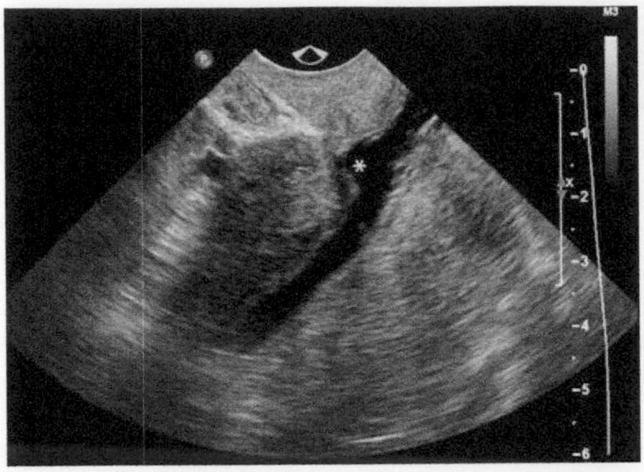

Fig. 13. Cesarean section niche. This 34-year-old woman presented with intermenstrual spotting. Sagittal TVUS shows fluid within the uterine cavity and a triangular defect in the lower uterine segment anterior myometrium (*asterisk*) associated with her cesarean section scar.

to obtain diagnostic information for the patient and her referring physician.

REFERENCES

1. American Institute of Ultrasound in Medicine. AIUM practice guideline for the performance of sonohysterography. Revised February 15, 2007. Published in Conjunction with ACR, ACOG. Available at: http://www.aium.org/publications/clinical/sonohysterography. Accessed January 4, 2010.
2. De Kroon CD, de Bock GH, Dieben SW, et al. Saline contrast hysterosonography in abnormal uterine bleeding: a systematic review and meta-analysis. Br J Obstet Gynaecol 2003;110:947–88.
3. Erdem M, Bilgin U, Bozkurt N, et al. Comparison of transvaginal ultrasonography and saline infusion sonohysterography in evaluating the endometrial cavity in pre- and postmenopausal women with abnormal uterine bleeding. Menopause 2007;14:846–52.
4. Berridge D, Winter T. Saline infusion sonohysterography: technique, indications and imaging findings. J Ultrasound Med 2004;23:97–112.
5. Parsons AK, Lense JJ. Sonohysterography for endometrial abnormalities: preliminary results. J Clin Ultrasound 1993;21:87–95.
6. O'Neill MJ. Sonohysterography. Radiol Clin North Am 2003;4(1):781–97.
7. Bonnamy L, Marret T, Perrotin F, et al. Sonohysterography: a prospective survey of results and complications in 81 patients. Eur J Obstet Gynecol Reprod Biol 2002;102:41–7.
8. Devore GR, Schwartz PE, Morris JM. Hysterography: a five year followup in patients with endometrial carcinoma. Obstet Gynecol 1982;60:369–72.
9. Spieldoch RL, Winter TC, Schouweiler C, et al. Optimal catheter placement during sonohysterography. Obstet Gynecol 2008;111(1):15–22.
10. Bates B. A guide to physical examination. Philadelphia: JB Lippincott Co; 1979. p. 230–48.
11. Lindheim SR, Sprague C, Winter TC. Hysterosalpingography and sonohysterography: lessons in technique. AJR Am J Roentgenol 2006;186:24–9.
12. Lindheim SR, Morales AJ. Comparison of sonohysterography and hysteroscopy: lessons learned and avoiding pitfalls. J Am Assoc Gynecol Laparosc 2002;9:223–31.
13. Cullinan J, Fleischer A, Kepple DM, et al. Sonohysterography: a technique for endometrial evaluation. Radiographics 1995;15(3):501–14.
14. Jeanty P, Besnard S, Arnold A, et al. Air-contrast sonohysterography as a first step assessment of tubal patency. J Ultrasound Med 2000;19:519–27.
15. Lindheim SR. Echosight Patton coaxial catheter guided hysteroscopy. J Am Assoc Gynecol Laparosc 2001;8:307–11.
16. Glanc P, Betel C, Lev-Toaff A. Sonohysterography: technique and clinical applications. Ultrasound Clin 2008;3:427–49.
17. Hajishafiha M, Zobairi T, Zanjani VR, et al. Diagnostic value of sonohysterography in the determination of fallopian tube patency as an initial step of routine infertility assessment. J Ultrasound Med 2009;28(12):1671–7.
18. Kupesic S, Kurjak A. Interventional ultrasound in human reproduction. In: Kupesic S, De Ziegler D, editors. Ultrasound and infertility. New York: Parthenon Publishing; 2000. p. 253–63.
19. Chenia F, Hofmeyr GJ, Moolla S, et al. Sonographic hydrotubation using agitated saline: a new technique for improving fallopian tube visualization. Br J Radiol 1997;70:833–6.
20. Campbell S, Bourne TH, Tan SL, et al. Hysterosalpingocontrast sonography (HyCoSy) and its future role within the investigation of infertility in Europe. Ultrasound Obstet Gynecol 1994;4:245–53.
21. Laifer–Narin S, Ragavendra N, Lu DS, et al. Transvaginal saline hysterosonography: characteristics distinguishing malignant and various benign conditions. AJR Am J Roentgenol 1999;172:1513–20.
22. Lev-Toaff AS, Pinheiro LW, Bega G, et al. Three-dimensional multiplanar sonohysterography. Comparison with conventional two-dimensional sonohysterography and x-ray hysterosalpingography. J Ultrasound Med 2001;20:295–306.
23. Ors F, Lev-Toaff A, Bergin D. Echogenic foci mimicking adenomyosis presumably due to air intravasation into the myometrium during sonohysterography. Diagn Interv Radiol 2007;13:26–9.
24. Verma SK, Lev-Toaff A, Baltarowich OH, et al. Adenomyosis: sonohysterography with MRI correlation. AJR Am J Roentgenol 2009;192:1112–6.

25. Bree RL, Bowerman RA, Bohm-Velez M, et al. US evaluation of the uterus in patients with postmenopausal bleeding: a positive effect on diagnostic decision making. Radiology 2000;216: 260–4.
26. Hann LE, Gretz EM, Lev-Toaff A, et al. Sonohysterography for evaluation of the endometrium in women treated with tamoxifen. AJR Am J Roentgenol 2001; 177:337–42.
27. Hann LE, Kim CM, Gonen M, et al. Sonohysterography compared with endometrial biopsy for evaluation of the endometrium in tamoxifen-treated women. J Ultrasound Med 2003;22:1173–9.
28. Goldstein SR. Unusual ultrasonic appearance of the uterus in patients receiving tamoxifen. Am J Obstet Gynecol 1994;170:447–51.
29. Achiron R, Lipitz S, Sivan E, et al. Sonohysterography for ultrasonographic evaluation of tamoxifen-associated cystic thickened endometrium. J Ultrasound Med 1995;14:685–8.
30. Jorizzo JR, Riccio GJ, Chen MY, et al. Sonohysterography: the next step in the evaluation of the abnormal endometrium. RadioGraphics 1999;19: S117–30.
31. Jorizzo JR, Chen MY, Martin D, et al. Spectrum of endometrial hyperplasia and its mimics on saline hysterosonography. AJR Am J Roentgenol 2002; 179:385–9.
32. Davis PC, O'Neill MJ, Yoder IC, et al. Sonohysterographic findings of endometrial and subendometrial conditions. RadioGraphics 2002;22:803–16.
33. Dessole S, Rubattu G, Farina M, et al. Risks and usefulness of sonohysterography in patients with endometrial carcinoma. Am J Obstet Gynecol 2006;194(2):362–8.
34. Alcazar JL, Errasti T, Zornoza A. Saline infusion sonohysterography in endometrial cancer: assessment of malignant cells dissemination risk. Acta Obstet Gynecol Scand 2000;79(4):321–2.
35. Lev-Toaff AS. Sonohysterography: evaluation of endometrial and myometrial abnormalities. Semin Roentgenol 1996;31(4):288–98.
36. Lev-Toaff AS, Toaff ME, Liu JB, et al. Value of sonohysterography in the diagnosis and management of abnormal uterine bleeding. Radiology 1996;201: 179–84.
37. Corson SL, Brooks PG. Resectoscopic myomectomy. Fertil Steril 1991;55:1041–4.
38. Monteagudo A, Carreno C. Saline infusion sonohysterography in nonpregnant women with previous caesarian delivery: the "niche" in the scar. J Ultrasound Med 2001;20:1105–15.
39. Kim AH, McKay H, Keltz MD, et al. Sonohysterographic screening before in vitro fertilization. Fertil Steril 1998;69:841–4.
40. Deutch TD, Abuhamad AZ. The role of 3-dimensional ultrasonography and magnetic resonance imaging in the diagnosis of Mullerian duct anomalies: a review of the literature. J Ultrasound Med 2008;27:413–23.
41. Kupesic S, Kurjak A. Ultrasound and Doppler assessment of uterine anomalies. In: Kupesic S, de Ziegler D, editors. Ultrasound and infertility. Pearl River (NY): Parthenon; 2000. p. 147–53.
42. Jurkovic D, Gelpel A, Gruboeck K, et al. Three-dimensional ultrasound for the assessment of uterine anatomy and detection of congenital anomalies: a comparison with hysterosalpingography and two-dimensional sonography. Ultrasound Obstet Gynecol 1995;5:233–7.
43. Ghate SV, Crockett MM, Boyd BK, et al. Sonohysterography: do 3D reconstructed images provide additional value? AJR Am J Roentgenol 2008;190:W227–33.

Ultrasound Evaluation of Gynecologic Causes of Pelvic Pain

Lawrence A. Cicchiello, MD[a,*], Ulrike M. Hamper, MD, MBA[b], Leslie M. Scoutt, MD[c]

KEYWORDS

• Pelvic pain • Ultrasound • Gynecologic • Obstetric

Acute pelvic pain, defined as noncyclic pain lasting for less than 3 months, is a common presenting symptom of premenopausal women in an emergency department or physician's office. Acute pelvic pain is a nonspecific symptom and there is a broad range of gynecologic and nongynecologic causes, including gastrointestinal, urologic, and musculoskeletal etiologies. Acute pelvic pain is often associated with other nonspecific signs and symptoms, including nausea, vomiting, and leukocytosis. Hence, imaging is frequently required to narrow the differential diagnosis, and endovaginal ultrasound (EVUS) is the most widely accepted initial imaging modality of choice if there is high clinical suspicion for obstetric or gynecologic etiologies.[1]

Chronic pelvic pain is defined as noncyclic pain lasting longer than 6 months. Approximately 14% of women in the United States report symptoms of chronic pelvic pain, but the cause is often undiagnosed.[2,3] The most common gynecologic causes of chronic pelvic pain include adenomyosis, endometriosis, leiomyomas, adhesions, and pelvic congestion syndrome.[4] Ultrasound (US) is most helpful in the diagnosis of leiomyomas, adenomyosis, and endometriosis. This article reviews the role of US in the evaluation of gynecologic causes of acute and chronic pelvic pain.

ACUTE PELVIC PAIN

Gynecologic causes of acute pelvic pain can be further categorized into obstetric and nonobstetric causes. Therefore, the first step in the evaluation of a premenopausal woman with acute pelvic pain is to establish if the patient is pregnant, with a β–human chorionic gonadotropion (hCG) level. Common gynecologic causes of pelvic pain in nonpregnant patients include large ovarian cysts, ruptured or hemorrhagic cysts, pelvic inflammatory disease (PID), ovarian or adnexal torsion, and malpositioned intrauterine devices (IUDs). Because many of these conditions may also occur during pregnancy, they should also be considered in pregnant patients with pelvic pain. Common gynecologic causes of pelvic pain associated with pregnancy include hemorrhagic corpus luteums (CL), spontaneous abortion (SAB), ectopic pregnancy (EP), subchorionic hemorrhage, pain associated with ovarian hyperstimulation syndrome (OHSS), and degenerated fibroids. Postpartum causes of pelvic pain include endometritis, retained products of conception (RPOCs), ovarian vein thrombophlebitis, and rupture of the uterus.[5]

[a] Department of Diagnostic Radiology, Yale University School of Medicine, 333 Cedar Street, PO Box 208042, New Haven, CT 06520-8042, USA
[b] Division of Ultrasound, Department of Diagnostic Radiology, The Johns Hopkins Medical Institutes, 600 North Wolfe Street, Baltimore, MD 21287, USA
[c] Ultrasound Service, Department of Diagnostic Radiology, Yale University School of Medicine, 333 Cedar Street, PO Box 208042, New Haven, CT 06520-8042, USA
* Corresponding author. Department of Diagnostic Radiology, Yale-New Haven Hospital, 20 York Street, New Haven, CT 06511.
E-mail address: lcicchiello@gmail.com

Ultrasound Clin 5 (2010) 209–231
doi:10.1016/j.cult.2010.03.005
1556-858X/10/$ – see front matter

ACUTE PELVIC PAIN IN NONPREGNANT PATIENTS

Simple Ovarian Cysts

Most ovarian follicles measure less than 1 cm in diameter. The dominant follicle typically measures less than 2.5 cm at the time of ovulation. A follicle that fails to release an oocyte or does not regress can enlarge into a follicular cyst and accounts for the vast majority of simple ovarian cystic structures. The term, *follicular cyst*, is reserved for lesions measuring greater than 3 cm, but these lesions can often grow larger, especially during pregnancy. Small ovarian cysts are common but usually asymptomatic and have been reported in up to 7% of asymptomatic premenopausal women.[6] Large or enlarging ovarian cysts, however, can be a source of pelvic pain, and cysts larger than 5 cm are believed to predispose to ovarian torsion. Sonographically, follicular cysts appear as unilocular anechoic intraovarian or exophytic ovarian masses with thin, imperceptible walls and posterior acoustic enhancement. When follicular cysts become large, it may be difficult to appreciate the adjacent ovarian parenchyma, which may be compressed or hidden from view (**Fig. 1**). In premenopausal women, the risk of malignancy in a simple ovarian cyst is low.[7] The current recommendation by the Society of Radiologists in Ultrasound is that asymptomatic simple ovarian cysts larger than 7 cm in premenopausal women should be referred for evaluation with MRI to ensure that mural nodularity is not missed due to sampling error with US.[8] Asymptomatic simple cysts greater than 5 cm but less than 7 cm in diameter are amenable to yearly follow-up with US. Follow-up is not necessary for asymptomatic simple cysts less than or equal to 5 cm in diameter in the reproductive age group.[8]

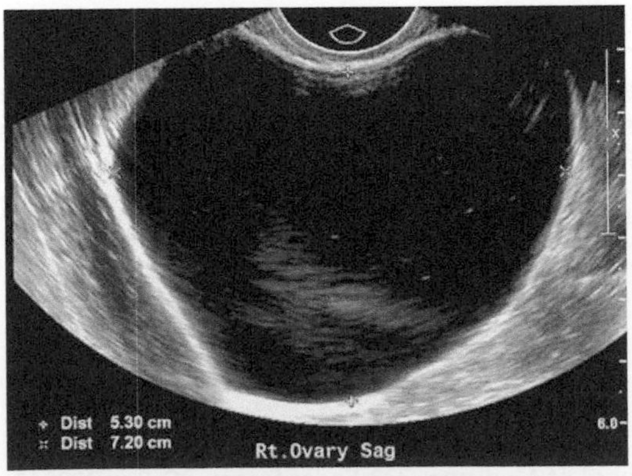

Fig. 1. Follicular cyst. This 19-year-old woman presented to the emergency department with acute pelvic pain. EVUS reveals a large right adnexal anechoic cystic structure (calipers) in the region of the patient's pain consistent with a follicular cyst. The wall is smooth and there is posterior wall enhancement. The origin of the pain is not certain in this patient and could be due to mass effect, stretching of the capsule of the cyst or ovary, torquing of the ovarian pedicle, or leakage.

Ruptured or Hemorrhagic Ovarian Cysts

The most common gynecologic cause of acute pelvic pain in nonpregnant, afebrile premenopausal women presenting to an emergency department is a ruptured or hemorrhagic ovarian cyst. Ruptured or hemorrhagic ovarian cysts typically present with acute-onset, severe, but self-limited, unilateral pelvic pain. Patients are most commonly afebrile with a normal white blood cell count. If the cyst is leaking, rebound tenderness may be present. If there is a large amount of intra-abdominal bleeding, patients may be hypotensive or present with syncope. A ruptured ovarian cyst may be a diagnosis of exclusion on US examination because the ovary may appear completely normal if the cyst has completely ruptured and the fluid resorbed or dispersed throughout the peritoneal cavity. A leaking ovarian cyst may have a crenated appearance, however, containing low-level echoes or clot. Adjacent free fluid may be noted (**Fig. 2**).[9] On US, hemoperitoneum, which is most commonly found in the cul-de-sac, is diagnosed by the presence of free intraperitoneal fluid containing low-level echoes. Free intraperitoneal fluid often has a triangular or pointed configuration as it interdigitates between loops of bowel and pelvic structures. If there is a large amount of bleeding, heterogeneous masses of clot may be observed within the fluid or surrounding the uterus and ovary (**Fig. 3**). Clot can be distinguished from adjacent bowel by the lack of vascularity on Doppler interrogation and absence of peristalsis. Bowel also has a tubular configuration. If there is a substantial amount of bleeding, hemoperitoneum extends from the pelvis into the upper abdomen. Hence, the hepatorenal recess, or Morison pouch, as well as the left upper quadrant should be evaluated transabdominally for the presence of blood (see **Fig. 2**).[10] This constellation of findings can mimic a ruptured EP, and a β-hCG level should be obtained in any premenopausal women presenting with acute pelvic pain, hemoperitoneum, or syncope.[11] The US findings of hemoperitoneum are nonspecific, however, and echoes within fluid can also be caused by debris or infection.

The sonographic appearance of hemorrhagic cysts is variable depending on when, in the evolution of the hemorrhage, patients are imaged.

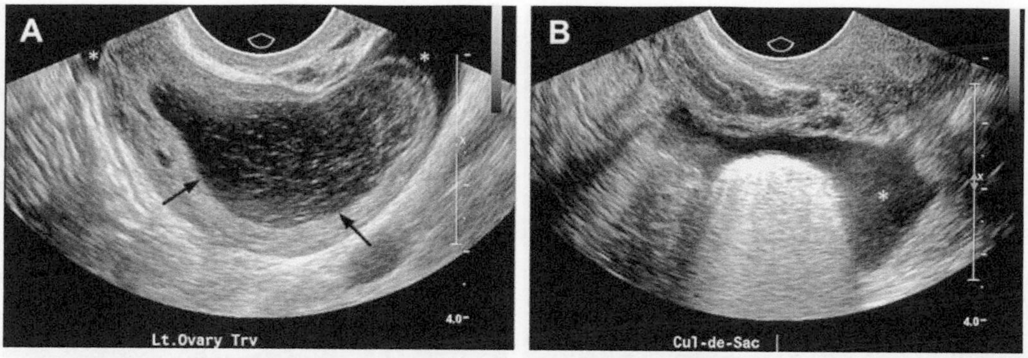

Fig. 2. Leaking hemorrhagic ovarian cyst. This 18-year-old woman presented to the emergency department with acute, left-sided, pelvic pain. (*A*) Transverse EVUS image of the left ovary reveals a collapsing, crenated hemorrhagic left ovarian cyst (*arrows*). Note adjacent free fluid (*) and fine reticular stranding within the cyst consistent with hemorrhage. (*B*) Image of the cul-de-sac reveals free fluid (*) containing low-level echoes consistent with hemoperitoneum.

Acutely, a hemorrhagic cyst on US examination demonstrates a pattern of diffuse, low-level, internal echoes; no internal vascularity; a thin wall; and increased through transmission. As the red blood cells lyse and fibrin strands form within the hemorrhagic cyst, a lace-like or fishnet reticular pattern of internal echoes is observed (**Fig. 4**). These strands should be thin, smooth, and avascular. Over time, echogenic thrombus coalesces within the cyst, forming a heterogenous avascular mass with retractile (angular or concave) margins (**Fig. 5**). Clot within a hemorrhagic cyst is

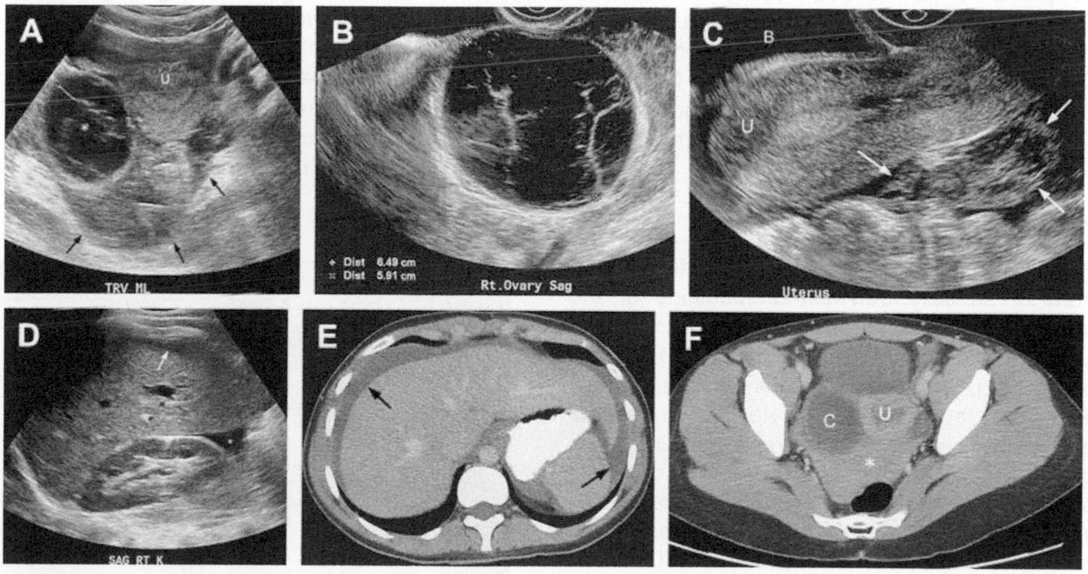

Fig. 3. Ruptured hemorrhagic ovarian cyst. This 33-year-old woman presented to the emergency department with syncope after abrupt onset of right-sided pelvic pain. (*A*) Transverse transabdominal image of the pelvis reveals a large right adnexal cystic structure (*) with internal septations. Note large amount of adjacent clot and complex free fluid consistent with hemoperitoneum (*arrows*). The uterus (U) has an arcuate configuration. (*B*) EVUS image reveals fine, irregular septations within the cyst (calipers) consistent with fibrin stranding. (*C*) Sagittal midline EVUS image reveals free fluid and clotted blood (*arrows*) in the cul-de-sac posterior to the uterus (U). Note small amount of free fluid superior to the uterine fundus underneath the bladder (B). (*D*) Transabdominal US image of the right upper quadrant reveals free fluid (*) in Morison pouch and also between the liver and the diaphragm (*arrow*). The presence of clotted blood in the cul-de-sac as well as fluid in the right upper quadrant suggests that there has been a large amount of bleeding. (*E*) CT scan of the upper abdomen reveals fluid around the liver and spleen (*arrows*). (*F*) CT scan of the pelvis reveals dense fluid (*) in the cul-de-sac consistent with hemorrhage. Note hemorrhagic right ovarian cyst (C) and uterus (U) posterior to the bladder.

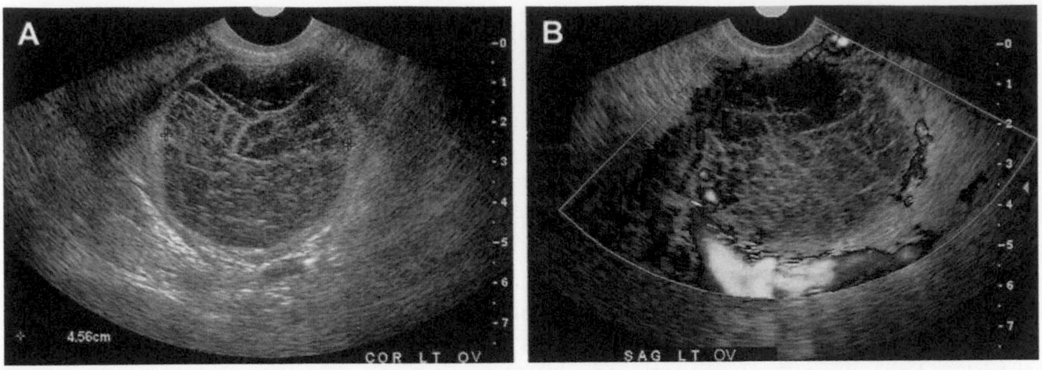

Fig. 4. Hemorrhagic ovarian cyst. This 24-year-old patient presented with acute, left-sided, pelvic pain. (*A*) EVUS of the left ovary reveals a 4.56-cm cystic mass (calipers) demonstrating a reticular lace-like pattern of internal echoes and strand-like septations. (*B*) Power Doppler EVUS image reveals a small amount of blood flow in the wall of the cyst but no evidence of internal vascularity.

usually dependent but can become adherent to the cyst wall as it evolves. Intraluminal clot can occasionally have a more rounded configuration and thereby mimic the US appearance of a mural nodule within a cystic ovarian neoplasm.[12] Although lack of vascularity on Doppler interrogation within a focal echogenic area in an ovarian cyst favors the diagnosis of hemorrhagic clot, Doppler US is not 100% sensitive for the depiction of tumor vascularity. Therefore, follow-up imaging in 6 to 8 weeks in such cases is recommended. Clots resolve or change in that time frame.[12] If vascularity develops or if the area increases in size or even stays the same, a tumor nodule should be strongly suspected.

Pelvic Inflammatory Disease

Pelvic inflammatory disease (PID) includes a spectrum of sexually transmitted infections of the cervix, uterus, fallopian tubes, and ovaries. The classic clinical symptoms of acute PID include pelvic pain, cervical motion tenderness, vaginal discharge, fever, and leukocytosis. The severity of the pain is variable, ranging from mild pelvic discomfort to severe bilateral lower quadrant pain. Most cases are caused by *Chlamydia trachomatis* or *Neisseria gonorrhoeae*, but coinfection with other bacteria is common.[13] PID is an ascending infection beginning as cervicitis, ultimately spreading upwards through the genital tract to involve first the endometrium (endometritis) and then the fallopian tubes (salpingitis). As the purulent material spills out into the peritoneal cavity from the fimbriated ends of the fallopian tubes, it typically coats the serosal surface of the uterus causing a serositis and eventually engulfs the adjacent ovary forming a tubo-ovarian abscess (TOA). PID is most commonly a bilateral process involving both adnexa, although sometimes to different degrees. Less commonly, TOAs can be the result of direct spread of infection to the adnexa from intra-abdominal infections, usually from the bowel, such as appendicitis or diverticulitis. Although endometritis most often occurs in the setting of PID, endometritis may also occur post partum or after instrumentation.

Because the symptoms of PID are frequently nonspecific, endovaginal sonography can be a useful adjunct to the clinical presentation in the diagnosis of PID. Although EVUS is most sensitive for detecting ovarian and tubal involvement of disease, with sensitivity of 90% and 93%, respectively, it is less sensitive for the detection of cervical or uterine involvement.[14] In early acute

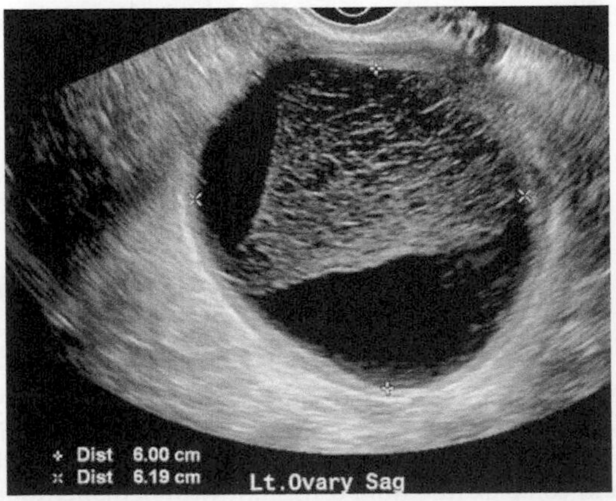

Fig. 5. Hemorrhagic ovarian cyst. This 34-year-old woman presented with acute, left-sided, pelvic pain for 2 days. EVUS reveals a cystic structure (calipers) in the left adnexa. Note moth-eaten appearance of the central area of internal echoes, which has straight/concave margins consistent with retractile clot. Doppler interrogation (not shown) revealed no internal vascularity.

PID, when only the cervix is involved, US examination is typically normal, and the diagnosis of cervicitis is usually made by visual inspection and culture. Sonographic findings of endometritis include the presence of fluid or gas within the endometrial canal, heterogeneous thickening of the endometrial stripe, and indistinctness of the endometrial stripe. Echogenic foci with distal shadowing may indicate the presence of air within the infected debris in the endometrial cavity (**Fig. 6**). Doppler interrogation may demonstrate increased, low-resistance vascularity. Inflammation of the fallopian tubes manifests as thickening of the tube with increased vascularity. Hydrosalpinx, or a dilated, fluid-filled fallopian tube, can develop secondary to obstruction from pelvic adhesions or post inflammatory scarring and appears sonographically as a tubular anechoic adnexal structure, often U- or S-shaped. It is common for a dilated tube to fold on itself. When this occurs, the inner walls of the tube along the fold compress together creating the appearance of an incomplete septation. The dilated tube can have a cogwheel appearance on transverse images with multiple tiny mural protrusions representing the inflamed folded/redundant tubal mucosa. In patients with chronic salpingitis, the tube may demonstrate a beads-on-a-string appearance.[15] The presence of low-level echoes or layering with a fluid-debris level in a dilated, fluid-filled tube suggests the diagnosis of pyosalpinx (**Fig. 7**). The presence of a thin hypoechoic rim, likely representing fluid and purulent material, surrounding the uterus suggests inflammation of the serosal surface of the uterus (uterine serositis). Finally, when the infection involves the fallopian tube and ovary, a tubo-ovarian complex or abscess develops, which manifests sonographically as a complex thick-walled, multilocular cystic collection in the adnexa. Typically, internal echoes or multiple fluid-fluid levels are observed within the locules (**Fig. 8**). The walls and septations of TOAs are usually hypervascular with a low-resistance arterial waveform pattern. Acute TOAs are usually bilateral and tender on US examination. TOA is used to describe lesions with complete breakdown of tubal and ovarian architecture.[14–16] If an ovarian capsule or some ovarian tissue is preserved, the term, *tubo-ovarian complex*, is used. Tubo-ovarian complexes usually respond better to antibiotic therapy than TOAs. Purulent fluid, with increased echogenicity and debris, can be seen in the cul-de-sac. Increased echogenicity of the pelvic fat also can be seen occasionally (**Fig. 9**) and is the sonographic correlate of fat stranding commonly seen on CT in patients with inflammatory disorders.[16]

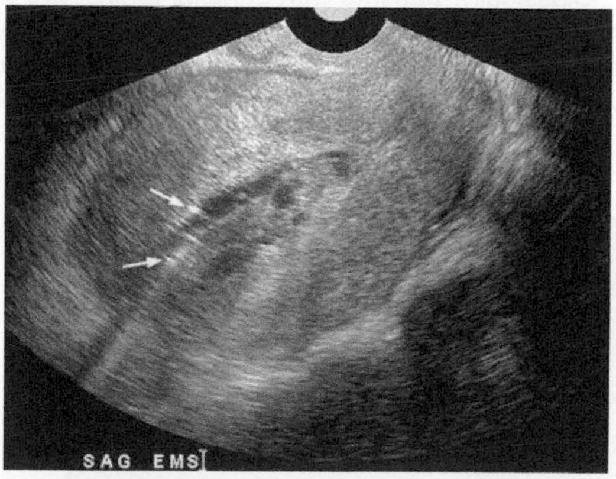

Fig. 6. Endometritis. This 23-year-old woman presented with pelvic pain, fever, and purulent discharge. Sagittal EVUS images of the uterus demonstrate a thick, heterogeneous, endometrial stripe consistent with the presence of debris, hemorrhage, or purulent material. The outer margins of the endometrial stripe are indistinct. Echogenic areas (*arrows*) with posterior shadowing and ring-down artifact are consistent with the presence of air.

Pelvic abscesses may occur after surgery or trauma or may develop secondary to bowel pathology. Patients most often present with acute pain, fever, and leukocytosis. Rebound tenderness may be present. The degree of pain may be variable and the presenting symptoms are nonspecific. Although CT is generally considered the imaging modality of choice in women with suspected pelvic abscess, US is an alternative imaging choice in pregnant or younger patients because it avoids the risk of radiation exposure. In addition, abscesses may be found when a patient is imaged with US for other suspected pathology.

On US, pelvic abscesses appear as complex, often irregularly marginated, multilocular fluid collections containing low-level echoes (**Fig. 10**). The internal echogenicity may range from hypoechoic to quite echogenic if air or subacute bleeding is present. The walls may be vascular with a low-resistance arterial waveform pattern. Adjacent purulent fluid containing low-level echoes may be noted. Pelvic hematomas may be indistinguishable (**Fig. 11**) and may also present with acute pelvic pain. Aspiration may be required to exclude superinfection although the wall of an abscess is typically more echogenic and vascular than the wall of a hematoma.

Ovarian Torsion

Ovarian torsion accounts for approximately 3% of all gynecologic emergencies.[17] It is defined as

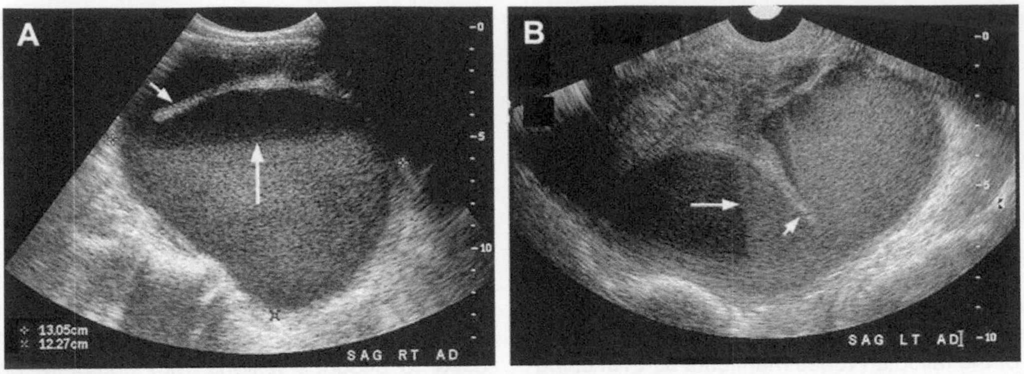

Fig. 7. Pyosalpinx. (*A, B*) EVUS images of the left adnexa in this 19-year-old woman with pelvic pain and fever demonstrate a dilated tubular structure (calipers in [*A*]) filled with debris/purulent material consistent with a pyosalpinx. Note fluid/fluid layering (*long arrow*) and incomplete septation (*short arrow*) where the tube folds on itself. Note that the fimbriated end of the tube is larger than the more medial portion.

partial or complete twisting of the ovary or fallopian tube around its vascular pedicle. Torsion of the vascular pedicle initially results in lymphatic and venous obstruction and, if not relieved, eventually progresses to compromise arterial flow. In up to 67% of cases, the ovary and fallopian tube are twisted together resulting in adnexal torsion.[18] The right adnexa is more commonly involved.[17] Adnexal torsion is a surgical emergency and timely diagnosis and intervention are required to preserve vascularity and prevent ovarian necrosis. The chance of salvaging viable ovarian tissue markedly decreases if symptoms have persisted for longer than 48 hours.[19] Risk factors for ovarian torsion include the presence of an ipsilateral adnexal mass, pregnancy, ovulation induction, prior tubal ligation, and hypermobility of adnexal structures.[17,18,20–22] An ipsilateral adnexal mass greater than 5 cm is the most common risk factor and is reported to be present in 22% to 73% of cases.[17,18,21,22] Dermoids are reportedly the most commonly associated lesion, present in up to 20% of cases.[18] Malignant lesions are less likely than benign lesions to cause adnexal torsion, with 1 series reporting less than 1% of cases involving a malignant lesion.[20] Larger masses (>10 cm) are less likely to undergo torsion probably due to the larger weight as well as compression or fixation in place by adjacent pelvic structures. Although adnexal torsion occurs most commonly in women of reproductive age, ovarian torsion is reported in all age groups, including in utero. Hypermobility of adnexal structures is believed to be the most common predisposing risk factor in children and adolescents. Isolated torsion of the fallopian tube is most common in the adolescent age group.

Classically, patients with adnexal torsion are of reproductive age and present with acute onset of excruciating pelvic pain associated with nausea, vomiting, and adnexal tenderness. The greater

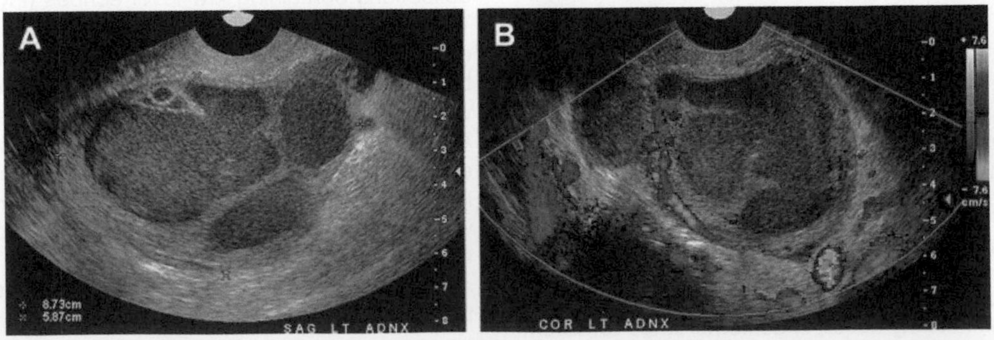

Fig. 8. Tubo-ovarian abscess. This 23-year-old woman presented with pelvic pain, fever, and purulent vaginal discharge. (*A*) Sagittal EVUS image of the left adnexal reveals a complex multilocular cystic mass (calipers) with thick irregular septations and low-level echoes within the cystic components consistent with debris, pus, or hemorrhage. (*B*) Color Doppler image demonstrating vascularity in the wall of the TOA. This mass was tender on physical examination.

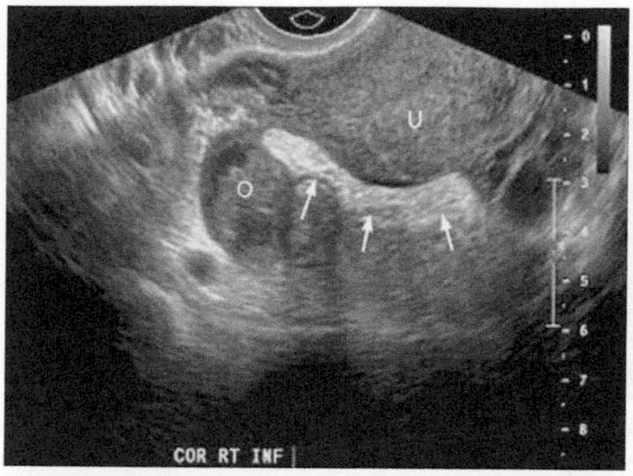

Fig. 9. Echogenic pelvic fat. Note increased echogenicity in the pelvic fat (*arrows*) between the uterus (U) and the right ovary (O) in this 23-year-old woman with PID. Increased echogenicity in the pelvic fat is a nonspecific finding indicative of inflammation or infection and may be seen on US examination in patients with Crohn disease, ulcerative colitis, diverticulitis, and appendicitis.

the pain, the higher the concern for ovarian torsion. In more than half of all patients with adnexal torsion, however, the pelvic pain is reported as mild or intermittent.[20–22] A pelvic or abdominal mass is a common presentation of adnexal torsion in children and adolescents. Although there is usually no accompanying fever or leukocytosis, occasionally a mildly elevated white blood cell count can be found. Because of the often confusing clinical picture and overlap of clinical presentation with other causes of pelvic pain, including gastrointestinal pathology and renal colic, a CT scan is often the first imaging study performed. If ovarian torsion is clinically suspected, however, EVUS should be the initial imaging modality of choice.

The sonographic findings of ovarian torsion are variable and often depend on the degree of twisting, the tightness of the torquing, the duration of the torsion, whether or not the fallopian tube has also undergone torsion, and whether or not the

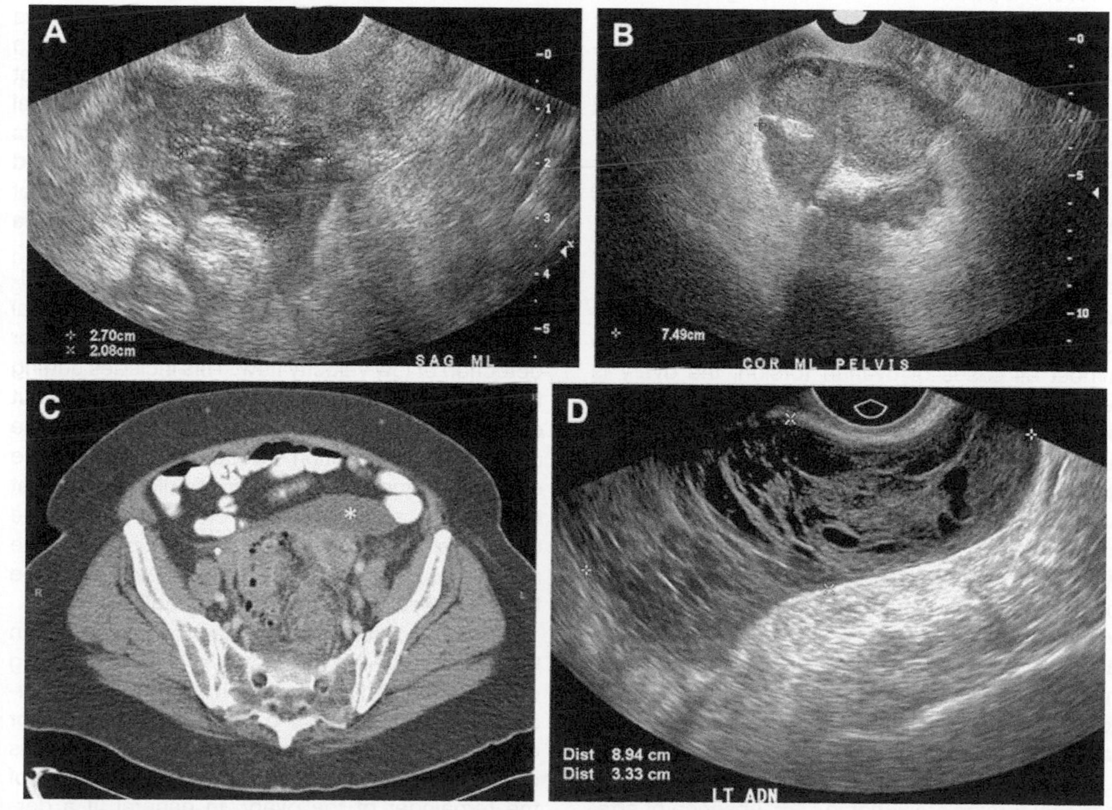

Fig. 10. Pelvic abscess. (*A*) Sagittal EVUS images in a patient status–post hysterectomy who presents with pelvic pain and fever. Note fluid collection (calipers) containing debris/purulent material in the midline superior to the vaginal cuff. (*B*) This second patient also presented with pelvic pain and fever. EVUS revealed a complex, irregular cystic mass (calipers) in the region of the patient's pain. (*C*) CT scan demonstrates diverticular abscess containing air and fluid. Note free intraperitoneal air and adjacent free fluid (*) as well as many diverticula arising from the sigmoid colon. (*D*) In this third patient with a pelvic abscess status–post hysterectomy, note fluid collection (calipers) with many fine reticular septations in the left adnexa.

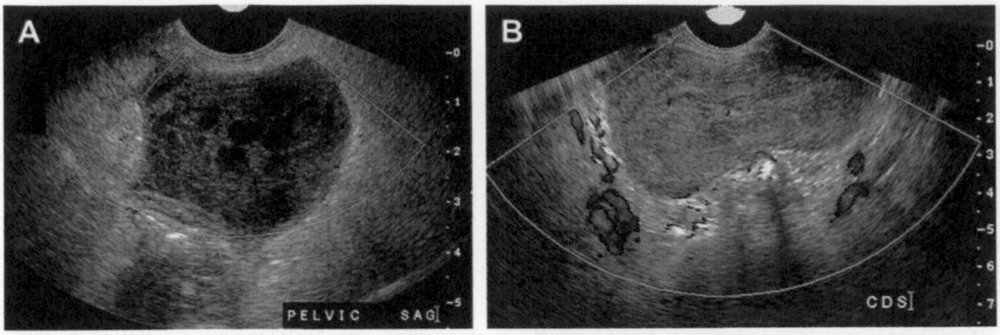

Fig. 11. Pelvic hematoma. There is a wide spectrum of sonographic appearance depending on the length of time since the hemorrhage occurred. The sonographic findings overlap with those of pelvic abscess and, depending on the clinical presentation, aspiration may be required to exclude superinfection of a hematoma. (*A*) Note avascular hypoechoic collection with coalescent anechoic spaces on this color Doppler image. The US appearance is reminiscent of a hemorrhagic cyst. Note triangular outer margins as the hematoma collects between loops of the bowel. (*B*) In this second patient, the hematoma is more echogenic with well-defined smooth margins similar to the US appearance of clotted blood. Power Doppler interrogation revealed no evidence of blood flow.

torsion is intermittent.[23] The ovarian pedicle may have multiple geometric twists, but if there is no pressure to pull the twisted vessels tight, the blood supply may not be compromised. The classic gray-scale US features of ovarian torsion are enlargement of the ovary, which is often found in a midline position; heterogeneity of the central stroma with echogenic areas representing hemorrhage and hypoechoic areas indicative of edema; and peripheral displacement of the ovarian follicles (**Fig. 12**).[19,23] These findings are not always seen, especially if the duration of symptoms has been long (**Fig. 13**). A longstanding infarcted ovary may have a more complex or amorphous morphologic appearance with cystic degeneration. In almost all cases of ovarian torsion, the ovary is tender. An underlying ovarian mass is often identified (**Fig. 14**). A thickened, swollen tubular structure between the ovary and uterus representing the twisted vascular pedicle may be seen. In cross section, this twisted vascular pedicle demonstrates a target appearance on gray-scale imaging with alternating hyperechoic and hypoechoic bands/circles.[24] On color Doppler, the twisted vessels within the vascular pedicle are described as a whirlpool sign.[25] Adjacent free fluid may be noted. If the fallopian tube alone has undergone torsion, a hydrosalpinx with beaking or angular tapering of the twisted end may be observed.

Spectral Doppler findings in women with adnexal torsion are variable.[26–28] Absence of arterial flow is a highly specific finding for ovarian torsion with a positive predictive value of 94% in 1 study.[26] This is a late finding of ovarian torsion, however, and often indicates that the ovary is not viable. Abnormal vascularity is frequently seen, including decreased or absent diastolic flow and absent venous flow.[28] Completely normal arterial and venous ovarian flow has been described, however, in surgically proven cases of ovarian torsion (see **Figs. 12** and **13**). Therefore, if the gray-scale appearance is suggestive of ovarian torsion, a normal Doppler examination does not exclude the diagnosis. One series reported normal Doppler US findings in up to 60% of cases.[27] This may be due to varying degrees of twisting and tightening of the twists, the intermittent nature of adnexal torsion, and the dual blood supply to the ovary from the ovarian and uterine arteries.

To accurately use Doppler interrogation to evaluate for arterial flow in suspected cases of adnexal torsion, the Doppler settings must be optimized for detection of low velocity flow. This includes setting the color/spectral gain as high as possible without causing noise and motion artifact. The color scale and pulse repetition frequency should be decreased and the wall filter should also be set to low.[29] A small straight color box should be used and attention should be focused on the area between the ovary and uterus near the uterine fundus to search for the twisted pedicle.

Pitfalls in sonographic diagnosis of ovarian torsion include the coexistence of an underlying complex ovarian mass, which can obscure visualization of the normal ovarian architecture. For example, acoustic attenuation from calcifications or fat in a dermoid cyst can limit evaluation of the remainder of the ovary. In general, if a dermoid is tender on examination, there must be concern for torsion or rupture (see **Fig. 14**). Also, in the presence of OHSS, the ovary becomes enlarged and the ovarian architecture is markedly distorted, making the diagnosis of ovarian torsion difficult.

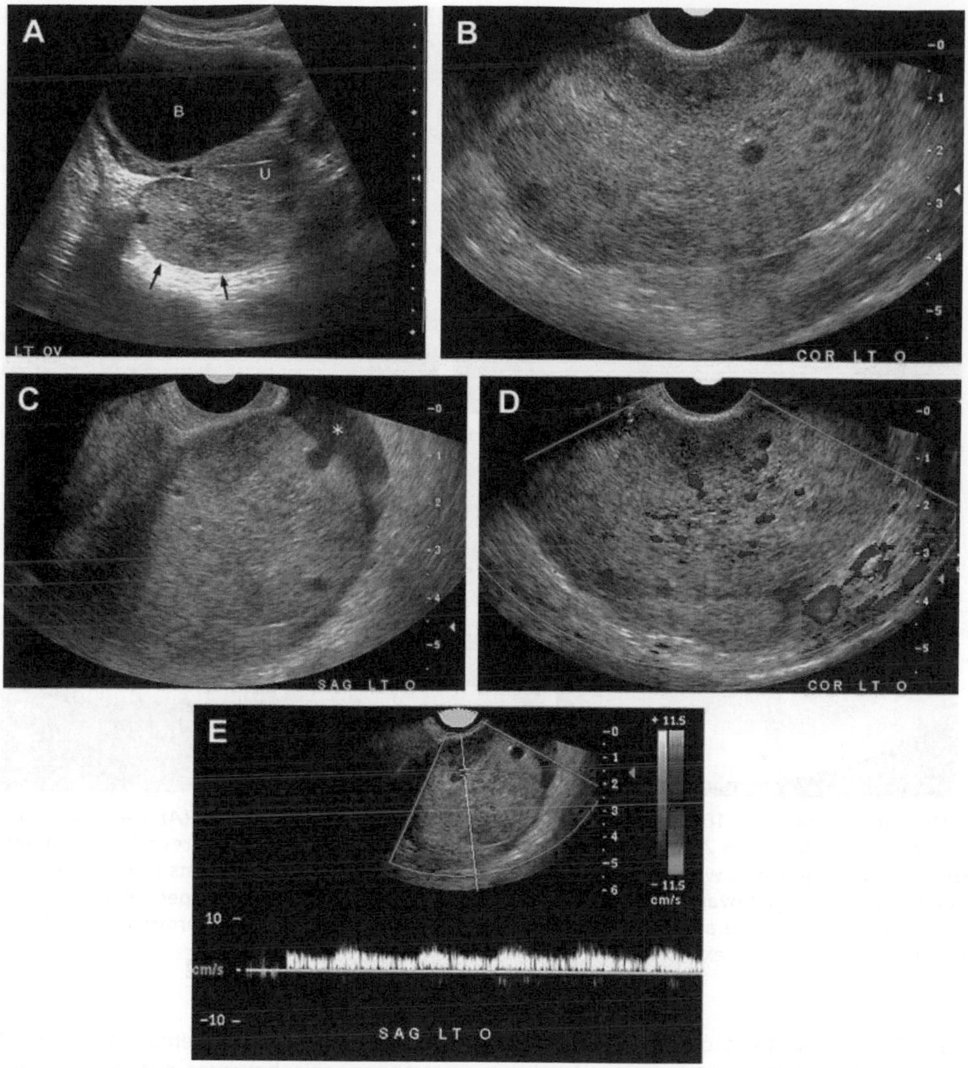

Fig. 12. Ovarian torsion. This 33-year-old woman presented with intermittent left pelvic pain. (*A*) Transabdominal image reveals a markedly enlarged left ovary (*arrows*) located midline in the cul-de-sac posterior to the uterus (U) and bladder (B). (*B, C*) EVUS gray-scale images show to better advantage the heterogenous central ovarian stroma and peripheral displacement of small follicles in the enlarged left ovary. No underlying mass is seen. (*C*) Note small amount of adjacent free fluid (*). (*D*) Color Doppler image demonstrates venous and arterial flow (red and blue). (*E*) Spectral Doppler tracing reveals a normal arterial waveform. The presence of normal arterial and venous flow does not exclude the diagnosis of ovarian torsion.

Malpositon of Intrauterine Devices

IUDs should be positioned in the center of the endometrial cavity in the uterine fundus. Localization of an IUD is most readily accomplished with EVUS. Penetration of the myometrium or perforation of the uterus is a rare complication of IUDs (**Figs. 15** and **16**). Such patients most often present with pelvic pain or loss of visualization of the string within the endocervical canal. Occasionally, penetration of the myometrium may be an incidental finding. Recent literature suggests that 3-D US is more accurate and sensitive than EVUS alone for identifying myometrial penetration of IUDs.[30]

ACUTE PELVIC PAIN ASSOCIATED WITH PREGNANCY

Corpus Luteum

A corpus luteum is the remnant of a mature ovarian follicle after ovulation and is frequently seen during the secretory phase of the menstrual cycle. If a patient becomes pregnant, the CL secretes progesterone, which serves to maintain the pregnancy until the placenta forms. Although usually

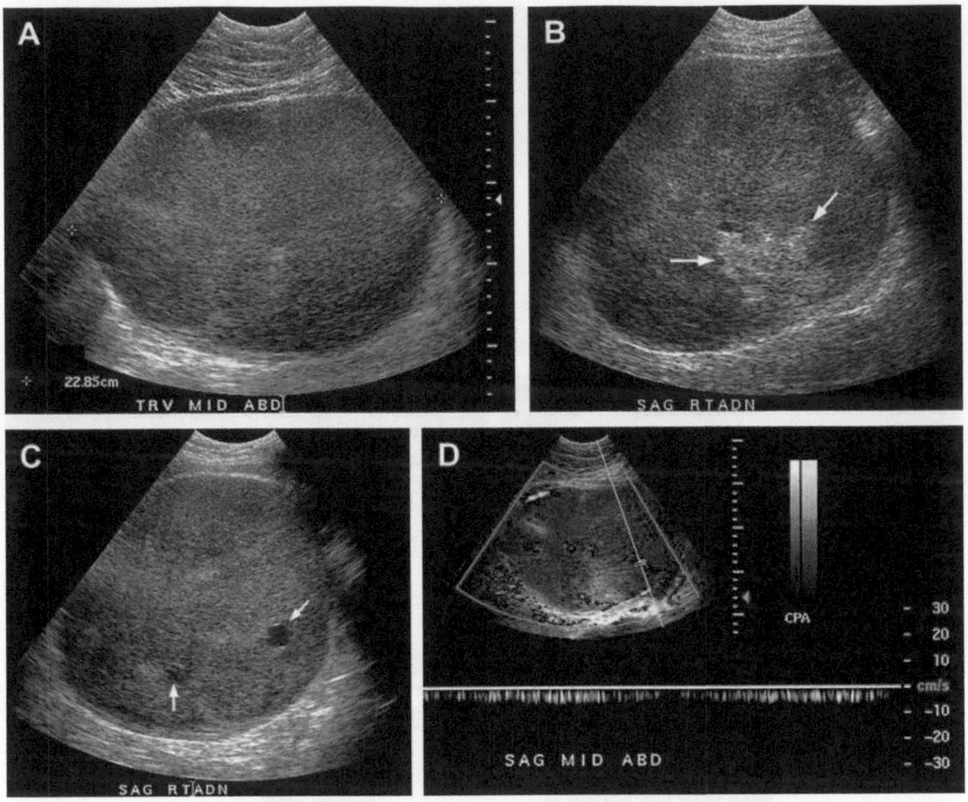

Fig. 13. Ovarian torsion. This 16-year-old girl presented with a large pelvic mass. (*A*) Transabdominal image reveals a largely homogeneous 22.8-cm pelvic mass (calipers). (*B*) Careful inspection reveals a geographic echogenic area (*arrows*) consistent with hemorrhagic infarction and (*C*) several small cysts (*arrows*), which confirm that this mass is an enlarged ovary. (*D*) Despite the presence of venous flow on this spectral and power Doppler image, the ovary was infarcted at surgery, which also revealed a large underlying fibrothecoma, which was not prospectively identified on US examination.

asymptomatic, leaking from or hemorrhage into the CL can cause unilateral pelvic pain or tenderness. Rarely, clinically significant hemoperitoneum can result from rupture of a CL (see **Fig. 3**). A normal CL has a variety of sonographic appearances. Most commonly on US, the CL appears as a round anechoic intraovarian or exophytic ovarian cystic mass with a homogeneous thick moderately echogenic wall, which may be highly vascular with a low-resistance arterial waveform (**Fig. 17**).[31] CLs are usually under 3 cm in size. Hemorrhage into a CL can create a sonographic pattern of internal echoes similar to a hemorrhagic follicular cyst (see **Figs. 4** and **5**) and rupture of the cyst can result in hemorrhage or clot surrounding the ovary or within the peritoneal cavity (see **Figs. 2** and **3**). Occasionally the CL has a diffusely homogeneous echotexture similar in echogenicity to the ovarian stroma and mimics the US appearance of a solid ovarian mass. Color Doppler interrogation may demonstrate marked vascularity in the wall, thereby separating the CL from the surrounding ovarian parenchyma. These findings are nonspecific, however, and in pregnant patients an exophytic CL may be difficult to differentiate from an EP. Great care must be taken to confirm the presence of an intrauterine pregnancy (IUP). Correlation with serum β-hCG levels may also be helpful in these cases.

Subchorionic Hemorrhage

Subchorionic hemorrhage is defined as separation of the chorion and the endometrial lining by blood, which collects within the subchorionic space. Small subchorionic hemorrhages are common and usually asymptomatic. Large collections may present with vaginal bleeding or abdominal pain or cramping. The echogenicity of a subchorionic hemorrhage varies over time. Acute hemorrhage typically appears more echogenic whereas subacute to chronic hemorrhages can appear hypoechoic (**Fig. 18**).[32] The outcome of subchorionic hemorrhage is likely related to the size of the

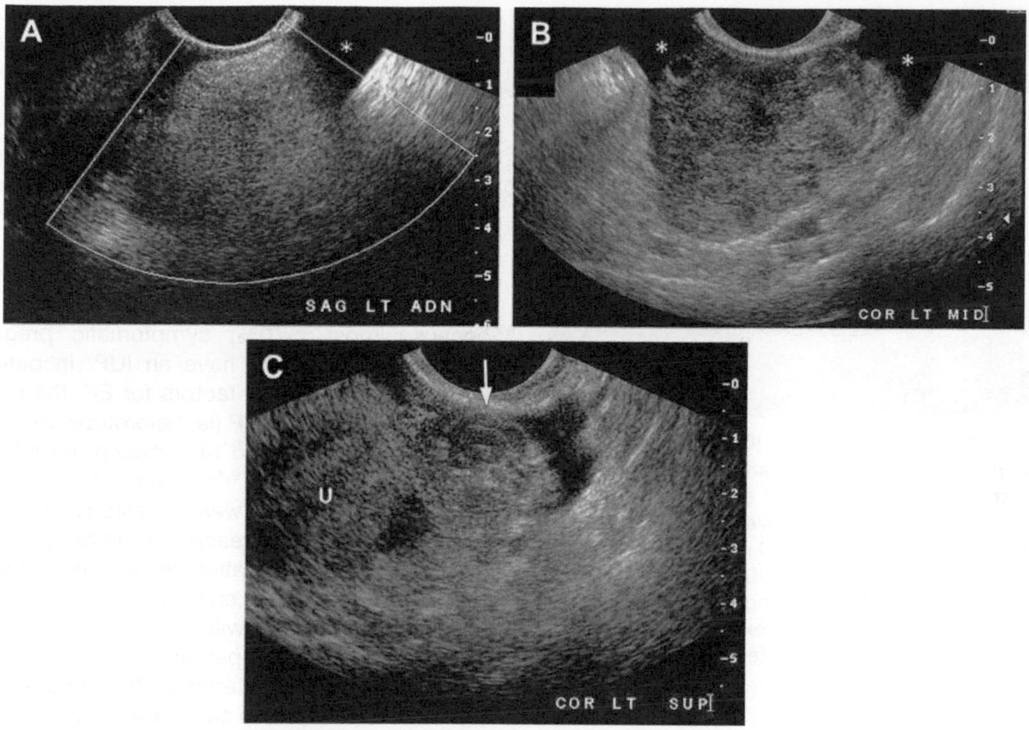

Fig. 14. Torsion of an ovarian dermoid. This 24-year-old woman presented with acute, left-sided, pelvic pain. (*A*) EVUS color Doppler image of the left adnexa reveals a homogeneously echogenic left adnexal mass with posterior attenuation in the region of the patient's pain. Findings are consistent with a dermoid. No color flow is identified. Because ovarian dermoids are primarily cystic, however, blood flow is rarely seen on color Doppler imaging. Tenderness on examination and adjacent free fluid (*) are clues to the possibility of torsion or rupture which can also cause pelvic pain. In a patient with a painful dermoid, every attempt should be made to look for the pedicle between the dermoid and the uterus as well as the adjacent ovarian parenchyma because of the clinical concern for torsion. (*B*) EVUS image slightly more superior and midline reveals the adjacent ovary, which is enlarged with heterogeneity of the central stroma. Note peripheral displacement of small follicles and adjacent free fluid (*), findings suggestive of ovarian torsion. (*C*) EVUS image more superiorly reveals the target sign (*arrow*) in a transverse plane through the swollen and twisted vascular pedicle between the ovary/dermoid below (not shown) and the uterus (U) confirming the diagnosis of torsion.

collection, maternal age, gestational age, and the presence or absence of pain.[32–34]

Spontaneous Abortion

SAB is defined as pregnancy loss before 20 weeks gestational age, but the majority of SABs occur during the first 16 weeks. Causes of SAB include genetic or fetal causes, structural uterine abnormalities, maternal endocrine causes, immunologic causes, and infectious causes.[35] The most common presenting symptoms are pelvic pain, cramping, or vaginal bleeding. The sonographic findings depend on the gestational age. In symptomatic pregnant patients, US examination has an important role in differentiating SAB or fetal demise from a viable IUP or EP. In patients with a suspected SAB, EVUS can be useful in determining whether or not macroscopic tissue remains, which may influence patient management. The presence of an abnormal distorted gestational sac or tissue demonstrating trophoblastic flow, characterized by increased diastolic and systolic velocity, suggests an incomplete abortion (**Fig. 19**).[36] The EVUS criterion for embryonic demise is the absence of cardiac activity as documented by 2 or more observers for 1 to 3 minutes in an embryo with a crown-rump length greater than 5 to 6 mm. A complete abortion is defined as complete expulsion of products. In this case, the endometrial cavity is empty or may contain hemorrhage or debris, but no products of conception or trophoblastic flow are seen.[35,36]

Ectopic Pregnancy

EP results when a fertilized oocyte implants outside the endometrial cavity. Although EPs are most commonly located in the ampullary segment of the fallopian tube, ectopic implantation can

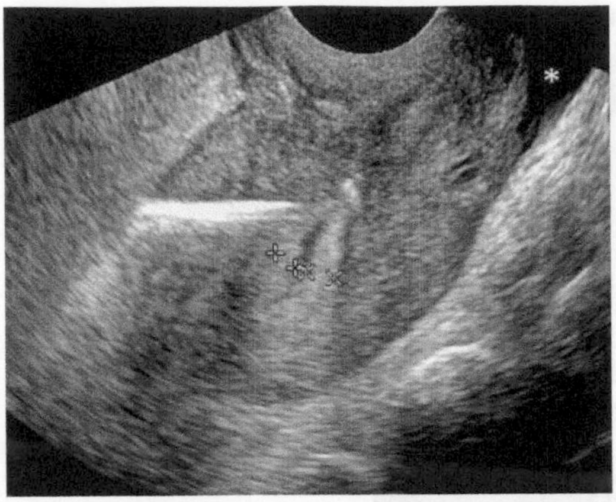

Fig. 15. Malposition of an IUD. This 26-year-old woman presented with pain and vaginal bleeding 2 years status–post placement of an IUD. Sagittal endovaginal image of the uterus reveals a small amount of fluid between the anterior and posterior layers of the endometrium (calipers). The IUD, an echogenic linear structure with distal shadowing, has penetrated the anterior myometrial wall and extends beyond the serosal surface of the uterus. Note small amount of free fluid (*) in the cul-de-sac.

occur, in order of decreasing frequency, in the isthmic, fimbrial, or interstitial portions of the fallopian tube, ovary, cervix, myometrial scars, and peritoneal cavity (intra-abdominal EP).[37] The possibility of EP should be considered in any woman of reproductive age who presents with acute pelvic pain and a positive β-hCG level. The most recent reports indicate that EPs account for approximately 2% of all pregnancies.[38] Although the mortality rate from EPs has declined in recent years, it remains the most common cause, accounting for 9%, of pregnancy-related deaths in the first trimester.[39] Risk factors for EP include history of prior EP, PID, infertility treatment, prior pelvic surgery, endometriosis, and pregnancy that occurs after placement of an IUD.[40] Although patients with EPs can be asymptomatic, EPs more commonly present with pelvic pain, vaginal bleeding, a palpable adnexal mass, or peritoneal signs. Evaluation for suspected EP should begin with a quantitative measurement of serum β-hCG levels and EVUS.[41,42]

The first step in an EVUS examination performed to evaluate for EP should be to assess for an IUP because most (>70%) symptomatic pregnant patients are found to have an IUP. In patients without significant risk factors for EP, the risk of a coexisting IUP and EP (ie, heterotopic pregnancies) is rare, estimated at between 1/7000 and 1/30,000 pregnancies.[9,43,44] An IUP should be seen on EVUS by 5 weeks gestational age or once the β-hCG level reaches 1000 to 2000 mIU/mL.[41] An eccentric location, within the anterior or posterior layer of the endometrium, of a round anechoic structure with an echogenic rim describes the initial appearance of an IUP on US examination and is termed, *the intradecidual sign*.[45] Once the mean sac diameter of an IUP is greater than or equal to 10 mm, the double decidual sac sign should be present.[46] This refers to the presence of 2 echogenic rings surrounding part of the anechoic gestational sac. The 2 echogenic rings represent the decidua capsularis and decidua parietalis. The hypoechoic area in-between the 2 layers represents a small amount of hypoechoic fluid in the endometrial cavity. If no IUP is seen in a pregnant woman, the diagnostic possibilities include an early IUP of less than 5 weeks' gestational age, embryonic demise or miscarriage, and EP. If the serum β-hCG level is greater than 2000 mIU/mL and no IUP is seen, an EP must be strongly considered even in the absence of adnexal

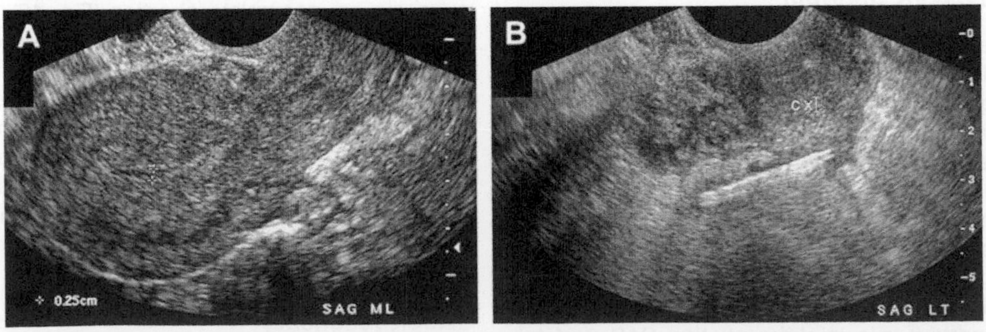

Fig. 16. Perforation of the myometrial wall by an IUD with extrusion into the peritoneal cavity. This 31-year-old woman presented with pelvic pain 5 years status–post insertion of an IUD. (*A*) Midline sagittal EVUS of the uterus reveals no evidence of an IUD within the endometrial cavity (calipers). (*B*) Sagittal EVUS reveals the linear echogenic IUD posterior to the cervix (cx) in the cul-de-sac surrounded by a small amount of complex fluid. It has been completely extruded through the myometrial wall.

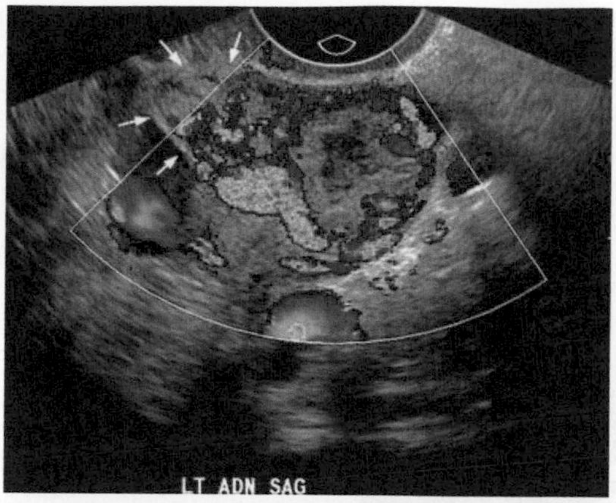

Fig. 17. Corpus luteum. Color Doppler EVUS image of the left adnexal reveals an exophytic CL arising from the left ovary (*arrows*). The wall is thick, homogenous, hypoechoic, and vascular. As the CL involutes, the central cystic component may develop a star-like configuration with internal echoes due to debris and hemorrhage.

findings, although the diagnostic possibilities include SAB or multiple IUPs.[9,47–50]

The most specific sonographic finding of an EP is the presence of an extrauterine gestational sac containing a yolk sac or embryo (**Fig. 20**).[49–51] An empty tubal ring is the next most specific finding. The wall of an EP is typically echogenic and vascular and EPs are most commonly found in the adnexa between the uterus and ovary. The next most common location is in the cul-de-sac. In the absence of an IUP and with a serum β-hCG level greater than 2000 mIU/mL, however, any extraovarian adnexal mass (except a simple cyst) raises suspicion for an EP.[48–51] A pseudogestational sac, caused by decidualized endometrium and fluid within the endometrial cavity, may be found in 10% to 20% of patients.[49,50,52] A pseudogestational sac is distinguished from an early IUP by the central location of the fluid between the anterior and posterior endometrial layers and by its elliptical shape.[52] Free fluid may be the only initial sonographic finding in 15% of cases.[51,53] One series reported that 63% of patients with EP had free fluid in the cul-de-sac. Low-level echoes within the free fluid correlates with hemoperitoneum and has been reported in 56% of patients with EP.[54]

It is often difficult to distinguish the empty tubal ring of an EP from an exophytic CL cyst. Both may have an echogenic, vascular wall (ring of fire) and a low-resistance arterial waveform.[31,53,55] Establishing an intraovarian location strongly favors the diagnosis of a CL cyst because intraovarian ectopic pregnancies are rare. Intraovarian location can be confirmed by synchronous movement of the structure with the ovary after manual compression of the ovary during the endovaginal examination or by the demonstration of a small rim of ovarian tissue surrounding the lesion (claw sign).[9] In addition, the wall of the CL tends to be thicker and more homogeneous and hypoechoic than the rim of an EP, although there is overlap in the US appearance.[55,56]

Ovarian Hyperstimulation Syndrome

OHSS is an iatrogenic condition that arises in women undergoing ovulation induction, and

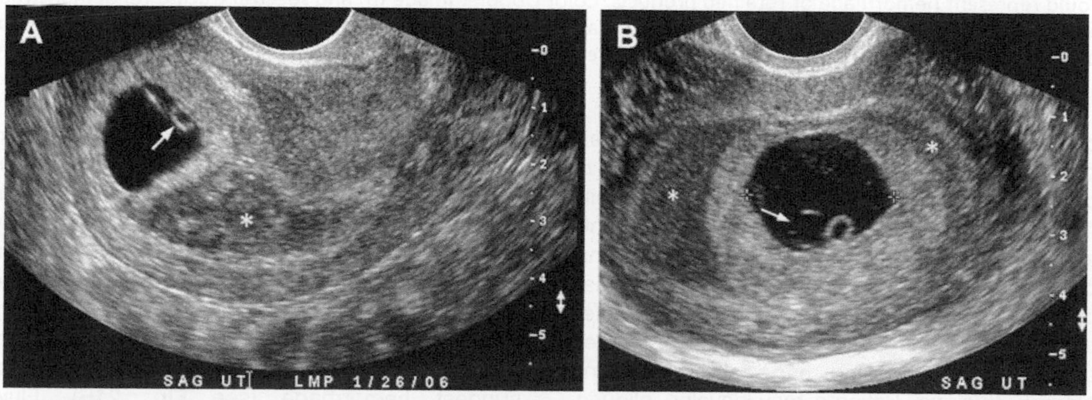

Fig. 18. Subchorionic hemorrhage. (*A*) Note echogenic subchorionic hemorrhage (*) in this asymptomatic patient. The subchorionic hemorrhage is adjacent to and slightly larger than the intrauterine gestational sac, which contains a yolk sac (*arrow*). Approximately 25% of the perimeter of the gestational sac is undermined by the subchorionic hemorrhage in this imaging plane. (*B*) This second patient presented with vaginal bleeding in the first trimester. The subchorionic hemorrhage (*) is hypoechoic and, although smaller in volume than the gestational sac (calipers), undermines close to 75% of the perimeter. Note empty amnion (*arrow*) without evidence of an embryo, another poor prognostic sign, next to the yolk sac.

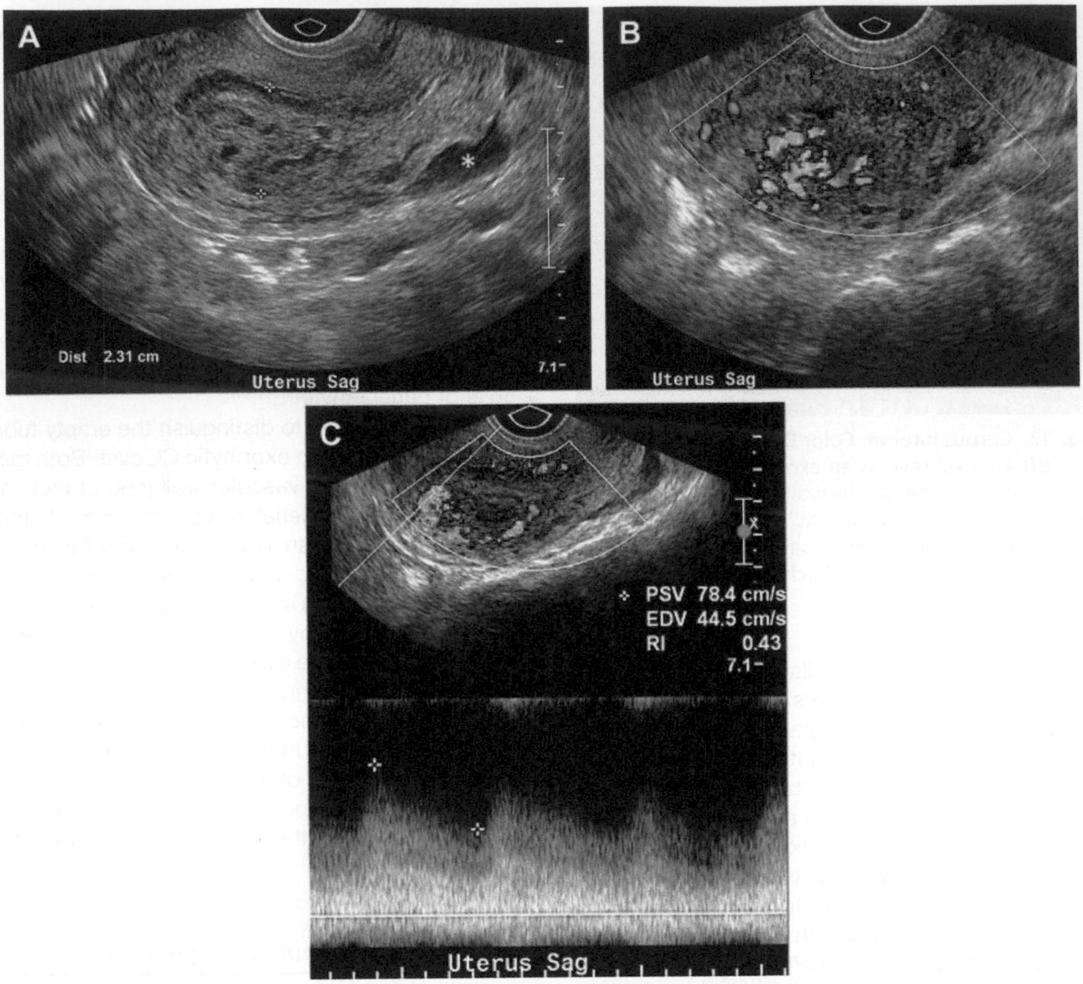

Fig. 19. Spontaneous abortion. This 29-year-old woman presented with pain and vaginal bleeding in the first trimester. (*A*) Sagittal EVUS images of the uterus. Note thickened (2.3-cm) heterogenous endometrial stripe (calipers) and a small amount of free fluid in the cul-de-sac (*). Findings are nonspecific on gray-scale imaging and could represent hemorrhage or retained products. Color Doppler image (*B*) and spectral tracing (*C*) demonstrate a large amount of vascularity with a low-resistance arterial waveform pattern within the heterogeneous material distending the endometrial canal consistent with retained trophoblastic tissue.

occurs during early pregnancy or during the luteal phase of the ovulatory cycle. The incidence of severe OHSS ranges from 0.5% to 5%.[57] In mild cases, both ovaries become enlarged and patients experience mild pelvic discomfort. Abdominal distention, nausea, and vomiting also may occur.[58] In advanced cases, multiple follicles develop and enlarge both ovaries accompanied by third spacing of fluid, especially ascites and pleural effusions. Patients may develop oliguria, tachypnea, and hypotension.[59] The ovaries can grow to more than 10 cm in diameter predisposing them to torsion. Acute pelvic pain in these patients can result from rapid enlargement of a follicle, stretching of the ovarian capsule, hemorrhage into or rupture of a follicle, or ovarian torsion. In 1 series, 60% of pregnant patients who developed ovarian torsion had undergone ovulation induction and had some degree of OHSS.[27] As the ovarian parenchyma is almost completely replaced by many enlarged follicles, the diagnosis of ovarian torsion is difficult in these patients. Sonographic findings in patients with OHSS include markedly enlarged multicystic ovaries (**Fig. 21**A). Debris, retractile clot, or fluid-fluid levels within a cyst suggest hemorrhage (see **Fig. 21**B). Fluid surrounding an ovary or change in shape of a cyst can suggest recent cyst rupture or leakage. Doppler interrogation should always be performed in symptomatic patients to help assess for torsion, although the presence of blood flow does not exclude the diagnosis. Asymmetric size and

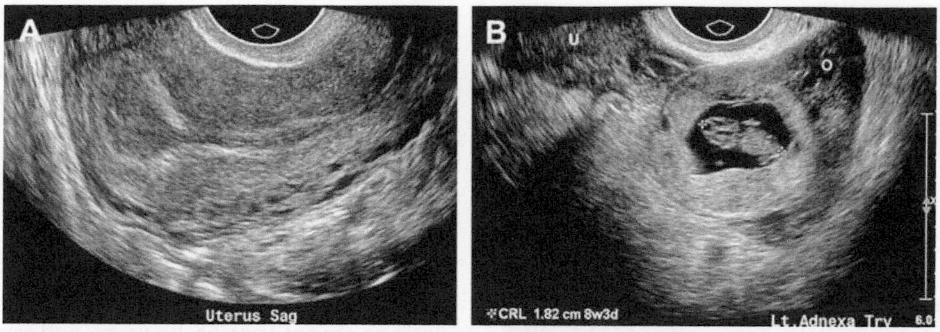

Fig. 20. Ectopic pregnancy. This 24-year-old woman presented with left-sided pelvic pain in the first trimester. (*A*) Sagittal EVUS image of the uterus reveals no evidence of an IUP. (*B*) Image of the left adnexa reveals an extra-uterine gestational sac with an echogenic rim containing an embryo (calipers). The EP is located between the uterus (U) and left ovary (O). M-mode Doppler revealed a heart rate of 124 beats per minute (not shown).

tenderness should be viewed with suspicion and follow-up MRI may be helpful in confirming the diagnosis of ovarian torsion in these patients. Pelvic ascites can be seen on EVUS, but transabdominal imaging should be performed to evaluate the extent of peritoneal fluid and to look for pleural effusions.

Leiomyomas

Uterine leiomyomas are benign smooth muscle neoplasms reported to occur in up to 40% of women over 30 years old.[60,61] They are commonly associated with dysmennorhea, menorrhagia, chronic pelvic pain and pressure, and infertility. Chronic pelvic pain is usually due to mass effect from large leiomyomas and compression of adjacent structures. Compression of the ureters by an enlarged fibroid uterus, for example, may cause hydronephrosis and flank pain. Leiomyomas are hormonally responsive, and acute pelvic pain can occur when a leiomyoma infarcts or undergoes degeneration, usually after a rapid change in size growing during pregnancy or involuting post partum. Most commonly, a leiomyoma appears as a well-defined hypoechoic mass arising from the myometrium, but the sonographic appearance is variable and leiomyomas can appear echogenic or heterogeneous on US examination. Leiomyomas often demonstrate posterior acoustic shadowing and edge refraction.[62–64] Leiomyomas that have undergone hemorrhagic degeneration during pregnancy tend to demonstrate anechoic cystic spaces and echogenic areas (**Fig. 22**).[65] Pedunculated subserosal leiomyomas can also undergo torsion and become necrotic, which can also be a source of pelvic pain.

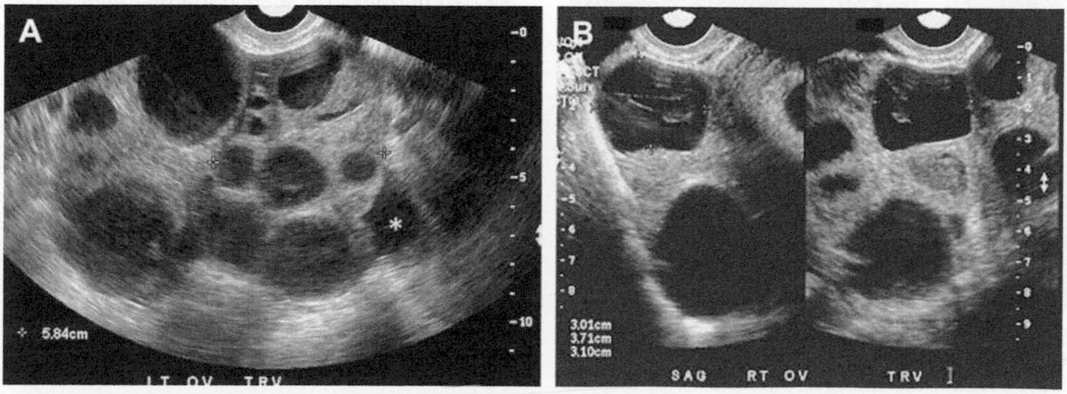

Fig. 21. Ovarian hyperstimulation syndrome. This 37-year-old woman presented with pelvic pain and fullness after ovulation induction. (*A*) Transverse EVUS reveals that both ovaries are massively enlarged (calipers = left ovary) and contain many anechoic cysts or follicles. A small amount of free fluid (*) is noted adjacent to the left ovary. (*B*) Two weeks later the patient experienced sudden onset of severe pain on the right. Note debris consistent with hemorrhage in one of the right ovarian follicles (calipers).

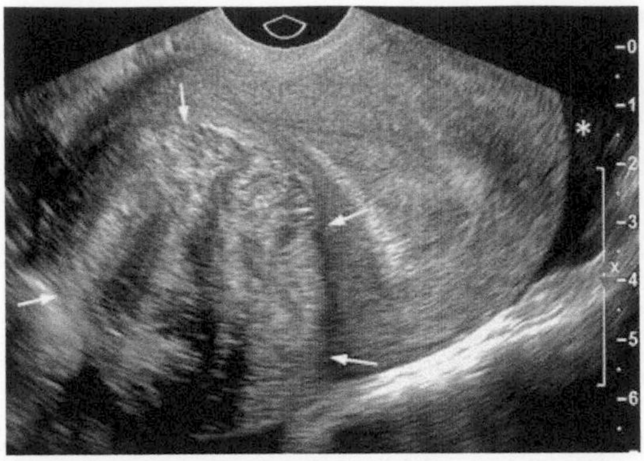

Fig. 22. Hemorrhagic infarction of a leiomyoma. This 28-year-old patient presented with acute, right-sided, pelvic pain in the first trimester. Sagittal EVUS reveals a retroverted uterus, empty endometrial canal, and a moderate amount of free fluid (*) near the fundus of the uterus. Note heterogeneous mass (*arrows*) in the anterior wall of the uterus in the region of the patient's pain with areas of increased echogenicity and shadowing. A shadowing myometrial mass most likely represents a leiomyoma. Although leiomyomas may be echogenic on US, in the setting of acute pain this likely represents hemorrhagic infarction. Under the hormonal stimulation of pregnancy, this leiomyoma likely grew rapidly, outstripping its blood supply and infarcting causing sudden-onset, severe, pelvic pain.

PELVIC PAIN IN THE POSTPARTUM PERIOD

Retained Products of Conception

RPOCs complicate approximately 1% of all deliveries but are more common after termination of pregnancy or miscarriage. Patients usually present with vaginal bleeding and pelvic pain or cramping.[66] Without treatment, not only do symptoms persist but also pelvic infection and sepsis may develop. Sonographically, RPOCs have a variable appearance, ranging from a heterogenous thick endometrial stripe with trophoblastic flow similar to the US appearance of a patient undergoing miscarriage with residual trophoblastic tissue (see **Fig. 19**) to the presence of an echogenic crescentic mass of placental tissue or fetal parts. The findings are not specific, however, and similar findings can be observed in the normal postpartum uterus.[67,68] Although the diagnosis is made clinically by plateauing of the serum β-hCG level, the finding of visible macroscopic tissue on EVUS can help direct patient management and is suggestive that surgical or pharmacologic completion may be preferable to observation.

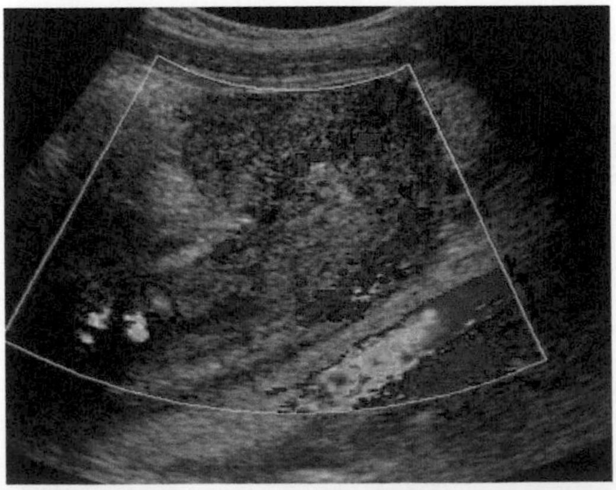

Fig. 23. Ovarian vein thrombophlebitis. This 34-year-old patient presented with abdominal pain and fever 2 days status–post cesarean section. Color Doppler image demonstrates a large tubular structure anterior to the iliac artery (red) and vein (blue) consistent with a massively dilated gonadal vein almost completely filled with thrombus. Minimal peripheral vascularity is noted.

Endometritis

Endometritis is a common cause of postpartum pelvic pain and fever and is usually accompanied by leukocytosis and vaginal discharge. Endometritis occurs after cesarean section more commonly than vaginal delivery. Risk factors include prolonged labor, premature rupture of membranes, and RPOCs. The sonographic appearance of endometritis is variable and nonspecific with overlap in the appearance of the normal postpartum endometrium and RPOCs. The endometrium can appear normal or thickened with increased vascularity. Fluid and echogenic debris consistent with hemorrhage or clot are common findings. Echogenic foci with distal shadowing or ring-down artifact may be seen in patients with air in the endometrial cavity, which is concerning for infection (see **Fig. 6**).[66] However, air can normally be seen in the endometrial cavity for up to 3 weeks post delivery up to 3 weeks post

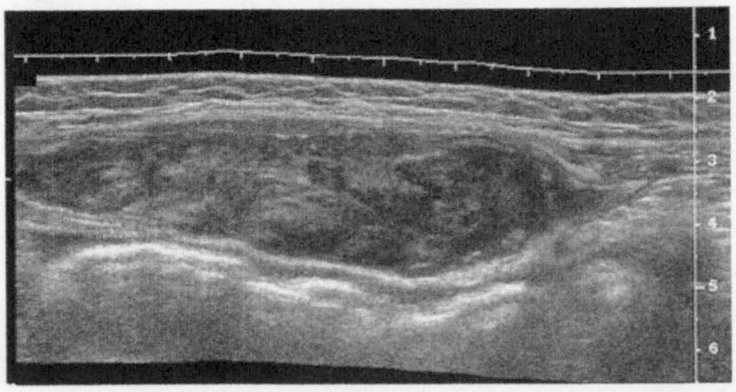

Fig. 24. Rectus sheath hematoma. This 29-year-old woman presented with pain in the anterior abdominal wall 3 days after a cesarean section. Extended field of view US demonstrates a heterogeneous, elliptical hematoma in the rectus muscle.

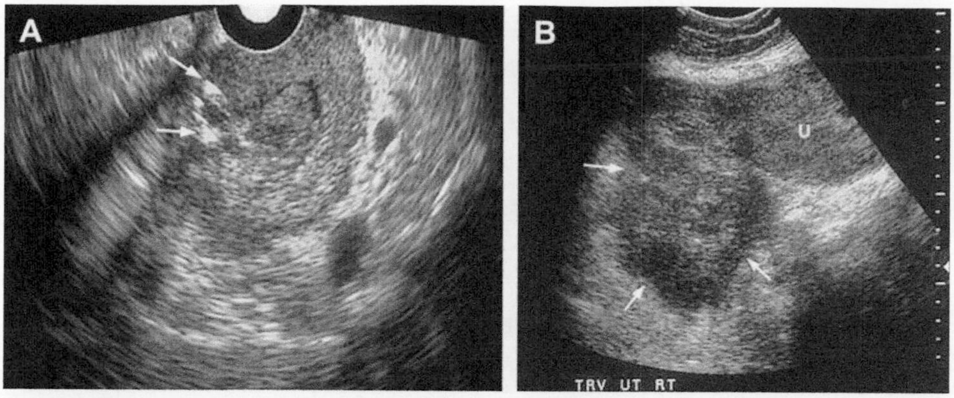

Fig. 25. Uterine rupture. This 25-year-old woman developed excruciating pain 12 hours after the vaginal delivery of her second child. Her first child had been delivered by cesarean section. (*A*) Transverse US image of the lower uterine segment reveals punctate echogenic foci with distal shadowing (*arrows*) in the myometrial wall on the right and debris/hemorrhage within the endometrial cavity. These findings suggest the presence of air and hemorrhage in the cesarean section scar. (*B*) Higher oblique image reveals hemorrhage (*arrows*) dissecting into the broad ligament on the right of the uterus (U). This patient had ruptured her uterus at the site of the cesarean scar.

delivery, particularly after cesarean section.[69] Hence, clinical correlation with the presence of fever and purulent vaginal discharge is important.

Unusual Causes of Postpartum Pelvic Pain

There are several other, less common, causes of acute pelvic pain in the postpartum period. Ovarian vein thrombophlebitis occurs in less than 2% of patients in the immediate postpartum period. It is more common on the right and after cesarean section. Patients usually present with fever and pain. Sonographic findings may include a tubular or serpiginous avascular mass in the region of the right adnexa and inferior vena cava, lack of color Doppler flow in the right ovarian vein (**Fig. 23**), and thrombus extending to the inferior vena cava, typically better seen with transabdominal imaging. The ovary may be enlarged.[70] Bladder flap hematomas occur in patients after cesarean section and usually appear as a solid complex mass between the posterior bladder wall and anterior wall of the lower uterine segment. These are best seen with transabdominal imaging.[71] Hematomas can also occur in the rectus sheath after cesarean section and are best seen with transabdominal technique using a linear array high-frequency transducer (**Fig. 24**).[72] Finally, uterine rupture is an unusual complication of vaginal delivery, most commonly observed in women who have had prior cesarean section. US usually fails to identify the uterine defect, but can demonstrate intra- or extraperitoneal hematoma and intrauterine hemorrhage (**Fig. 25**).[73]

CHRONIC PELVIC PAIN

Adenomyosis

Adenomyosis is defined as the ectopic location of endometrial glands within the uterine myometrium, usually the inner one-third, with surrounding smooth muscle hyperplasia. Patients present with dysfunctional uterine bleeding, dysmenorrhea, infertility, or pelvic pain. Adenomyosis is a difficult diagnosis to make clinically because the signs and symptoms are nonspecific and often mimic endometriosis or leiomyomas. The reported frequency of adenomyosis in hysterectomy specimens varies, but the largest series reports an incidence of approximately 20%.[74–76] Adenomyosis

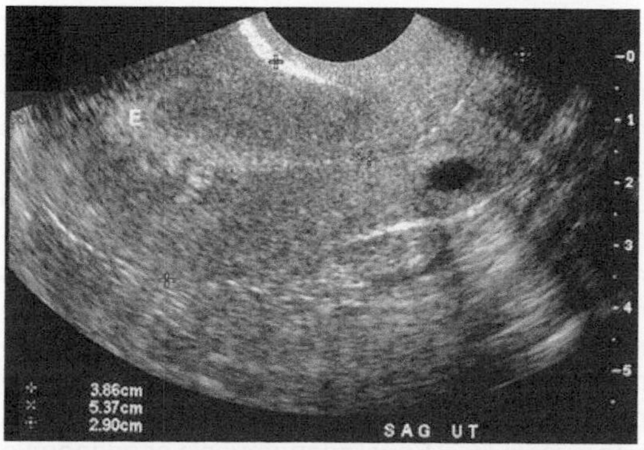

Fig. 26. Adenomyosis. Sagittal EVUS image of the uterus in a 48-year-old woman with menorrhagia reveals nodular and linear echogenic areas extending from the endometrium (E) into the subjacent myometrium consistent with adenomyosis. There is a nabothian cyst in the cervix. Calipers indicate craniocaudad and anteroposterior measurement of the uterus.

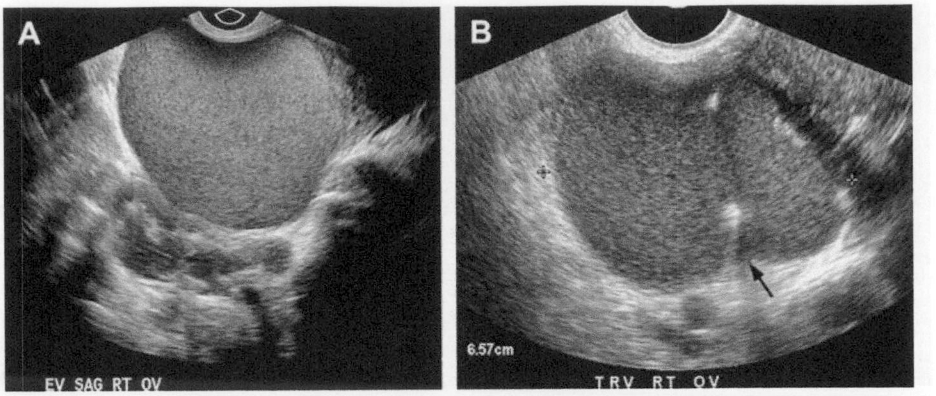

Fig. 27. Endometrioma. This 42-year-old woman presented with chronic pelvic pain. (*A*) Large right adnexal mass with homogeneous low-level echogenicity, the most classic US appearance of an endometrioma. Hypoechoic band anteriorly that gradually becomes more echogenic inferiorly has been described as shading, which is most likely due to gradual settling of blood products and RBCs in the thick viscous fluid within the endometrioma. (*B*) Another patient with endometriosis demonstrates 2 adjacent endometriomas (calipers) in the right adnexa. Note angular margins (*arrow*) likely due to scarring or adhesions. Small echogenic linear mural foci are a specific US feature of endometriomas, although the histologic/pathologic correlate is not known.

occurs more frequently in multiparous women and there is evidence to suggest that it is associated with SAB and dilatation and curettage.[77]

The reported accuracy of EVUS in the detection of adenomyosis varies greatly with sensitivities ranging from 80% to 85% and specificities ranging from 50% to 96%.[78–80] The sonographic appearance of diffuse adenomyosis includes enlargement of the uterus, heterogeneity of the myometrium with poorly marginated heterogeneous hypoechoic or echogenic areas, thickening (especially asymmetric thickening) of the subendometrial halo, asymmetry of the thickness of the anterior and posterior myometrial walls, subendometrial myometrial cysts, echogenic nodules or linear striations extending from the endometrium into the myometrium, and poor definition of the endometrial-myometrial junction (**Fig. 26**). Most studies describe myometrial cysts, which are most commonly visualized in the second half of the menstrual cycle, as the most specific finding on US for adenomyosis.[80–83] These likely represent the dilated or hemorrhagic endometrial glands. Another study reported that subendometrial echogenic nodules/radiating striations, representing the ectopic endometrial tissue (see **Fig. 26**), and asymmetric myometrial thickness had the highest positive predictive value in the sonographic diagnosis of adenomyosis.[82,83] Focal adenomyosis or adenomyomas are a less common form of adenomyosis and on US are described as poorly defined myometrial masses with internal vascularity. Rarely, adenomyomas may be cystic. Adenomyosis usually does not alter the outer contour of the uterus.[84,85] Intramural leiomyomas, alternatively, are typically avascular and hypoechoic with well-defined margins. Peripheral vascularity may be noted, especially if the leiomyoma is large.[86] In cases where US is equivocal, MRI increases the

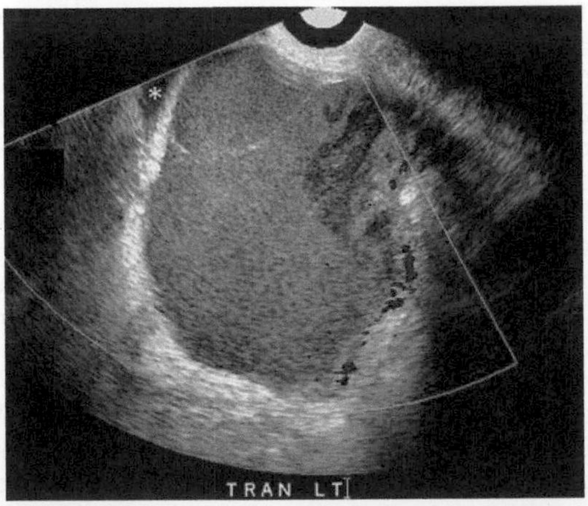

Fig. 28. Rupture of an endometrioma. This patient with known endometriosis presented with sudden onset of severe abdominal pain after a car accident. Endometriomas may be fixed in the pelvis due to scarring and adhesions and large endometriomas therefore may be at risk to rupture after direct trauma. EVUS color Doppler image of the left adnexal demonstrates a mass that is largely homogenous with low-level echoes consistent with the diagnosis of an endometrioma. Note, however, the irregular contour and adjacent free fluid (*). More echogenic free fluid, consistent with hemoperitoneum was noted in the cul-de-sac (not shown). At surgery the endometrioma had ruptured, leaking its contents into the peritoneal cavity.

diagnostic accuracy.[87,88] Transient myometrial contractions, however, may mimic on US and MRI examination some of these findings, especially thickening of the subendometrial halo/junctional zone, ill-defined focal hypoechoic areas within the myometrium, and asymmetry in the thickness of the anterior and posterior walls of the uterus.

Endometriosis

Endometriosis is defined as the presence of ectopic endometrial tissue outside of the uterus, most commonly implanted on the surface of the ovary, uterine suspensory ligaments, uterus, or fallopian tube and on the peritoneal surfaces of the pouch of Douglas. Less common sites include

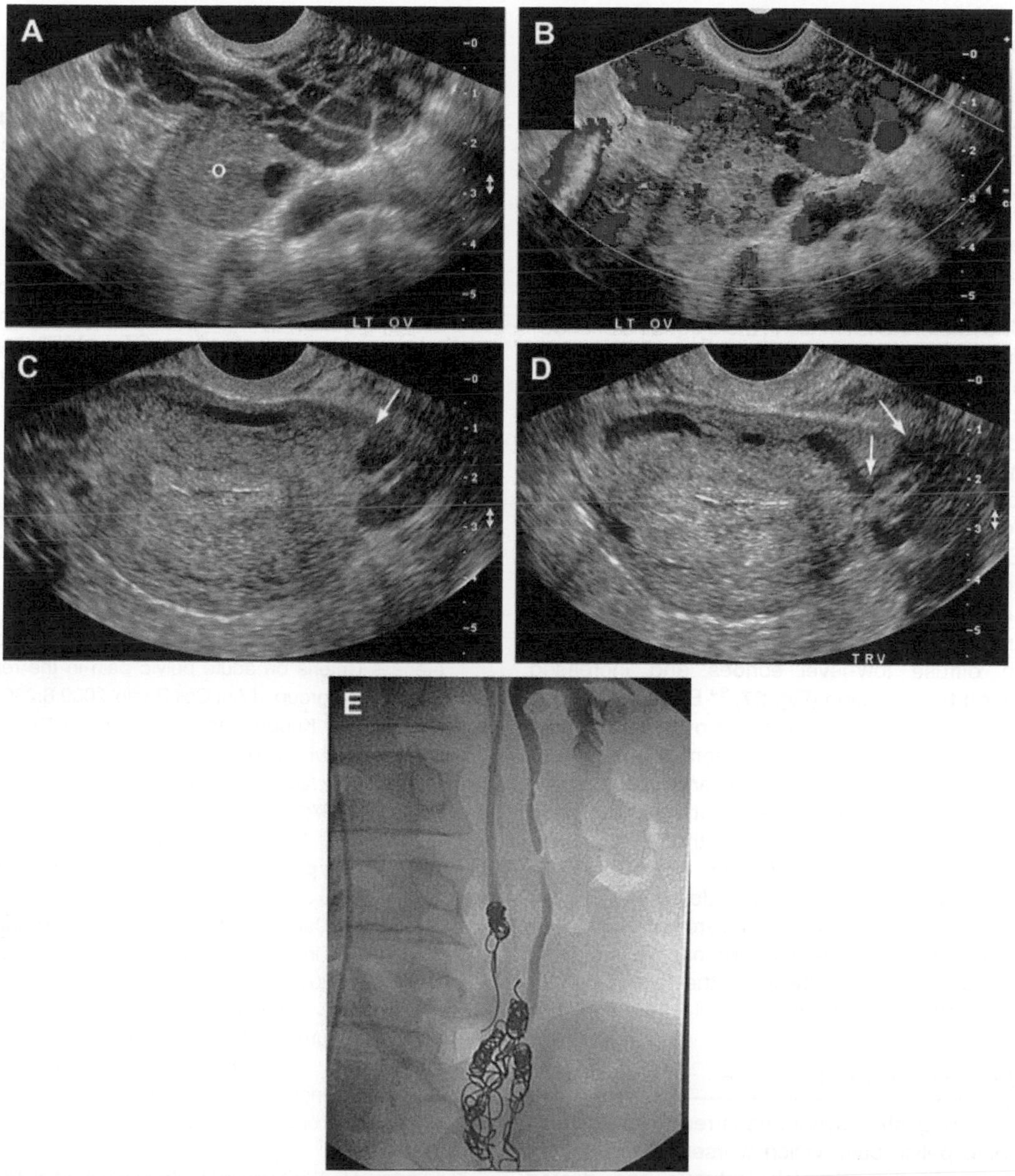

Fig. 29. Pelvic congestion syndrome. This 45-year-old woman presented with chronic pelvic pain. Gray-scale (*A*) and color Doppler image (*B*) reveal many dilated veins in the left adnexa. Left ovary (O). (*C, D*) The enlarged pelvic veins directly communicated with the arcuate veins (*arrows*) within the myometrium. Pelvic venogram demonstrated reflux in the gonadal vein consistent with pelvic congestion syndrome. The patient underwent coil embolization and sclerotherapy of the pelvic varices and gonadal veins (coils in the *left* gonadal veins shown in [*E*]) with relief of her symptoms.

the vagina, bladder, cervix, cesarean section scars, abdominal scars, or the inguinal ligament.[86] Under hormonal stimulation, the ectopic endometrium undergoes repeated cycles of hemorrhage, resorption, and fibrosis, resulting in the formation of endometriomas, scarring, and adhesions. Endometriosis has a reported prevalence of 10% in women of reproductive age and has been found in approximately 20% of women undergoing laparoscopy for chronic pelvic pain.[89,90] Risk factors for the development of endometriosis include short menstrual cycles, longer menstrual flow, intermenstrual spotting, and hormone replacement therapy. One half to 80% of patients are symptomatic. Symptoms include dysmenorrhea, dysfunctional uterine bleeding, dyspareunia, infertility, and chronic pelvic pain.[91] Endometriosis is hormonally responsive and pain can be cyclic, related to the menstrual cycle. The degree of pain is not related to the macroscopic extent of disease.

The role of US is limited in the diagnosis of endometriosis because small implants and adhesions are difficult to visualize on US examination. The reported sensitivity of US for the detection of small implants is as low as 11%.[92] Although pelvic MRI is more sensitive than US in the detection of small implants and adhesions, laparoscopy remains the gold standard for diagnosis and staging.[93]

EVUS, however, plays an important role in the diagnosis of endometriomas. On US examination, an endometrioma classically appears as a unilocular homogeneously hypoechoic cystic structure with diffuse low-level echoes and increased through transmission (**Fig. 27**).[94] Echogenic mural foci and shading within a cystic ovarian mass are highly suggestive of endometrioma (see **Fig. 27**).[94] Mural or septal nodularity is worrisome for malignancy because clot occurs less commonly in an endometrioma than in a hemorrhagic cyst. Therefore, further evaluation with MRI or surgery should be considered. Rarely, endometriomas can cause severe pain due to rupture (**Fig. 28**). As endometriomas may be fixed within the pelvis by adhesions, they are at risk for rupture after direct trauma.

Pelvic Congestion Syndrome

Pelvic congestion syndrome is reported to cause chronic pelvic pain, which worsens on standing. Retrograde flow through tortuous and dilated pelvic veins that develop secondary to incompetent valves in the ovarian vein is considered the most likely cause.[86,95–97] It is estimated that up to 60% of patients with pelvic varices have symptoms related to the varicosities.[1] EVUS demonstrates multiple dilated veins surrounding the pelvic organs.[97] Direct connection to the arcuate veins in the myometrium, low velocity flow, and increase in diameter after the Valsalva maneuver all are associated with symptoms (**Fig. 29**).[96] The treatment of pelvic congestion syndrome remains controversial, but bilateral transcatheter embolization with sclerotherapy is reported to successfully improve symptoms in some cases, although the durability of the symptomatic improvement is highly variable.

SUMMARY

US should be considered the first-line imaging modality of choice in women presenting with acute or chronic pelvic pain of suspected gynecologic or obstetric origin because many, if not most, gynecologic/obstetric causes of pelvic pain are easily diagnosed on US examination. Since the clinical presentation of gynecologic causes of pelvic pain overlaps with gastrointestinal and genitourinary pathology, however, referral to CT or MRI, especially in pregnant patients, should be considered if the US examination is nondiagnostic.

ACKNOWLEDGMENTS

The authors would like to thank Ms Geri Mancini for her expert help with image preparation.

REFERENCES

1. Andreotti RF, Lee SI, Choy G, et al. ACR Appropriateness Criteria on acute pelvic pain in the reproductive age group. J Am Coll Radiol 2009;6:235–41.
2. Mathias SD, Kuppermann M, Liberman RF, et al. Chronic pelvic pain: prevalence, health-related quality of life, and economic correlates. Obstet Gynecol 1996;87(3):321–7.
3. Howard FM. The role of laparoscopy in chronic pelvic pain: promise and pitfall. Obstet Gynecol Surv 1993;48:357–87.
4. Sharma D, Dahiya K, Duhan N, et al. Diagnostic laparoscopy in chronic pelvic pain. Arch Gynaecol Obstet Jan 2010. [online].
5. Burnett LS. Gynecologic causes of the acute abdomen. Surg Clin North Am 1988;68:385–516.
6. Borgfeldt C, Andolf E. Transvaginal sonographic ovarian findings in a random sample of women 25–40 years old. Ultrasound Obstet Gynecol 1999; 13:345–50.
7. Ekerhovd E, Wienerroith H, Staudach A, et al. Preoperative assessment of unilocular adnexal cysts by transvaginal ultrasonography: a comparison between ultrasonographic morphologic imaging and histopathologic diagnosis. Am J Obstet Gynecol 2001; 184(2):48–54.

8. D.Levine D.Brown Report from the SRU Consensus Conference on Management of asymptomatic ovarian and other adnexal cysts imaged on ultrasound. Radiology, in press.
9. Scoutt LM. Sonographic evaluation of acute pelvic pain in women. In State-of- the-art emergency and trauma radiology: ARRS categorical course syllabus; 2008. p. 229–40.
10. Hertzberg BS, Kliewer MA, Paulson EK. Ovarian cyst rupture causing hemoperitoneum: imaging features and the potential for misdiagnosis. Abdom Imaging 1999;24:304–8.
11. Hertzberg BS, Kliewer MA, Bowie JD. Adnexal ring sign and hemoperitoneum caused by hemorrhagic ovarian cyst: pitfall in the sonographic diagnosis of ectopic pregnancy. Am J Roentgenol 1999;173: 1301–2.
12. Jain KA. Sonographic spectrum of hemorrhagic ovarian cysts. J Ultrasound Med 2002;21:879–86.
13. Barret S, Taylor C. A review on pelvic inflammatory disease. Int J STD AIDS 2005;16:715–21.
14. Patten RM, Vincent LM, Wolner-Hanssen P, et al. Pelvic inflammatory disease. Endovaginal sonography with laparoscopic correlation. J Ultrasound Med 1990;9:681–9.
15. Timor-Tristsch IE, Lerner JP, Mongeagudo A, et al. Transvaginal sonographic markers of tubal inflammatory disease. Ultrasound Obstet Gynecol 1998; 12:56–66.
16. Horrow M. Ultrasound of pelvic inflammatory disease. Ultrasound Q 2004;20:171–9.
17. Hibbard LT. Adnexal torsion. Am J Obstet Gynecol 1985;152:456–61.
18. Albayram F, Hamper UM. Ovarian and adnexal torsion: spectrum of sonographic findings with pathologic correlation. J Ultrasound Med 2001;20:1063–9.
19. Chen M, Chen C, Yang Y. Torsion of the previously normal uterine adnexa. Evaluation of the correlation between the pathologic changes and the clinical characteristics. Acta Obstet Gynecol Scand 2001; 80:58–61.
20. Argenta PA, Yeagley TJ, Ott G, et al. Torsion of the uterine adnexa. Pathologic correlations and current management trends. J Reprod Med 2000;45:831–6.
21. Houry D, Abbott JT. Ovarian torsion: a fifteen-year review. Ann Emerg Med 2001;38:156–9.
22. White M, Stella J. Ovarian torsion: 10-year perspective. Emerg Med Australas 2005;17:231–7.
23. Graif M, Shalev J, Strauss J, et al. Torsion of the ovary: sonographic features. Am J Roentgenol 1984;143:1331–4.
24. Lee EJ, Kwon HC, Joo HJ, et al. Diagnosis of ovarian torsion with color Doppler sonography: depiction of twisted vascular pedicle. J Ultrasound Med 1998; 17:83–9.
25. Vijayaraghavan SB. Sonographic whirlpool sign in ovarian torsion. J Ultrasound Med 2004;23:1643–9.
26. Ben-Ami M, Perlitz Y, Haddad S. The effectiveness of spectral and color Doppler in predicting ovarian torsion. A prospective study. Eur J Obstet Gynecol Reprod Biol 2002;104:64–6.
27. Pena J, Ufberg D, Cooney N, et al. Usefulness of Doppler sonography in the diagnosis of ovarian torsion. Fertil Steril 2000;73:1047–50.
28. Fleischer AC, Stein SM, Cullinan JA, et al. Color Doppler sonography of adnexal torsion. J Ultrasound Med 1995;14:523–8.
29. Pellerito JS, Troiano RN, Quedens-Case C, et al. Common pitfalls of endovaginal color Doppler flow imaging. Radiographics 1995;15:37–47.
30. Benacerraf BR, Shipp TD, Bromley B. Three-dimensional ultrasound detection of abnormally located intrauterine contraceptive devices which are a source of pelvic pain and abnormal bleeding. Ultrasound Obstet Gynecol 2009;34: 110–5.
31. Durfee SM, Frates MC. Sonographic spectrum of the corpus luteum in early pregnancy: gray-scale, color, and pulsed Doppler appearance. J Clin Ultrasound 1999;27:55–9.
32. Abu-Yousef MM, Bleicher JJ, Williamson RA, et al. Subchorionic hemorrhage: sonographic diagnosis and clinical significance. Am J Roentgenol 1987; 149:737–40.
33. Bennett GL, Bromley B, Lieberman E, et al. Subchorionic hemorrhage in first- trimester pregnancies: prediction of pregnancy outcome with sonography. Radiology 1996;200:803–6.
34. Sauerbrei EE, Pham DH. Placental abruption and subchorionic hemorrhage in the first half of pregnancy: US appearance and clinical outcome. Radiology 1986;160:109–12.
35. Dighe M, Cuevas C, Moshiri M, et al. Sonography in first trimester bleeding. J Clin Ultrasound 2008;36: 352–66.
36. Nyberg DA, Laing FC, Filly RA. Threatened abortion: sonographic distinction of normal and abnormal gestation sacs. Radiology 1986;158:397–400.
37. Bouyer J, Coste J, Fernandez H, et al. Sites of ectopic pregnancy: a 10 year population-based study of 1800 cases. Hum Reprod 2002;17: 3224–30.
38. Centers for disease control and prevention. Ectopic pregnancy—United States, 1990–1992. MMWR Morb Mortal Wkly Rep 1995;44:46–8.
39. Chang J, Elam-Evans JD, Berg CJ, et al. Pregnancy related mortality surveillance—United States, 1991–1999. MMWR Surveill Summ 2003;52:1–9.
40. Barnhart KT, Sammel MD, Gracia CR, et al. Risk factors for ectopic pregnancy in women with symptomatic first-trimester pregnancies. Fertil Steril 2006; 86:36–43.
41. Carson SA, Buster JE. Ectopic pregnancy. N Engl J Med 1993;329:1174–81.

42. Barnhart KT. Ectopic pregnancy. N Engl J Med 2009;361:379–87.
43. Hann LE, Bachman DM, McArdle CR. Coexistent intrauterine and ectopic pregnancy: a reevaluation. Radiology 1984;152:151–4.
44. Anastasakis E, Jetti A, Macara L, et al. A case of heterotopic pregnancy in the absence of risk factors. A brief literature review. Fetal Diagn Ther 2007;22:285–8.
45. Yeh HC, Goodman JL, Carr L, et al. Intradecidual sign: is it effective in diagnosis of an early intrauterine pregnancy? Radiology 1997;204:655–60.
46. Bradley WG, Friske CE, Filly RA. The double decidual sac sign of early intrauterine pregnancy: use in exclusion of ectopic pregnancy. Radiology 1982;143:223–6.
47. Cacciatore B, Stenman UH, Ylostalo P. Diagnosis of ectopic pregnancy by vaginal ultrasonography in combination with discriminatory serum beta-hCG level of 1000 IU/l IRP. Br J Obstet Gynaecol 1990; 97:904–8.
48. Atri M, Leduc C, Gillett P, et al. Role of endovaginal sonography in the diagnosis and management of ectopic pregnancy. Radiographics 1996;16:755–74.
49. Lin EP, Bhatt S, Dogra VS. Diagnostic clues to ectopic pregnancy. Radiographics 2008;28:1661–71.
50. Levine D. Ectopic pregnancy. Radiology 2007;245: 385–97.
51. Brown DL, Doubilet PM. Transvaginal sonography for diagnosing ectopic pregnancy: positivity criteria and performance characteristics. J Ultrasound Med 1994;13:259–66.
52. Dillon EF, Feyock AL, Taylor KJ. Pseudogestational sacs: Doppler differentiation from normal or abnormal intrauterine pregnancies. Radiology 1990;176:359–64.
53. Pellerito JS, Taylor KJ, Quedens-Case C, et al. Ectopic pregnancy: evaluation with endovaginal color flow imaging. Radiology 1992;183:407–11.
54. Nyberg DA, Hughes MP, Mack LA, et al. Extrauterine findings of ectopic pregnancy at transvaginal US: importance of echogenic fluid. Radiology 1991; 178:823–6.
55. Frates MC, Visweswaran A, Laing FC. Comparison of tubal ring and corpus luteum echogenicities; useful differentiating characteristics. J Ultrasound Med 2001;20:27–31.
56. Stein MW, Ricci ZJ, Novak L, et al. Sonographic comparison of the tubal ring of ectopic pregnancy with the corpus luteum. J Ultrasound Med 2004;23: 57–62.
57. Delvigne A, Rozenberg S. Epidemiology and prevention of ovarian hyperstimulation syndrome (OHSS): a review. Hum Reprod Update 2002;8:559–77.
58. Practice Committee of the American Society for Reproductive Medicine. Ovarian hyperstimulation syndrome. Fertil Steril 2008;90:S188–93.
59. Bergh PA, Navot D. Ovarian hyperstimulation syndrome: a review of pathophysiology. J Assist Reprod Genet 1992;9:429–38.
60. Wallach EE, Vlahos NF. Uterine myomas: an overview of development, clinical features, and management. Obstet Gynecol 2004;104:393–406.
61. Stewart EA. Uterine fibroids. Lancet 2001;357:293–8.
62. Sheth S, Macura K. Sonography of the uterine myometrium: myomas and beyond. Ultrasound Clin 2007;2:267–95.
63. Mayer DP, Shipilov V. Ultrasonography and magnetic resonance imaging of uterine fibroids. Obstet Gynecol Clin North Am 1995;22:667–725.
64. Karasick S, Lev-Toaff AS, Toaff ME. Imaging of uterine leiomyomas. Am J Roentgenol 1992;158: 799–805.
65. Lev-Toaff AS, Coleman BG, Arger PH, et al. Leiomyomas in pregnancy: sonographic study. Radiology 1987;164:375–80.
66. Zukerman J, Levine D, McNicholas MM, et al. Imaging of pelvic postpartum complications. Am J Roentgenol 1997;168:663–8.
67. Sadan O, Golan A, Girtler O, et al. Role of sonography in the diagnosis of retained products of conception. J Ultrasound Med 2004;23:371–4.
68. Dufree SM, Frates MC, Luong A, et al. The sonographic and color Doppler features of retained products of conception. J Ultrasound Med 2005;24:1181–6.
69. Brown DL. Pelvic ultrasound in the postabortion and postpartum patient. Ultrasound Q 2005;21:27–37.
70. Savader SJ, Otero RR, Savader BL. Puerperal ovarian vein thrombosis: evaluation with CT, US, and MR imaging. Radiology 1988;167:637–9.
71. Baker ME, Bowie JD, Killam AP. Sonography of post-cesarian-section bladder-flap hematoma. Am J Roentgenol 1985;144:757–9.
72. Wiener MD, Bowie JD, Baker ME, et al. Sonography of subfascial hematoma after cesarean delivery. Am J Roentgenol 1987;148:907–10.
73. Has R, Topuz S, Kalelioglu I, et al. Imaging features of postpartum uterine rupture: a case report. Abdom Imaging 2008;33:101–3.
74. Azziz R. Adenomyosis: current perspectives. Obstet Gynecol Clin North Am 1989;16:221–35.
75. Vercellini P, Parazzini F, Oldani S, et al. Adenomyosis at hysterectomy: a study on frequency distribution and patient characteristics. Hum Reprod 1995;10: 1160–2.
76. Vercellini P, Vigano P, Somigliana E, et al. Adenomyosis: epidemiological factors. Best Pract Res Clin Obstet Gynaecol 2006;20:465–77.
77. Levgur M, Abadi MA, Tucker A. Adenomyosis: symptoms, histology, and pregnancy terminations. Obstet Gynecol 2000;95:688–91.
78. Bromley B, Shipp TD, Benacerraf B. Adenomyosis: sonographic findings and diagnostic accuracy. J Ultrasound Med 2000;19:529–34.

79. Dueholm M. Transvaginal ultrasound for diagnosis of adenomyosis: a review. Best Pract Res Clin Obstet Gynaecol 2006;20:569–82.
80. Reinhold C, Tafazoli F, Mehio A, et al. Endovaginal US and MR imaging features with histopathologic correlation. Radiographics 1999;19:S147–60.
81. Bazot M, Cortez A, Darai E, et al. Ultrasonography compared with magnetic resonance imaging for the diagnosis of adenomyosis: correlation with histopathology. Hum Reprod 2001;16:2427–33.
82. Atri M, Reinhold C, Mehio A, et al. Adenomyosis: US features with histologic correlation in an in-vitro study. Radiology 2000;215:783–90.
83. Reinhold C, Tafazoli F, Wang L. Imaging features of adenomyosis. Hum Reprod Update 1998;4:337–49.
84. Andreotti RF, Fleischer AC. The sonographic diagnosis of adenomyosis. Ultrasound Q 2005;21:167–70.
85. Bostis D, Kassanos D, Antoniou G, et al. Adenomyoma and leiomyoma: differential diagnosis with transvaginal sonography. J Clin Ultrasound 1998;26:21–5.
86. Kuligowska E, Deeds L, Lu K. Pelvic pain: overlooked and underdiagnosed gynecologic conditions. Radiographics 2005;25:3–20.
87. Ascher SM, Arnold LL, Patt RH, et al. Adenomyosis: prospective comparison of MR imaging and transvaginal sonography. Radiology 1994;190:803–6.
88. Dueholm M, Lundorf E. Transvaginal ultrasond or MRI for diagnosis of adenomyosis. Curr Opin Obstet Gynecol 2007;19:505–12.
89. Mahmood TA, Templeton A. Prevalence and genesis of endometriosis. Hum Reprod 1991;6:544–9.
90. El-Yahia AW. Laparoscopic evaluation of apparently normal infertile women. Aust N Z J Obstet Gynaecol 1994;34:440–2.
91. Rawson JM. Prevalence of endometriosis in asymptomatic women. J Reprod Med 1991;36:513–5.
92. Friedman H, Vogelzang RL, Mendelson EB, et al. Endometriosis detection by US with laparoscopic correlation. Radiology 1985;157:217–20.
93. Dubela AJ. Diagnosis of endometriosis. Obstet Gynecol Clin North Am 1997;24:331–46.
94. Patel MD, Feldstein VA, Chen DC, et al. Endometriomas: diagnostic performance of US. Radiology 1999;210:739–45.
95. Beard RW, Reginald PW, Wadsworth J. Clinical features of women with chronic lower abdominal pain and pelvic congestion. Br J Obstet Gynaecol 1988;95:153–61.
96. Park SJ, Lim LW, Ko YT, et al. Diagnosis of pelvic congestion syndrome using transabdominal and transvaginal sonography. Am J Roentgenol 2004;182:683–8.
97. Ganeshan A, Upponi S, Hon LQ, et al. Chronic pelvic pain due to pelvic congestion syndrome: the role of diagnostic and interventional radiology. Cardiovasc Intervent Radiol 2007;30:1105–11.

Ultrasound for Pelvic Pain II: Nongynecologic Causes

Susan J. Ackerman, MD*, Abid Irshad, MD, Munazza Anis, MD

KEYWORDS

- Appendicitis • Diverticulitis • Mesenteric adenitis
- Ureteral calculus • Bowel obstruction
- Inflammatory bowel disease

Acute pelvic pain in women is a common presenting complaint that can result from various conditions. Because these conditions can be of gynecologic or nongynecologic origin, they may pose a challenge to the diagnostic acumen of physicians, including radiologists. A thorough workup should include clinical history, physical examination, laboratory data, and appropriate imaging studies, all of which should be available to the radiologist for evaluation. Ultrasound is the primary imaging modality in women with acute pelvic pain because of its high sensitivity, low cost, wide availability, and lack of ionizing radiation, particularly when a gynecologic disorder is suspected as the underlying cause. However, other modalities such as computed tomography (CT) and magnetic resonance imaging (MRI) may be very helpful, especially when a nongynecologic condition is suspected.

Nongynecologic causes of acute pelvic pain include appendicitis, diverticulitis, ureteral calculi, mesenteric adenitis, bowel obstruction, inflammatory bowel disease, and metastatic disease.

APPENDICITIS

Appendicitis is one of the most common nongynecologic causes of acute pelvic pain and right lower quadrant pain. Typically, these patients also present with nausea, vomiting, and anorexia. Physical examination and laboratory test results usually show abdominal tenderness and leukocytosis. However, the diagnosis can often be made on clinical evaluation alone. Ultrasound, CT, and MRI have proven to be useful examinations in avoiding unnecessary surgeries, especially in patients with atypical clinical presentations, particularly when the appendix is located at an unusual position, such as retrocecal, retroileal, or pericolic gutter (15% of cases)[1] or located behind a gravid uterus. Negative laparotomy findings have been reported in 35% to 45% of women of reproductive age who were suspected to have appendicitis.[2] When the clinical picture is unclear, the imaging can not only aid in the diagnosis but also reduce the frequency of unnecessary surgical intervention.

Ultrasound compares favorably with CT in diagnosing appendicitis, with sensitivities of 75% to 90% and specificities of 86% to 100%. A positive diagnosis can be made when a distended, noncompressible tubular blind-ending structure with a wall-to-wall diameter greater than 7 mm is visible or if the individual wall is greater than 3 mm in thickness (**Figs. 1 and 2**).[3,4] In the transverse section, the inflamed appendix usually appears as a double concentric ring like a target sign. Although an inflamed appendix is noncompressible, the inflamed bowel can also be noncompressible. One can use graded compression to displace normal gas-containing loops of bowel to get a better look at the structure.

Department of Radiology, Medical University of South Carolina, 96 Jonathan Lucas Street, Charleston, SC 29425, USA
* Corresponding author.
E-mail address: ackerman@musc.edu

Ultrasound Clin 5 (2010) 233–243
doi:10.1016/j.cult.2010.03.002

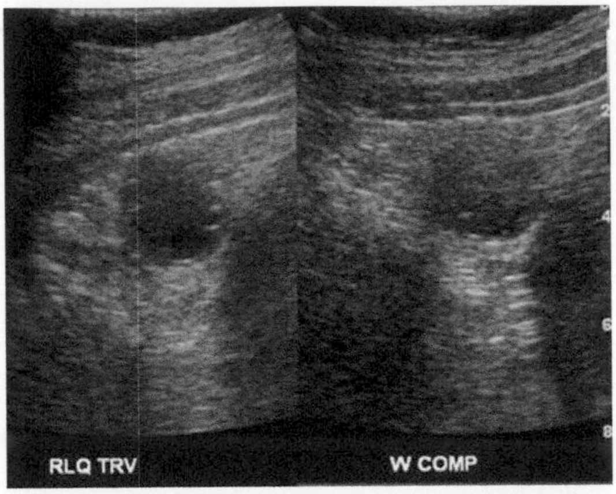

Fig. 1. Appendicitis showing non compressibility. Two transverse ultrasouns images through the right lower quadrant obtained without compression (*left image*) and with transducer compression (*right image*) show the appendix as a rounded fluid-filled structure. This structure is noncompressible because it shows no significant change in shape or height between images without and with compression. (*From* Angle R, Irshad A, Ackerman S. Practical imaging of acute pelvic pain in premenopausal women. Contemp Diagn Radiol 2010;33(1):4; with permission.)

Identifying the appendix in its entirety is important because appendicitis can be limited to the distal end.

Other findings suggesting appendicitis include inflammation of the adjacent mesenteric or omental fat and a shadowing appendicolith (see **Fig. 2**). In appendices measuring 5 to 7 mm, the diagnosis may be confirmed by the nonuniformity of the mural wall layers and the presence of increased blood flow in the appendix on color Doppler imaging. Once an inflamed appendix has been identified, ultrasound has a high specificity for diagnosing acute appendicitis.

However, the spontaneous resolution of appendicitis among other factors may contribute negatively toward its specificity.[5] Ultrasound may just show localized free fluid in the periappendiceal region when the appendix is not clearly seen on ultrasound, such as in cases of advanced-stage pregnancy (**Fig. 3**A, B). In these cases, a noncontrast MR (T2-weighted sequence) may be used for further evaluation (**Fig. 3**C, D). A periappendiceal abscess will appear on ultrasound as a hypoechoic fluid collection and may display a mass effect. Inflamed bowel may be difficult to distinguish from acute appendicitis, but can be differentiated through assessing the maximum thickening of the muscle layer of adjacent bowel and the appearance of the mucosal/submucosal complex.[6]

When the appendix is not visualized at all, the radiologist should carefully review the cecal tip and iliac vessels before reporting the study as normal. Limitation of sonography in diagnosing acute appendicitis could be secondary to an unusual location of the appendix (such as a retrocecal location), ruptured appendicitis, and obesity.[7] Additionally, a gas-filled appendix may be mistaken for small bowel, or a perforated appendix may become deflated. Occasionally, the inflammation may resolve secondary to spontaneous movement of the appendicolith relieving the obstruction.

DIVERTICULITIS

Diverticulitis is the inflammation of an outpouching of the colon. Left-sided diverticulosis is marked by multiplicity, associated muscular hypertrophy, and dysfunction, whereas right-sided diverticuli are predominantly solitary. It usually presents with symptoms of fever,

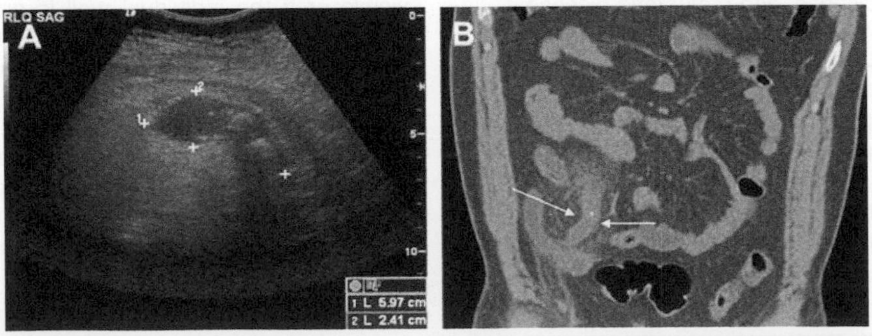

Fig. 2. Appendicitis with appendicolith. (*A*) Utrasound image through the right lower quadrant showing a fluid-filled elongated structure (*calipers*). This structure is 2.4 cm thick and contains internal fluid, debris, and calcifications, suggesting appendicolith. (*B*) Noncontrast coronal CT slice through the abdomen of the same patient showing a dilated appendix (*arrows*) with internal calcification. Moderate fat stranding is noted around the appendix, suggesting periappendiceal inflammation. (*From* Angle R, Irshad A, Ackerman S. Practical imaging of acute pelvic pain in premenopausal women. Contemp Diagn Radiol 2010;33(1):4; with permission.)

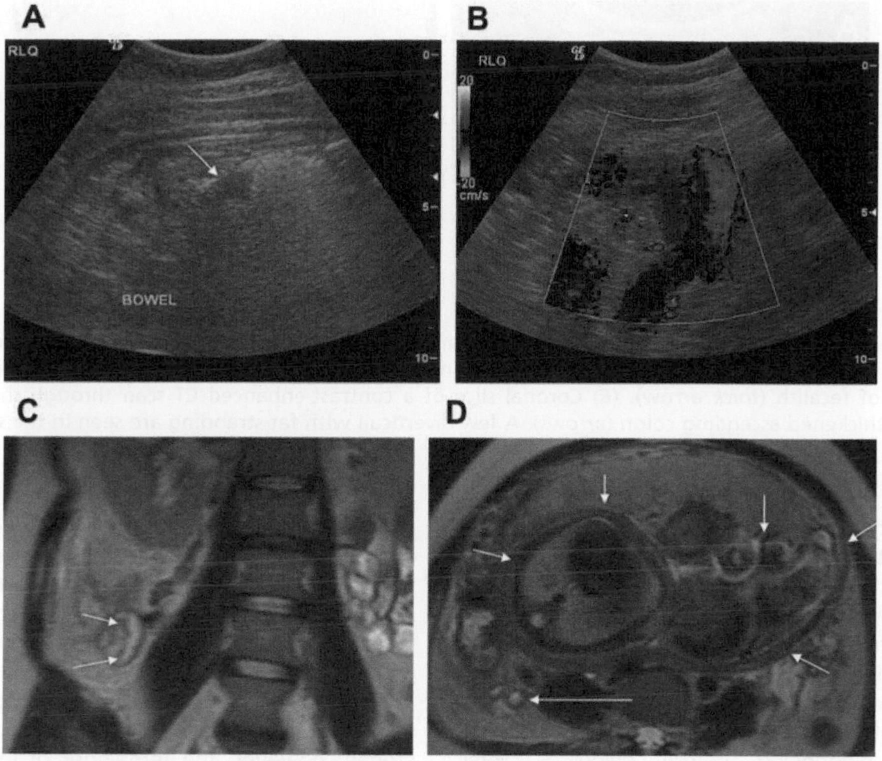

Fig. 3. Appendicitis in pregnancy. (*A*) Transverse ultrasound image through the right lower quadrant showing an anechoic triangular fluid pocket between the bowel loops (*arrow*). (*B*) Color Doppler image through the same area showing fluid adjacent to the vessels. (*C*) T2-weighted coronal MR image through the abdomen showing fluid-filled thickened appendix (*arrows*) with mild stranding in the fat. (*D*) Axial T2-weighted image showing a fluid-filled thickened appendix (*long arrow*). A fetus is noted in the central abdomen (*small arrows*).

anorexia, lower abdominal/pelvic pain, and obstination. Like epiploic appendagitis, it usually occurs in the left lower quadrant but can occur in the right lower quadrant.

The role of imaging is primarily to distinguish diverticulitis from other entities and to assess its severity to determine if surgery or interventional management will be required. Although CT is the preferred imaging modality for diverticulitis, ultrasound can also aid in the diagnosis. Endovaginal sonography can be particularly useful in diagnosing diverticulitis if it involves the pelvis. Endorectal or endovaginal scanning for diagnosing diverticulitis has shown the sensitivity of sonography to be approximately 94%.[8,9]

Three sonographic findings are generally used to diagnose diverticulitis: a segmental area of thickened bowel wall, an inflamed diverticulum, and inflamed pericolic fat. Abscesses and fistulas can also be seen with ultrasound. Although bowel wall thickening can be asymmetric, it usually retains its normal three layers. Preservation of the colonic wall layers distinguishes uncomplicated diverticulitis from cancer of the colon.[7] An inflamed diverticulum is visible as either a hypoechoic or hyperechoic outpouching of the bowel wall surrounded by a hypoechoic border. The diverticulum may contain gas or a fecalith, and therefore dirty or clean shadowing may be associated (**Fig. 4**). The pericolic fat will appear as a hyperchoic tissue adjacent to the bowel wall around the inflamed diverticulum. Although abscesses generally appear as hypoechoic masses, they may also be hyperechoic. The fistulas generally appear as hypoechoic bands.[10]

URETERAL CALCULUS

Women with ureteral calculi typically present with flank pain that radiates to the ipsilateral groin and vulva. Commonly, the patient will have hematuria, dysuria, and urgency. CT is currently the preferred imaging modality in the evaluation of renal colic. Ultrasound may not be sensitive for detecting ureteral calculi but is still considered very useful in evaluating ureteral obstruction because of its high sensitivity to detect hydronephrosis (**Fig. 5**). Yilmaz and colleagues[11] showed that although ultrasound had a specificity of 97%, it only had

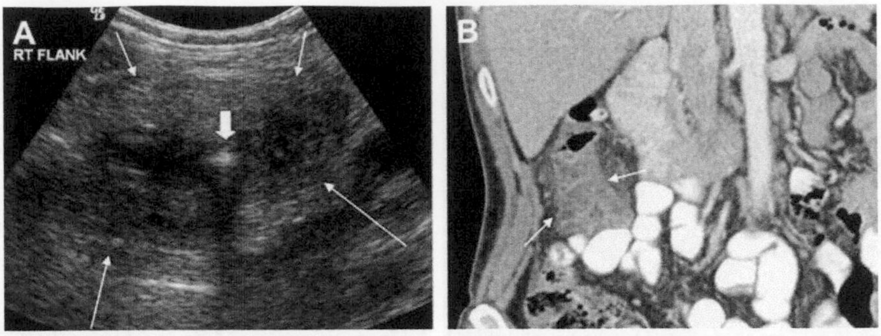

Fig. 4. Diverticulitis. (*A*) Transverse ultrasound image through the right flank that shows a thick-walled structure (*arrows*) in the area of the ascending colon. A small amount of fluid is present in the lumen with calcification suggestive of fecalith (*thick arrow*). (*B*) Coronal slice of a contrast-enhanced CT scan through the abdomen showing a thickened ascending colon (*arrows*). A few diverticuli with fat stranding are seen in the surrounding tissue.

a sensitivity of 19% for detecting ureteral calculi. However, they did not include transvaginal sonography in their study. In comparison, the same study showed the sensitivity and specificity of a noncontrast spiral CT to be 97% and 94%, respectively.

In another study by Patlas and colleagues, ultrasound showed a 93% sensitivity and 95% specificity for diagnosing ureteral calculi.[12] Distal ureteric stones close to the ureterovesical junction may be seen easily on ultrasound secondary to improved visibility of the distal ureteric regions when using the bladder as a window (**Fig. 6**A, C). A ureteral calculus is seen as an echogenic focus that shows posterior acoustic shadowing. Ultrasound has a special role in evaluating acute pain in pregnant women.[6] Transvaginal ultrasound can also be useful in detecting ureterovesical junction stones; however, the remainder of the ureter is usually difficult to assess secondary to bowel gas.

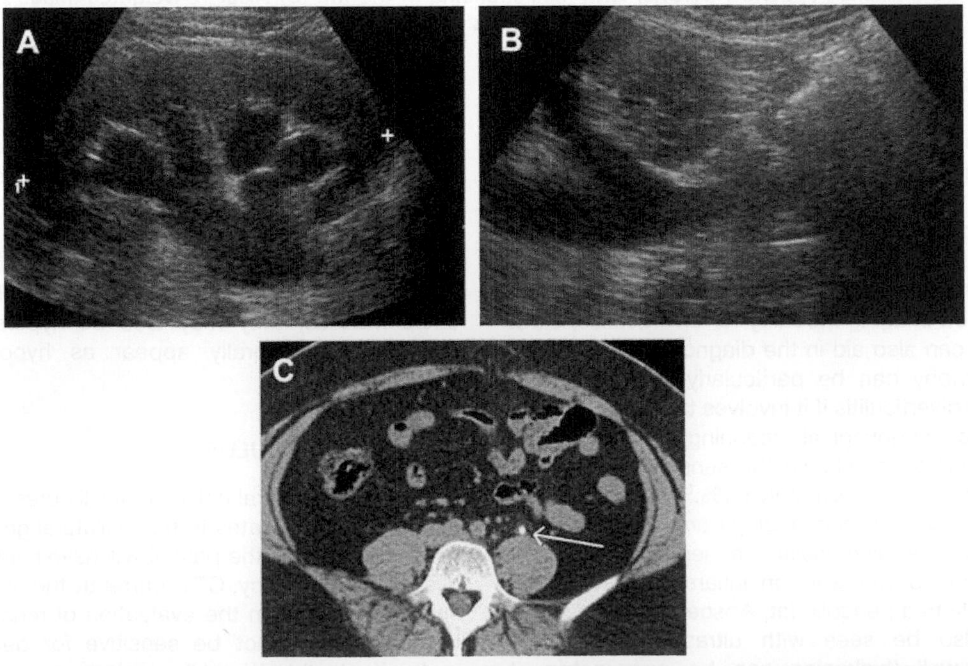

Fig. 5. Left mid ureteric calculus. (*A*) Ultrasound image through the left kidney showing moderate hydronephrosis. (*B*) Sagittal image through the left proximal ureter showing dilated upper ureter. The mid ureter is obscured by the bowel gas. (*C*) Axial slice of a noncontrast CT scan through the lower abdomen of the same patient that shows a small calculus (*arrow*) in the line of left mid ureter. (*From* Angle R, Irshad A, Ackerman S. Practical imaging of acute pelvic pain in premenopausal women. Contemp Diagn Radiol 2010;33(1):4; with permission.)

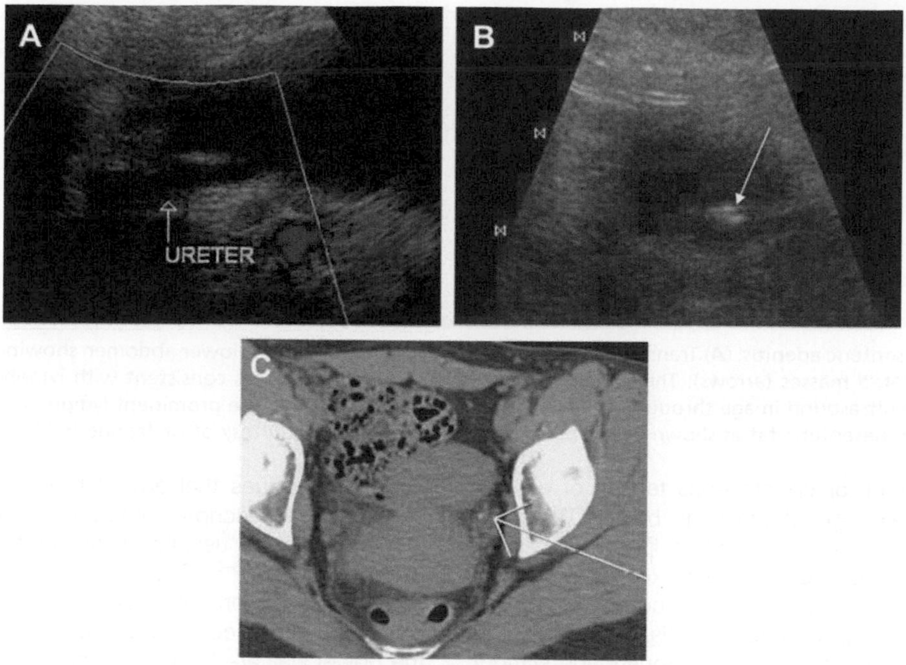

Fig. 6. Left distal ureteric stone. (*A*) Oblique color Doppler ultrasound image through the distal left ureter and bladder showing dilated left distal ureter (*arrow*). (*B*) Transverse image through the urinary bladder showing a small echogenic focus (*arrow*) in the area of the left distal ureter/ureterovesical junction with posterior acoustic shadowing suggestive of a stone. (*C*) Noncontrast CT scan; axial slice through the pelvis shows a small calcific density in the area of the left distal ureter (*arrow*) consistent with distal ureteric stone. (*From* Angle R, Irshad A, Ackerman S. Practical imaging of acute pelvic pain in premenopausal women. Contemp Diagn Radiol 2010;33(1); with permission.)

In the early phase of acute ureteral obstruction, the hydronephrosis may not be evident and the calculus may not be visible. However, one may see indirect signs of acute ureteral obstruction, including perirenal fluid, abnormally increased echotexture of the central renal sinus, and elevation of the arterial resistive index in the affected kidney. Asymmetry in the ureteral jets, with absent or less-frequent ureteral jet on the affected side, has also been identified with ureteral obstruction.[13]

Although appendicitis, diverticulitis, and ureteral calculus are some of the more common nongynecologic causes of pelvic pain, other less-common entities should also be considered. These entities include mesenteric adenitis, epiploic appendagitis, enteric duplications cysts, inguinal hernia, hydrocele, and bowel obstruction.

MESENTERIC ADENITIS

High-frequency transducers in the evaluation of lower abdominal pain may be able to detect enlarged abdominal lymph nodes. The term *mesenteric lymphadenitis* is used to describe an inflammatory process of the abdominal lymph nodes when the sole finding is enlarged lymph nodes and the patient presents with abdominal pain. It is usually a self-limiting process. A recent study by Simanovsky and Hiller[14] reports that enlarged abdominal lymph nodes of 10 mm or greater in the short axis in the clinical setting of abdominal pain may represent mesenteric lymphadenitis (**Fig. 7**).

Although mesenteric adenitis is predominantly seen in the pediatric population, it can occur in adults as a cause of lower quadrant/pelvic pain. In the pediatric literature, *mesenteric adenitis* is a term used for specific inflammation of mesenteric lymph nodes, caused by *Yersinia*, *Staphylococcus*, *Salmonella*, and other types of mycobacteria and viruses.[14] In the older population, multiple enlarged pelvic or mesenteric lymph nodes may occur in malignancy, appendicitis, or other inflammatory bowel conditions.

EPIPLOIC APPENDAGITIS

Epiploic appendagitis usually occurs on the left side but can mimic appendicitis when it occurs in the right lower quadrant. Epiploic appendages are visceral peritoneal outpouchings containing fat and blood vessels. Normally these appendages are invisible at sonography because their density is similar to that of surrounding fatty tissue. Epiploic appendagitis occurs from ischemia,

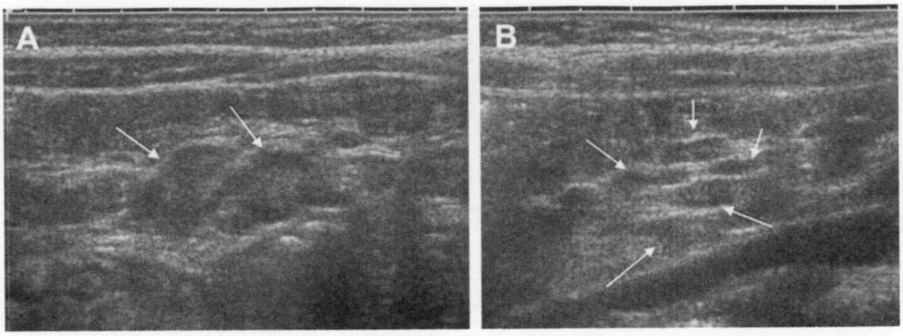

Fig. 7. Mesenteric adenitis. (*A*) Transverse ultrasound image through the right lower abdomen showing two adjacent lobulated masses (*arrows*). These masses show internal echogenic areas consistent with lymph nodes. (*B*) Transverse ultrasound image through the lower abdomen also shows multiple prominent lymph nodes (*arrows*) within the mesenteric fat as shown by surrounding echogenic areas. (*Courtesy of* Dr Jeanne Hill.)

inflammation, or spontaneous torsion of an epiploic appendage of the large bowel. The most common clinical presentation is pelvic pain in young patients after strenuous exercise or stretching. Typically, the pain is not associated with fever.

Primary epiploic appendagitis is inflammation and infarction of the epiploic appendage without an underlying cause.[15] The sonographic features include a small, usually echogenic, noncompressible, ovoid mass, located deep to the abdominal wall in the area of maximal tenderness.[16] Sometimes, a thin, hypoechoic rim may surround the mass.[16]

An important feature that distinguishes epiploic appendagitis from diverticulitis is the absence of thickening of the adjacent bowel wall and the absence of air within the echogenic nodule.[16] Segmental omental infarction (SOI) is caused by thrombosis of omental vessels, resulting in infarction. Ultrasound usually shows a solid, hyperechoic, and noncompressible mass deep to the area of maximal tenderness. The mass may become partly heterogeneous if necrosis from infarction is present; however, abnormal echogenic fat is usually seen around the lesion (**Fig. 8**). The clinical presentations of epiploic appendagitis and SOI are similar and both should be considered in the differential diagnosis of right lower quadrant pain. Both of these entities are self-limiting and resolve spontaneously with conservative management.

COLITIS

Colitis usually shows on ultrasound as a diffuse bowel wall thickening. Thickening of the terminal ileum and the cecum is seen in Crohn's disease. Other findings that may be seen on ultrasound include decreased peristalsis, lack of compressibility, strictures, and hyperemia of the bowel loops. Inflammation and proliferation of the surrounding fat and mesentery leads to noncompressible, echogenic tissues that are seen adjacent to the bowel.[17] This description has been referred to as *creeping fat* and usually occurs at the terminal ileum or cecum.[18–20] The earliest reported finding on ultrasound is presence of small echolucencies within the submucosa. Because all the layers of the bowel wall are thickened, there is loss of the normal striated gut signature. Echogenic foci within the hypoechoic muscularis layer represent ulceration.[17] Complex fluid collections or solid-appearing masses with air may represent abscesses or fistulas around the bowel.

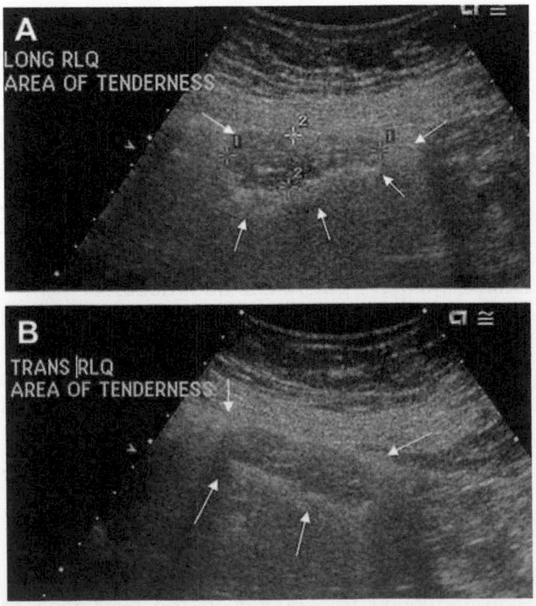

Fig. 8. Epiploic appendagitis. Longitudinal (*A*) and transverse (*B*) ultrasound images through the right lower quadrant show an elongated soft tissue mass seen posterior to the anterior abdominal wall that has heterogeneous texture. A rim of echogenic fat is seen around the lesion (*arrows*). (*Courtesy of* Dr Monser Abu-Yousef.)

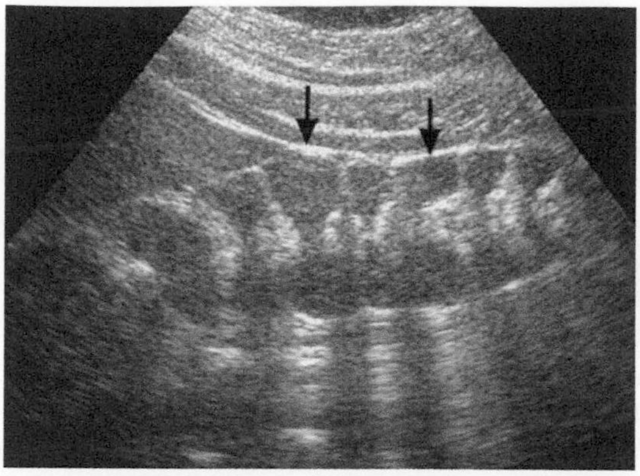

Fig. 9. Pseudomembranous colitis. Longitudinal image of the transverse colon shows thickening of the haustra. (*From* Scoutt LM, Swayers SR, Bokhari J, et al. Ultrasound evaluation of the acute abdomen. Ultrasound Clin 2007;2(3):512; with permission.)

In patients with ulcerative colitis, the rectum is involved first and then the disease extends proximally. Typhlitis is seen as wall thickening predominantly involving the cecum and ascending colon and usually occurs in neutropenic patients with secondary infections. Pseudomembranous colitis causes edema and diffuse wall thickening of the entire colon (**Fig. 9**), usually from *Clostridium difficile* infection in patients on antibiotic therapy. Ischemic colitis usually occurs in the region of splenic flexure and descending colon and is manifested by bowel wall thickening seen in these areas.

BOWEL OBSTRUCTION

Although sonography is not the gold standard for imaging the bowel, occasionally it can help diagnose bowel obstruction. In the cases of suspected bowel obstruction, sonographic assessment includes evaluation of caliber differences of various parts of bowel from the stomach to the rectum, exaggerated peristaltic activity, or any findings of intussusception. Occasionally, a large gallstones or a foreign body may be seen at the point of obstruction. The fluid in the dilated bowel serves as contrast medium and distends the bowel loops, making them readily detectable on ultrasound. Peristalsis with a to-and-fro bowel fluid movement may also be noted. Small bowel can be distinguished from colon by the presence of valvulae conniventes and absence of the thick haustral markings of the colon (**Fig. 10**). Sonography has a reported sensitivity of 89% for diagnosing small bowel obstruction.[8,21] Massively distended bowel loops with wall thickening and absent color flow on Doppler ultrasound may indicate bowel infarction. Sonography can also be used to evaluate colonic obstruction and has a reported sensitivity of 88%.[8,21,22] However, CT and plain films remain the preferred imaging modalities for the clinical suspicion of bowel obstruction.

METASTATIC DISEASE

Peritoneal metastatic disease or peritoneal carcinomatosis is defined as metastatic disease to the omentum, peritoneal surface, peritoneal ligaments, or mesentery. The ultrasound findings are better shown in the presence of ascites and include hypoechoic or hyperechoic nodular omental masses seen through the anechoic ascites (**Fig. 11**). Nodular masses may be present on the omentum (omental cake), parietal peritoneum, or serosal surface of the bowel walls. In the absence of ascites, detection of peritoneal implants smaller than 3 mm is difficult. Color Doppler ultrasound may detect vascularity in omental/peritoneal deposits. Thickening of the mesenteric side of the terminal ileum may be seen secondary to desmoplastic reaction.[23]

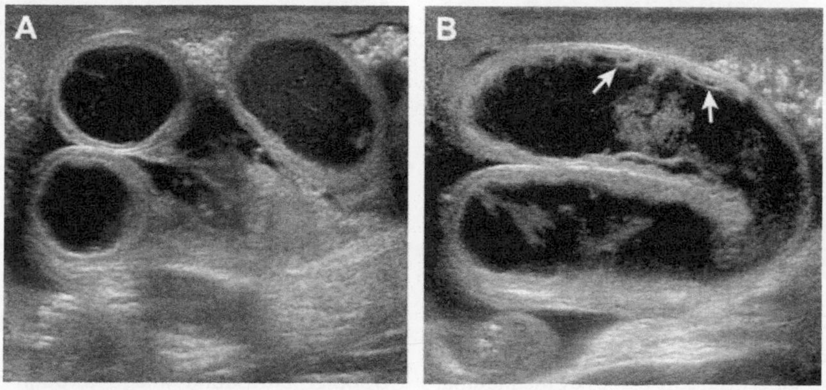

Fig. 10. Small bowel obstruction. Transverse (*A*) and longitudinal (*B*) of multiple dilated loops of small bowel in a patient with distal small bowel obstruction. (*From* Scoutt LM, Sawyers SR, Bokhari J, et al. Ultrasound evaluation of the acute abdomen. Ultrasound Clin 2007;2(3):513; with permission.)

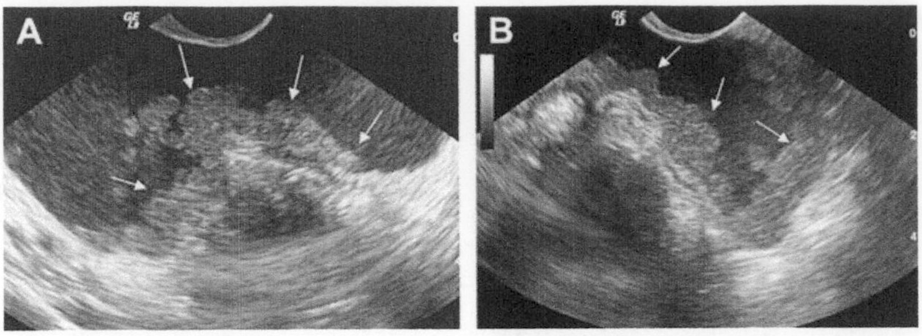

Fig. 11. Peritoneal metastasis. Transverse (*A*) and longitudinal (*B*) ultrasound image through the lower abdomen. Multiple solid irregular masses are seen overlying the peritoneal surface in the lower abdomen (*arrows*). Surrounding ascitic fluid shows internal echoes from hemorrhage.

INGUINAL HERNIAS

Although most inguinal hernias are diagnosed in childhood, they can also present in adulthood as the cause of acute pelvic pain. Ultrasound is considered the primary imaging modality for evaluating inguinal hernias (**Fig. 12**). Color Doppler sonography can be used to differentiate indirect versus direct inguinal hernias.[24] In direct hernias, the hernial defect is seen medial to the inferior epigastric artery, whereas indirect hernias occur through the inguinal canal. Ultrasound is helpful in distinguishing hernias from other groin masses, such as a varicocele, hematoma, or hydrocele.[25]

HYDROCELE

A hydrocele of the canal of Nuck is a rare cause of pain and sometimes can cause inguinal swelling in women. It is embryologically related to an indirect inguinal hernia because it develops in women who have a patent processus vaginalis accompanying the round ligament of the uterus.[26–28] The sonographic appearance is that of a cystic mass with a well-defined echogenic margin (**Fig. 13**). Occasionally, the mass may contain septa or cystic internal structures. Hammond[26] reported a case in which the use of pressure from the ultrasound transducer caused the cyst to be reduced into the peritoneal cavity.

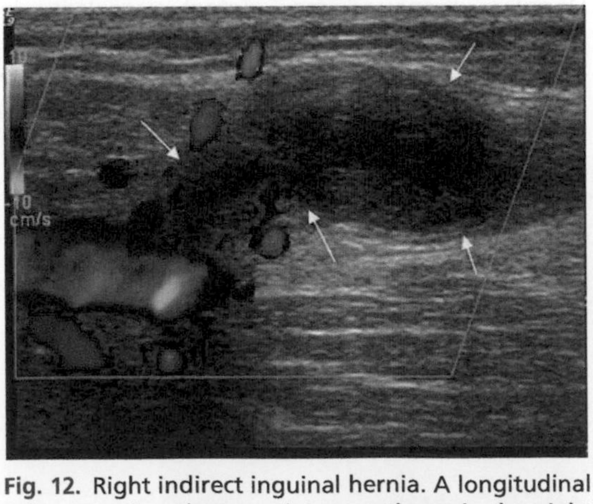

Fig. 12. Right indirect inguinal hernia. A longitudinal color Doppler ultrasound image through the right inguinal region shows an elongated hypoechoic mass within the superficial soft tissues of the inguinal canal (*arrows*). The mass shows a narrow neck (adjacent to the vessel), and the hernial sac mostly contains fat. No flow is noted within the mass.

VARICOCELE

A varicocele of the round ligament or labial varicocele is a rare entity that can cause pelvic pain and swelling. The round ligament passes from the pelvis, through the internal inguinal ring, and along the inguinal canal to the labia majora.[29] The varicocele is usually associated with pregnancy and worsens progressively until delivery. It usually resolves after delivery. Most cases present in the third trimester of pregnancy. Gray-scale sonography shows prominent anechoic

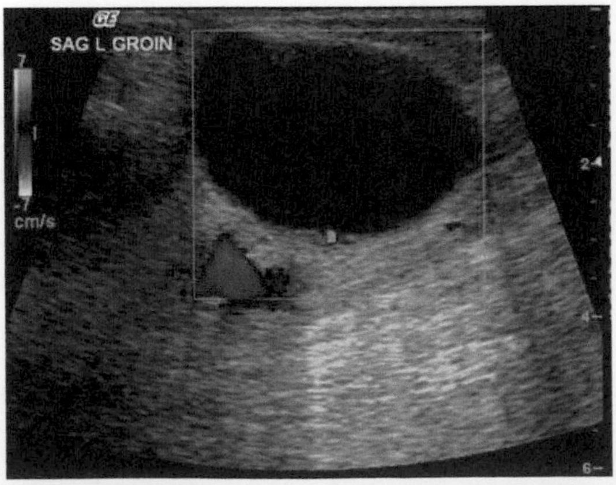

Fig. 13. Hydrocele in the canal of Nuck. An oblique Doppler ultrasound image through the left groin shows an anechoic fluid collection in the left inguinal region. The collection does not show thick walls or color flow.

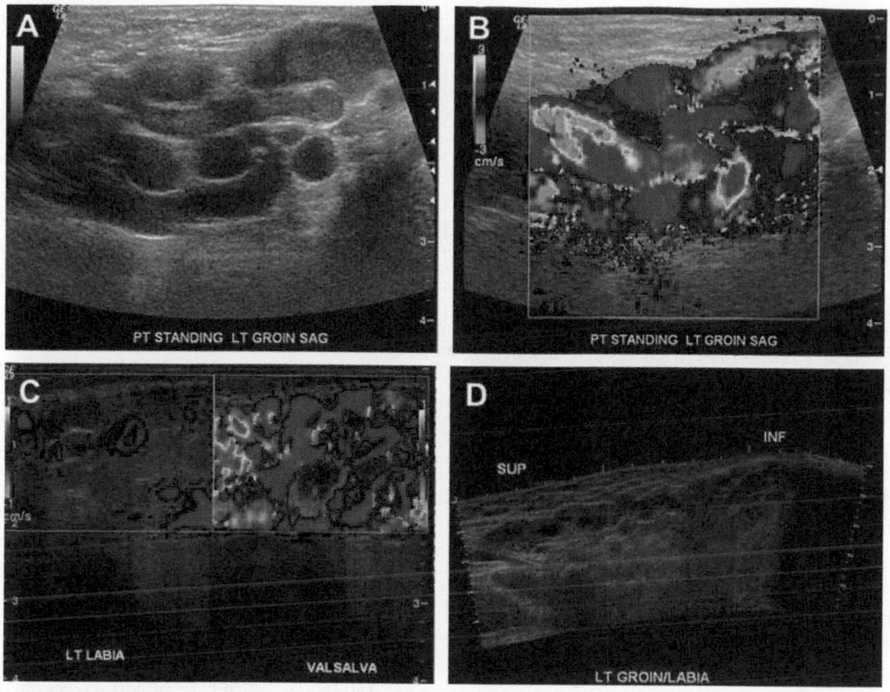

Fig. 14. Left varicocele. (*A*) Ultrasound image through the left groin in standing position that shows multiple anechoic tubular structures. (*B*) Color Doppler image through the same area showing vascular flow in these consistent with varices. (*C*) Dual image through the left labia without (*left*) and with (*right*) Valsalva maneuver. (*D*) Extended-view image through the left groin showing the extent of the varicocele.

tubular channels that reveal venous flow on color Doppler. Augmentation using valsalva maneuvers is helpful because venous flow at rest can be subtle. Sometimes having the patient stand can accentuate the findings (**Fig. 14**A, D).[30]

DUPLICATION CYSTS

Enteric duplication cysts are rare congenital anomalies arising anywhere along the gastrointestinal tract[31] that may cause abdominal or pelvic pain, especially when complicated by hemorrhage, infection, or torsion. Complicated cysts may present with symptoms similar to appendicitis or ovarian torsion. Duplication cysts are defined by their histologic appearance. Similar to the native gastrointestinal tract, these cysts contain an inner mucosa–submucosa layer surrounded by an outer smooth-muscle layer.[31,32] On imaging, the double wall or "muscular rim" sign has been suggested to be characteristic of duplication cysts.[31,32] The characteristic sonographic appearance includes

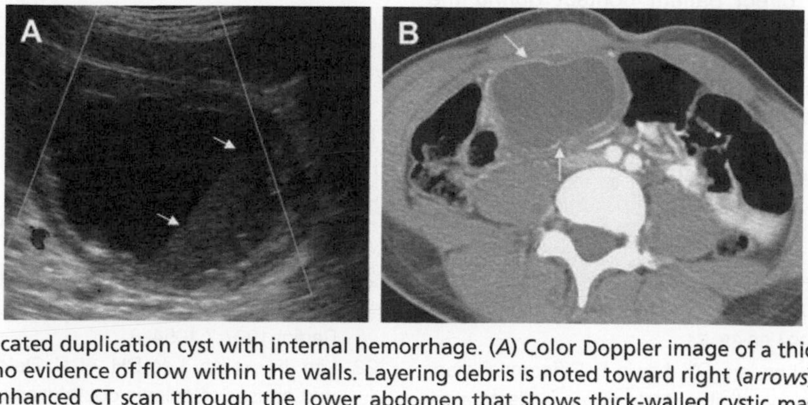

Fig. 15. Complicated duplication cyst with internal hemorrhage. (*A*) Color Doppler image of a thick-walled cystic mass showing no evidence of flow within the walls. Layering debris is noted toward right (*arrows*). (*B*) Axial slice of a contrast-enhanced CT scan through the lower abdomen that shows thick-walled cystic mass with slightly enhanced walls (*arrows*).

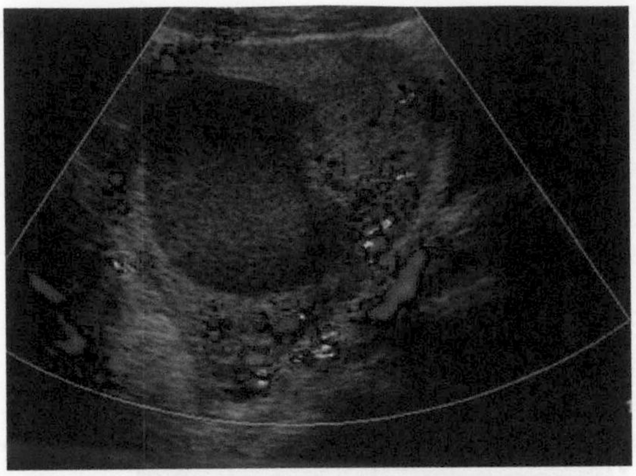

Fig. 16. Infected mesenteric cyst. Color Doppler ultrasound image through the right lower abdomen shows a large thick-walled cystic structure. The fluid shows internal echoes from infection. Increased vascularity is present in the thick walls, suggesting hyperemia.

visualization of an inner hyperechoic rim correlating to the mucosa–submucosa and an outer surrounding hypoechoic layer reflecting muscularis propria.[32–35] Occasionally, these cysts may become infected or show internal hemorrhage (**Figs. 15** and **16**).

SUMMARY

Ultrasound is a valuable noninvasive diagnostic tool for evaluating female patients who present with acute pelvic pain. Although gynecologic conditions constitute most causes of acute pelvic pain, particularly in women of childbearing age; nongynecologic conditions should also be considered. These conditions may be easily overlooked and delay diagnosis. Sometimes ultrasound can help diagnose nongynecologic disorders. Not only is sonography helpful from an imaging standpoint but also one can take advantage of direct patient contact during the examination to correlate the point of maximal tenderness with the underlying imaging findings. Ultrasound should be used as the primary imaging modality in children and pregnant women in whom appendicitis or ureteral calculi is clinically suspected.

REFERENCES

1. Guidry SP, Poole GV. The anatomy of appendicitis. Am Surg 1994;60:68–71.
2. Bongard F, Landers DV, Lewis F. Differential diagnosis of appendicitis and pelvic inflammatory disease. Am J Surg 1985;150:90–6.
3. Puylert JB. Acute appendicitis: US evaluation using graded compression. Radiology 1986;158:355–60.
4. Jeffrey RB, Jain KA, Nghiem HV. Sonographic diagnosis of acute appendicitis: interpretive pitfalls. Am J Roentgenol 1994;162:55–9.
5. Migraine S, Atri M, Bret PM, et al. Spontaneously resolving acute appendicitis: clinical and sonographic documentation. Radiology 1997;205:55–8.
6. Bau A, Atri M. Acute female pelvic pain: ultrasound evaluation. Semin Ultrasound CT MR 2000;2(1):78–93.
7. Angle R, Ackerman S, Irshad A. Practical imaging of acute pelvic pain in premenopausal women. Contemp Diagn Radiol 2010;33(1):1–6.
8. Kuzmich S, Howlett D, Andi A. Transabdominal sonography in assessment of the bowel in adults. Am J Roentgenol 2009;192:197–212.
9. Hollerweger A, Rettenbacher T, Macheiner P, et al. Sigmoid diverticulitis: value of transrectal sonography in addition to transabdominal sonography. Am J Roentgenol 2000;175:1155–60.
10. Hollerweger A. Colonic diseases: the value of US examination. Eur J Radiol 2007;64:239–49.
11. Yilmaz S, Sindel T, Arslan G, et al. Renal colic: comparison of spiral CT, US and IVU in the detection of ureteral calculi. Eur Radiol 1998;8:212–7.
12. Patlas M, Farkas A, Fisher D, et al. Ultrasound vs CT for the detection of ureteric stones in patients with renal colic. Br J Radiol 2001;74:901–4.
13. Platt JF. Doppler ultrasound of the kidney. Semin Ultrasound CT MR 1997;18:22–32.
14. Simanovsky N, Hiller N. Importance of sonographic detection in enlarged abdominal lymph nodes in children. J Ultrasound Med 2007;26:581–4.
15. McClure M, Khalili K, Sarrazin J, et al. Radiological features of epiploic appendagitis and segmental omental infarction. Clin Radiol 2001;56:819–27.
16. Rioux M, Lanigs P. Primary epiploic appendagitis: clinical, US, and CT findings in 14 cases. Radiology 1994;191:523–6.
17. Scoutt L, Sawyers S, Bokhari J, et al. Ultrasound evaluation of the acute abdomen. Ultrasound Clin 2007;2(3):493–523.
18. Puylaert JB. Ultrasonography of the acute abdomen: gastrointestinal conditions. Radiol Clin North Am 2003;41:1227–42.
19. Sarrazin J, Wilson S. Manifestations of Crohn's disease at US. Radiographics 1996;84:385–8.
20. Maconi G, Radice E, Greco A, et al. Bowel ultrasound in Crohn's disease. Best Pract Res Clin Gastroenterol 2006;20:93–112.
21. Schmutz G, Benko A, Fournier L, et al. Small bowel obstruction: role and contribution of sonography. Eur Radiol 1997;7:1054–8.
22. Lim JH, Yt Ko, Lee DH, et al. Determining the site and causes of colonic obstruction with sonography. Am J Roentgenol 1994;163:1113–7.

23. Lolge S. Peritoneal carcinomatosis. In: Ahuja A, editor. Diagnostic imaging: ultrasound. 1st edition. Salt Lake City (UT): Amirsys; 2007. p. 14–7.
24. Atri M, Migraine S, Nazari A, et al. Impact of endovaginal sonography on the evaluation of patients with clinical diagnosis of diverticulitis. Radiology 1997; 205:193.
25. Korenkov M, Paul A, Troidl H. Color duplex sonography: diagnostic tool in the differentiation of inguinal hernias. J Ultrasound Med 1999;18(8):565–8.
26. Hammond I. Letter to the editor: cyst of the canal of Nuck. J Ultrasound Med 2007;26:147.
27. Stickel WH, Manner M. Female hydrocele: sonographic appearance of a rare and little known disorder. J Ultrasound Med 2004;23:429–32.
28. Yigit H, Tuncbilek I, Fitoz S, et al. Cyst of the canal of Nuck with demonstration of the proximal canal: the role of the compression technique in sonographic diagnosis. J Ultrasound Med 2006;25: 123–5.
29. Murphy IG, Heffernan EJ, Gibney RG, et al. Groin mass in pregnancy. Br J Radiol 2007;80:588–9.
30. Nguyen Q, Gruenewald M. Doppler sonography in the diagnosis of round ligament varicosities during pregnancy. J Clin Ultrasound 2008;36(3):177–9.
31. Cheng G, Soboleski D, Daneman A, et al. Sonographic pitfalls in the diagnosis of enteric duplication cysts. Am J Roentgenol 2005;184:521–5.
32. Ros PR, Olmsted WW, Moser RP, et al. Mesenteric and omental cysts: histologic classification with imaging correlation. Radiology 1987;164:327–32.
33. Segal SR, Sherman NH, Rosenberg HK, et al. Ultrasonographic features of gastrointestinal duplications. J Ultrasound Med 1994;13:863–70.
34. Kangarloo H, Sample WR, Hansen G, et al. Ultrasonic evaluation of abdominal gastrointestinal tract duplication in children. Radiology 1979;131:191–4.
35. Moccia W, Astacio J, Kauge J, et al. Ultrasonographic demonstration of gastric duplication in infancy. Pediatr Radiol 1981;11:2–54.

Dysfunctional Uterine Bleeding: Diagnostic Approach and Therapeutic Options

Natasha Brasic, MD[a,*], Vickie A. Feldstein, MD[b]

KEYWORDS

- Dysfunctional uterine bleeding • Endometrium
- Endometrial polyp • Sonohysterography

Abnormal uterine bleeding accounts for 20% of gynecologic visits,[1] and approximately 70% of perimenopausal and postmenopausal visits are for this indication. The patient should first be clinically categorized as premenopausal, perimenopausal, or postmenopausal. In premenopausal women, following the exclusion of pregnancy, the most common cause for dysfunctional uterine bleeding is dysfunctional anovulatory bleeding. With age, the likelihood of pathology such as uterine leiomyomas, endometrial polyps, endometrial hyperplasia, or endometrial carcinoma as the cause for abnormal bleeding increases. Knowledge of the timing of the bleeding relative to the menstrual cycle is also useful. Intermenstrual or postcoital bleeding may be secondary to cervicitis, cervical lesions, endometritis, or other endometrial lesion. Menorrhagia is often linked to myomatous disease or adenomyosis. Menometrorrhagia may be secondary to anovulation, submucosal myomas, adenomyosis, hyperplasia, or carcinoma.

In perimenopausal or postmenopausal women, the differential diagnosis includes the cervical and endometrial pathology mentioned above, and also includes endometrial atrophy. The Society of Radiologists in Ultrasound (SRU) consensus statement[2] defines postmenopausal bleeding as any vaginal bleeding in a postmenopausal woman other than expected cyclic bleeding that occurs with sequential hormone replacement therapy. Postmenopausal bleeding is associated with a risk of endometrial cancer ranging from 1% to 10% depending on age and risk factors.[3,4]

The purpose of evaluating patients with abnormal bleeding is to differentiate those bleeding as a result of anovulatory cycles or endometrial atrophy from those with underlying structural pathology in a safe way that minimizes pain, inconvenience, and cost. Clinical assessment and pelvic examination with Pap smear may be used to exclude infection or cervical carcinoma as causes for bleeding. For other causes of vaginal bleeding, the use of endometrial biopsy or transvaginal sonography have been advocated as initial testing methods. In 2000, a multidisciplinary panel of physicians convened by the SRU discussed the role of sonography in women with postmenopausal bleeding.[2] The panelists agreed that either endometrial biopsy or transvaginal sonography could be used as a first diagnostic step depending on the physician's assessment of patient risk, the nature of the physician's practice, availability of high-quality sonography, and patient preference.

Several studies have suggested that undirected sampling, whether by curettage or suction/aspiration, results in an unacceptable number of false

The authors have nothing to disclose.
[a] Ultrasound and Breast Imaging, Department of Radiology and Biomedical Imaging, University of California, San Francisco, 505 Parnassus Avenue, Box 0628, San Francisco, CA 94143-0628, USA
[b] Gynecology and Reproductive Sciences, Department of Radiology and Biomedical Imaging, University of California, San Francisco, 505 Parnassus Avenue, Box 0628, San Francisco, CA 94143-0628, USA
* Corresponding author.
E-mail address: natasha.brasic@radiology.ucsf.edu

Ultrasound Clin 5 (2010) 245–256
doi:10.1016/j.cult.2010.03.007
1556-858X/10/$ – see front matter

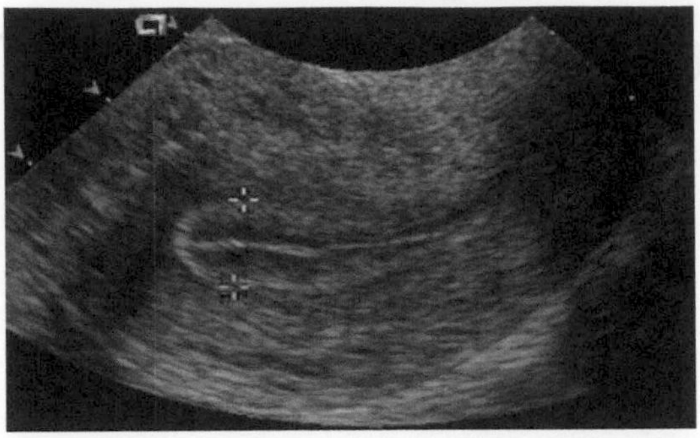

Fig. 1. Sagittal transvaginal sonographic image of the uterus shows normal endometrial stripe measurement (*calipers*) of 5 mm.

negatives, especially when the cause of bleeding is focal.[5–9] Because of these findings and because at least 90% of cases of postmenopausal bleeding have a benign cause,[3] the appropriateness of invasive tissue sampling with its associated inaccuracy, cost, risk, and inconvenience has been called into question as an initial diagnostic step. Several multicenter trials have established transvaginal ultrasound as a reliable means of identifying women with vaginal bleeding who are unlikely to have endometrial disease such that endometrial sampling is unnecessary.[10–15] Transvaginal sonography is thus advocated as a first step for distinguishing patients at a higher risk of malignancy who would benefit from tissue sampling from those with benign causes for bleeding.

The purpose of this article is to describe an algorithm for workup of abnormal vaginal bleeding and to propose appropriate use of transvaginal ultrasonography (TVUS) and saline-infused sonohysterography (SIS) in this workup. Subsequent referrals for blind endometrial sampling versus visually directed endometrial sampling are also discussed.

TRANSVAGINAL SONOGRAPHY

Standards have been set regarding the use of TVUS to exclude endometrial cancer as a cause of abnormal vaginal bleeding.[2] Sonography should be performed transvaginally with a 5- to 10-MHz transducer and an empty bladder for resolution of the endometrial morphology, margins, and double-layer thickness measurement. Transverse/coronal (short axis) and longitudinal/sagittal (long axis) images of the uterus should be obtained during each examination and should also include images of the cervix, as well as cornual and fundal portions of the endometrium. All portions of the uterus must be assessed (**Fig. 1**). The adnexae should also be included in the examination, keeping in mind that ovaries are not always seen in postmenopausal patients. If the entire endometrium is not assessed, the examination is nondiagnostic for workup of uterine bleeding. Often fibroids, adenomyosis, obesity, or unusual uterine orientation can prohibit complete assessment of the endometrium. In these cases, ultrasound cannot be used to exclude pathology. SIS or hysteroscopy are appropriate next steps for workup of abnormal uterine bleeding in these patients.[16]

Endometrial thickness should be measured on a sagittal image of the uterus, and the measurement should be performed on the thickest portion of the endometrium, excluding the hypoechoic inner myometrium. This is a double-layer thickness measurement from basalis to basalis layers. If fluid is present, then the layers are measured separately and should be symmetric.[17] The presence of endometrial fluid is usually a result of cervical stenosis and atrophy (**Fig. 2**).[18]

In premenopausal patients, the endometrial thickness may range from 1 to 18 mm depending on the phase of the menstrual cycle. The endometrium is thinnest in the postmenstrual phase, and is characteristically a thin echogenic line (**Fig. 3**A).

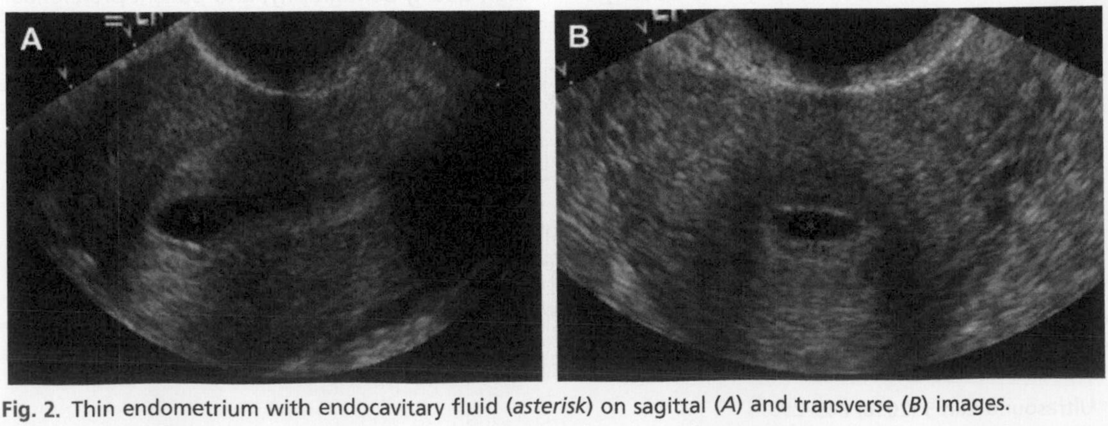

Fig. 2. Thin endometrium with endocavitary fluid (*asterisk*) on sagittal (*A*) and transverse (*B*) images.

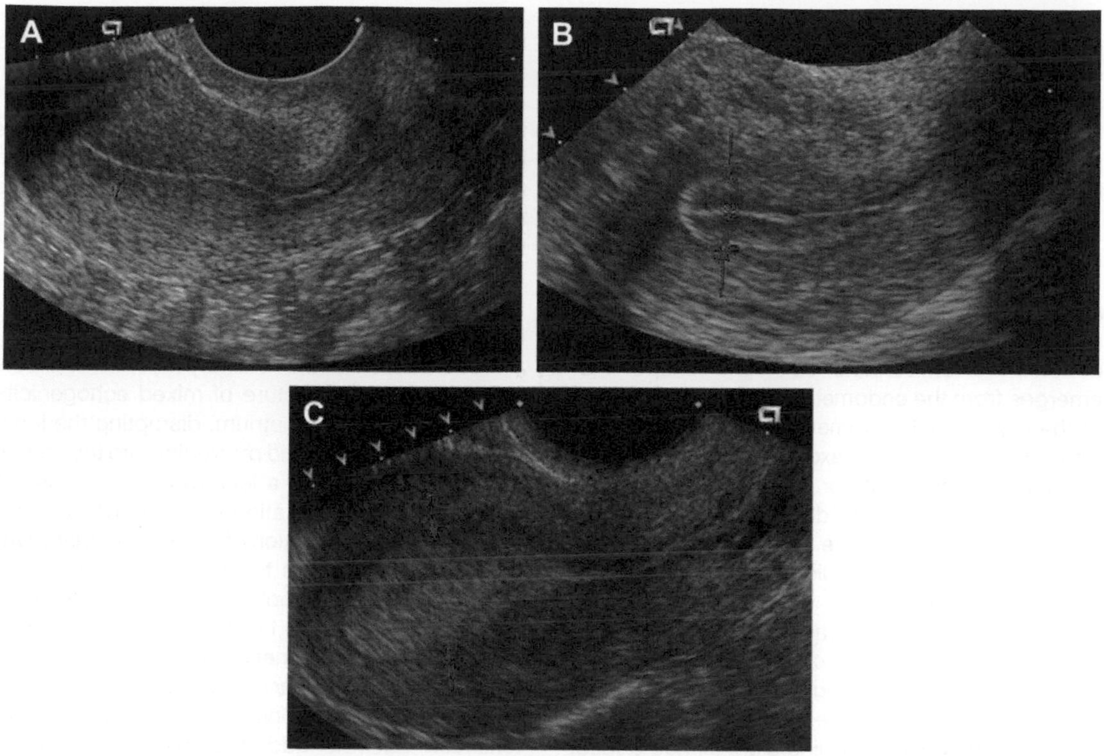

Fig. 3. (*A*) Postmenstrual endometrium (*arrow*) appears as a uniform, thin, echogenic line. (*B*) Proliferative endometrium is manifest as the triple line sign; the deep hyperechoic basalis layer (*arrows*) is separated by the hypoechoic, internal functionalis layer of endometrium. The site of apposed anterior and posterior functionalis layers appears as a thin, hyperechoic central line (*asterisk*). (*C*) In the secretory phase of the menstrual cycle, the functionalis layer becomes hyperechoic and indecipherable from the basalis layer. The endometrium is thicker and diffusely hyperechoic (*arrows*).

During the proliferative phase, the endometrium is hypoechoic with a hyperechoic central component (where the anterior and posterior walls meet), and typically demonstrates the triple line sign (**Fig. 3**B). The functional layer becomes more diffusely hyperechoic and thick in the secretory phase, with posterior acoustic enhancement (**Fig. 3**C). Sensitivity for detection of endometrial pathology is diminished with this physiologic endometrial thickening and hyperechogenicity, and thus, evaluation is best performed in the first half of the menstrual cycle.

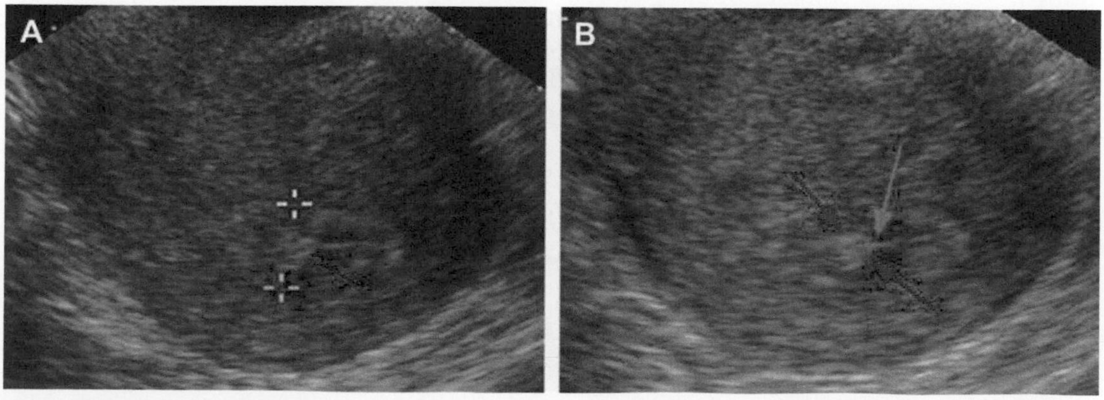

Fig. 4. (*A*) Sagittal transvaginal sonographic image of a retroflexed uterus shows a thickened endometrium measuring 9 mm (*calipers*) with a central hyperechoic mass (*arrow*). (*B*) Similar image of the same patient without calipers reveals a hyperechoic line (*red arrows*) circumscribing the endometrial polyp. Also, the polyp contacts the apposed innermost functionalis layers (*blue arrow*), providing additional confirmation of endometrial location.

Any focal endometrial discontinuity, deformation, absence of the central echogenic line, or focal expansion of the endometrium should be interpreted as abnormal. Moreover, an endometrial thickness greater than 5 mm in a postmenopausal woman with vaginal bleeding should prompt further workup.[10]

FOCAL PROCESSES

An endometrial polyp appears as a smoothly marginated, echogenic mass with a homogeneous echotexture of variable size and shape that emerges from the endometrium without disruption of the myometrial-endometrial interface (**Fig. 4**A). Endometrial polyps are excresent overgrowths of endometrial tissue with or without cystic spaces. Baldwin and colleagues[19] described a hyperechoic line circumscribing the central endometrial complex at TVUS as predictive of focal intracavitary disease, particularly when associated with cystic spaces in the central endometrial complex. This hyperechoic circumscribed line correlates to the separation of the echogenic endometrial basalis layers by a central process. Of 25 patients in the study with a hyperechoic line sign, all had a focal endometrial process, prompting targeted hysteroscopic resection rather than blind endometrial biopsy (**Fig. 4**B).[19]

Another marker for intracavitary polyps by transvaginal sonography is the pedicle artery sign as defined by Timmerman and colleagues.[20] The detection of a feeding blood vessel reaching the central endometrial complex by color Doppler has a sensitivity and specificity for endometrial polyps of 76% and 95%, respectively (**Fig. 5**). Endometrial polyps may be sessile or pedunculated, with preservation of the endometrial-myometrial interface in both instances.

Antunes and colleagues[21] found a low prevalence (3.8%) of malignancy in endometrial polyps and that only advanced age and postmenopausal bleeding were associated with malignancy; in these cases hysteroscopic removal of polyps is recommended. Another study by Ben-Arie and colleagues[22] of more than 400 patients also concluded that age, postmenopausal status, and size greater than 1.5 cm had a higher association with polyp malignancy. It was found, however, that the presence of postmenopausal or irregular bleeding did not correlate with malignancy.[22]

A submucosal or intracavitary myoma manifests as a solid round structure of mixed echogenicity arising from the myometrium, disrupting the inner circular muscle layer and protruding into the uterine cavity. Pathologically, a leiomyoma is a mass of smooth muscle proliferation surrounded by a pseudocapsule. The disruption of the endometrial-myometrial interface helps to distinguish submucous myomas from sessile polyps, although the distinction may nevertheless be difficult. Myomas often have characteristic venetian blind shadowing and tend to be hypovascular and predominantly hypoechoic (**Fig. 6**). Use of sonohysterography in characterization has the added benefit of estimating percent circumference adjacent to and within the uterine cavity. If surgical removal is planned, then at least 50% projection into the uterine cavity suggests hysteroscopic removal may be considered rather than hysterotomy and myomectomy.[23] Hysteroscopic removal also requires sufficient intervening myometrium (>1 cm) at the serosal surface.

Focal endometrial thickening may easily be confused with an endometrial polyp or submucosal fibroid. Such thickening is most easily distinguished by recognizing a broad attachment to the

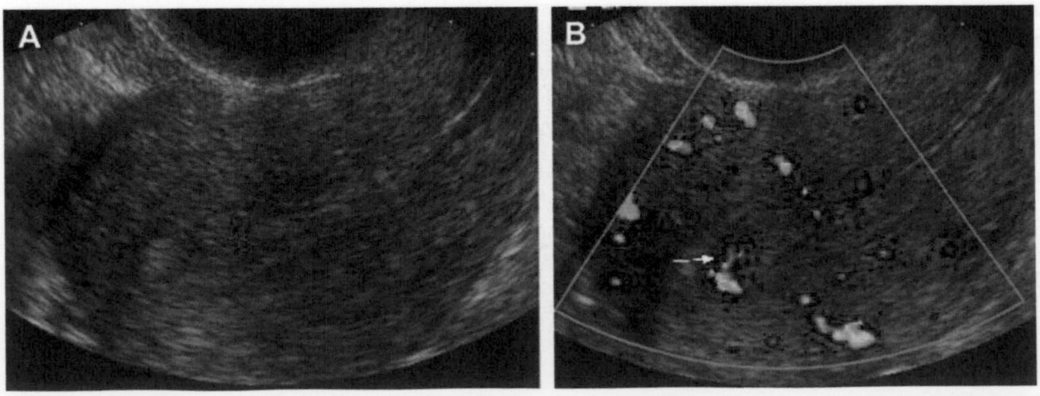

Fig. 5. (*A*) Longitudinal transvaginal sonogram demonstrating an endometrial hyperechoic mass (*asterisk*). (*B*) Color Doppler interrogation of this lesion demonstrates a feeding vascular pedicle (*arrow*). The presence of a vessel reaching the endometrial complex is abnormal and in the presence of a focal endometrial mass, polyp should be suspected.

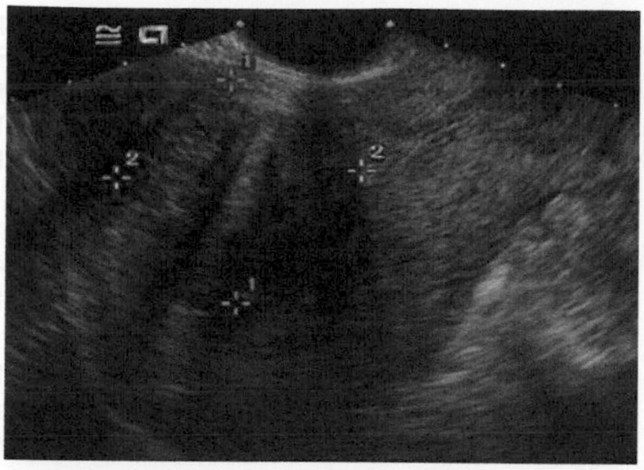

Fig. 6. Sagittal image from a transvaginal sonogram showing a solid mass of mixed echogenicity in the anterior myometrial body, representing a myoma, causing obscuration of the endometrium with venetian blind posterior acoustic shadowing artifact.

myometrium, hyperechogenicity, and lack of an endometrial rim. This differentiation is usually not possible without sonohysterography.

In premenopausal women, there is little consensus about an endometrial thickness threshold that excludes intracavitary pathology. In fact, a study of 206 patients concluded that sonographic evaluation of premenopausal abnormal uterine bleeding should include sonohysterography or equivalently accurate testing regardless of stripe thickness.[24] It has been argued that TVUS may miss submucosal fibroids and small intracavitary polyps that are detected on subsequent sonohysterography or hysteroscopy.[25–27] In a study of 114 patients by Laifer-Narin and colleagues,[28] 14% of patients with abnormal vaginal bleeding showed polyps and submucosal myomas on SIS despite normal transvaginal sonography. Possible reasons for this include the long narrow morphology of some polyps, which precludes recognition as focal thickening of the endometrium. Also, certain endometrial processes do not demonstrate the hyperechoic line sign or pedicle artery sign described earlier.

SONOHYSTEROGRAPHY

SIS is a diagnostic procedure in which sterile saline is infused into the uterine cavity during simultaneous transvaginal sonography, permitting distention of the cavity and an acoustic window by which the endometrium may be imaged. Compared with transvaginal sonography, sonohysterography is more accurate in the detection of focal endometrial lesions.[8,25,26,28] Farquhar and colleagues published a review of 19 studies looking at the diagnostic accuracy of transvaginal sonography, sonohysterography, and hysteroscopy for the investigation of abnormal bleeding in premenopausal women and found the sensitivities for detection of any intrauterine pathology by transvaginal sonography and sonohysterography ranged from 46% to 100% and 85% to 100%, respectively. Specificities for the 2 examinations ranged from 12% to 100% and 81% to 100%, respectively.[25] Erdem and colleagues[26] looked at the evaluation of bleeding in pre- and postmenopausal women and found sensitivity and specificity for detection of any endometrial lesion by sonohysterography to be 98% and 82%, respectively.

Ideally sonohysterography should be scheduled during the phase of the menstrual cycle when the endometrium is thin. This is during the postmenstrual or early proliferative phase, if performed in a premenopausal patient. Absolute contraindications include pregnancy and current pelvic infection. Ongoing vaginal bleeding may diminish the accuracy of the examination because of the presence of clot in the endometrial cavity, but this is not a contraindication to the study.

Adverse effects of the procedure are uncommon and include inability to complete the procedure (7%), pelvic pain (3.8%), vagal symptoms (3.5%), nausea (1%), and postprocedure fever (0.8%).[29] Causes of early examination termination or incomplete evaluation include inability to canulate the cervix, insufficient cervical seal causing backflow of saline, and difficulty distending the uterine cavity because of myomas or adhesions.[29] Mild discomfort is common, and usually abates at the termination of the examination. Severe discomfort is unusual, and if anticipated, the patient may be advised to take ibuprofen or acetaminophen before the examination. Endometritis is a serious but rare complication (<1%).[25] The authors do not recommend routine antibiotic prophylaxis but would advise it in situations of indolent or previous pelvic inflammatory disease, or for those patients who routinely get dental prophylaxis.[30]

The authors prefer routine preliminary transvaginal sonography before sonohysterography for assessment of the uterus and adnexae, and to assess for adnexal tenderness. Following bladder re-emptying, informed consent is obtained and the patient is placed in the lithotomy position. A 5 or 7 French preflushed sonohysterography catheter is inserted into the cervix under sterile speculum examination conditions. The balloon (if a straight catheter is not used) is gently inflated in the endocervical canal, and stable positioning is confirmed with gentle pulling on the catheter. Inflation of the balloon in the cervix is preferable to permit full visualization of the lower uterine

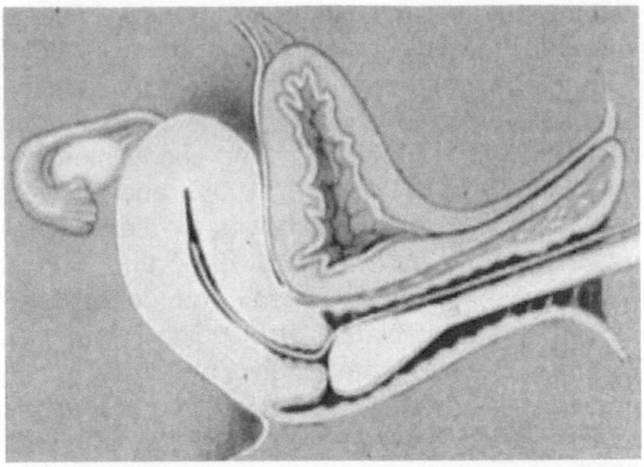

Fig. 7. Midline sagittal pelvis with sonohysterography catheter and transvaginal sonographic probe in place. (*From* Cullinan JA, Fleischer AC, Kepple DM, et al. RadioGraphics 1995;15(3):501–14; with permission.)

segment, but this is potentially more uncomfortable for the patient. The speculum is subsequently removed and the transvaginal ultrasound probe, with a sterile cover, is inserted (**Fig. 7**). Gentle infusion of sterile saline occurs with simultaneous real-time sonography. Coronal and sagittal imaging of the entire uterine canal is performed. The balloon is then deflated and withdrawn to just above the endocervical os (if initially inflated in the uterine cavity). Sonography of the lower uterine segment and endocervix is performed with simultaneous slow infusion of saline during slow withdrawal of the catheter. The catheter and endovaginal probe are removed (**Fig. 8**A, B).

In some cases, three-dimensional sonography may be helpful during saline infusion, but some have argued that true benefit over conventional two-dimensional sonography has not been shown.[31,32] Another study stated that coronal three-dimensional imaging either added information not seen in two-dimensional imaging or allowed more confident diagnosis of an abnormality in 25% of cases reviewed.[33] Overall, three-dimensional sonography is a relatively novel technique that may offer benefit over conventional two-dimensional imaging.

The main role of sonohysterography is for determination of the presence or absence of endometrial pathology, and assessing if endometrial pathology is focal or diffuse. If the endometrium is normal, no further workup may be needed. If disease is focal, sonohysterography is valuable for determination of location. Direct hysteroscopic evaluation and guided biopsy may be warranted in the setting of focal disease. Detection and characterization of a focal lesion does not obviate the need for biopsy, as polyps and fibroids may not be easily differentiated (**Fig. 9**A–E). If the disease process is diffuse, undirected endometrial biopsy may suffice for adequate tissue sampling (**Fig. 10**A, B).

DIFFUSE ENDOMETRIAL THICKENING

Transvaginal sonography should be interpreted as abnormal in postmenopausal bleeding when the endometrial thickness is more than 5 mm.[2,10] A 5-mm cutoff does not apply to asymptomatic or premenopausal women. If the endometrium is more than 11-mm thick in a postmenopausal asymptomatic woman, the risk of cancer is approximately 7%, comparable with that in a woman with bleeding and an endometrial thickness of more than 5 mm (**Fig. 11**).[34]

On TVUS, well-defined or cystic endometrial thickening may both be seen in endometrial hyperplasia. Histopathologically, endometrial hyperplasia is divided into 2 categories: hyperplasia with and without cytologic atypia. In hyperplasia

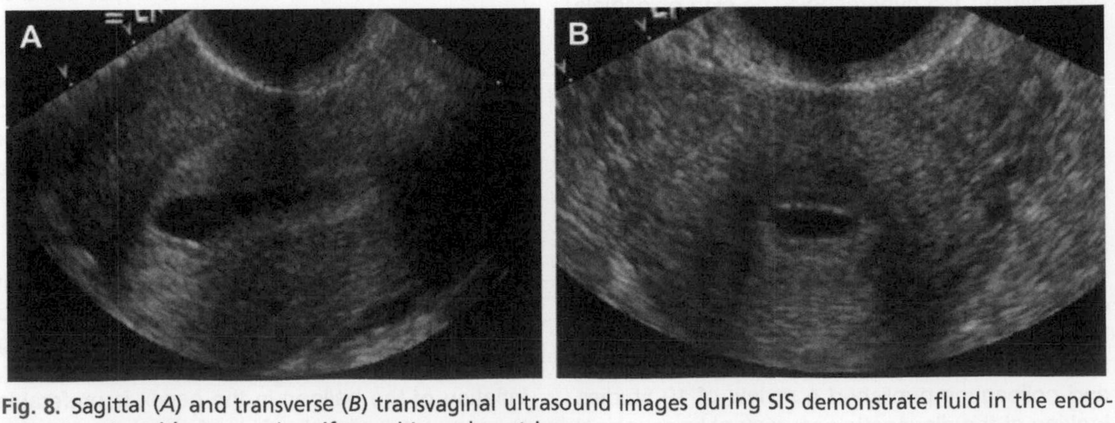

Fig. 8. Sagittal (*A*) and transverse (*B*) transvaginal ultrasound images during SIS demonstrate fluid in the endometrial cavity with a normal, uniform, thin endometrium.

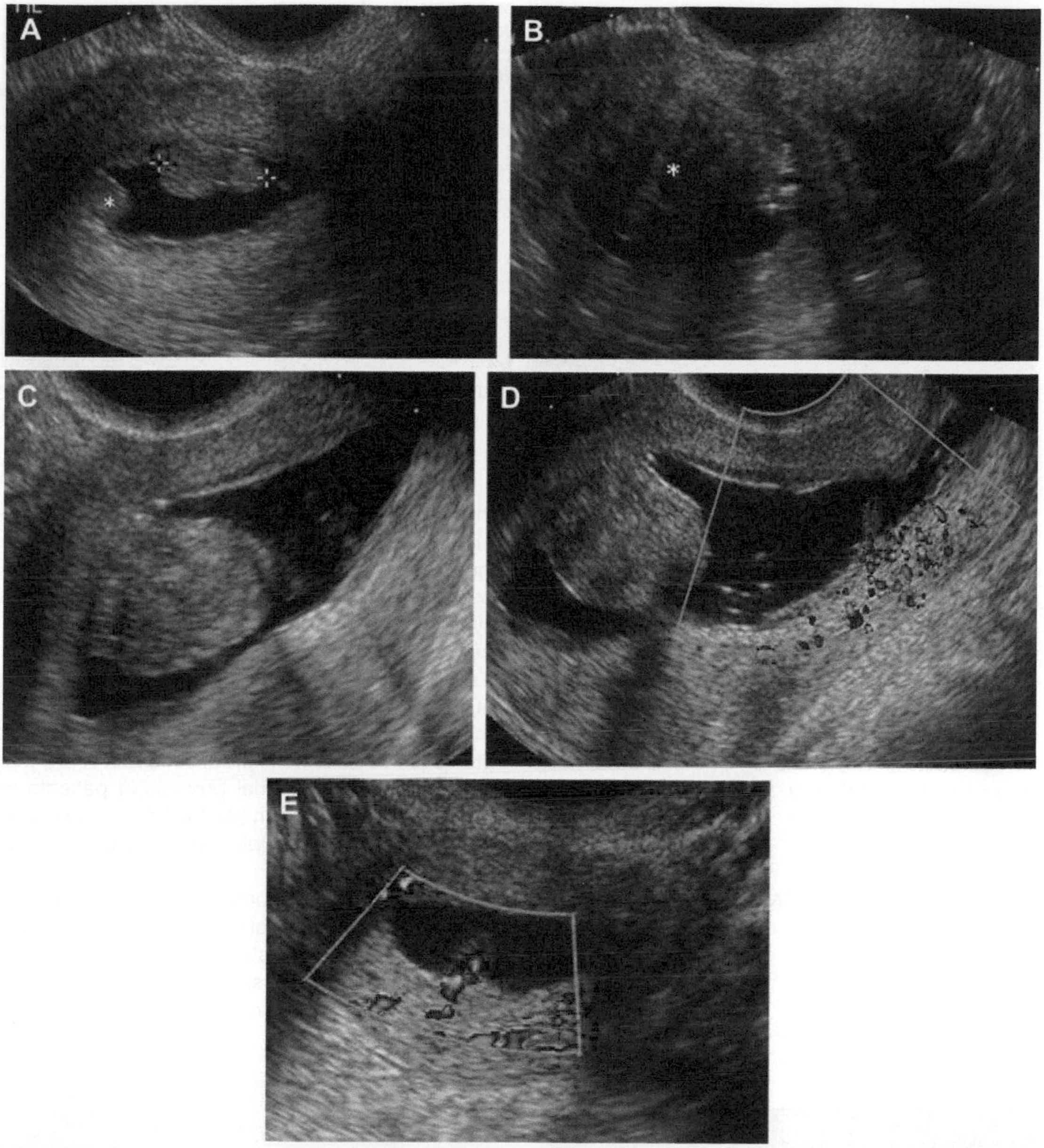

Fig. 9. (*A*) Sagittal sonohysterogram demonstrating 2 adjacent endometrial polyps (*calipers*) and a third fundal focal solid abnormality (*asterisk*). Imaging could not definitively differentiate whether this fundal lesion was a myoma or polyp. (*B*) Sagittal sonohysterogram showing submucosal fibroid (*asterisk*) with less than 50% intracavitary extension. Sonohysterographic assessment of submucosal myomas allows for estimation of the intraluminal component. This is important for determination of potential candidacy for hysteroscopic removal. (*C*) Sagittal sonohysterogram showing an anterior fundal submucosal myoma with at least 80% intracavitary component. In the same patient, a polyp is seen along the posterior uterine cavity (*D*) with color Doppler imaging showing a vascular pedicle (*E*).

without atypia, 2% are believed to progress to endometrial carcinoma versus 23% of cases with cytologic atypia.[35] Smooth, diffuse endometrial thickening and focal thickening may be caused by hyperplasia. Hyperplasia may be homogeneous or have cysts. On sonohysterography, endometrial surface irregularity may be present.

Endometrial cystic atrophy, also referred to as cystic degeneration, can be confused with cystic

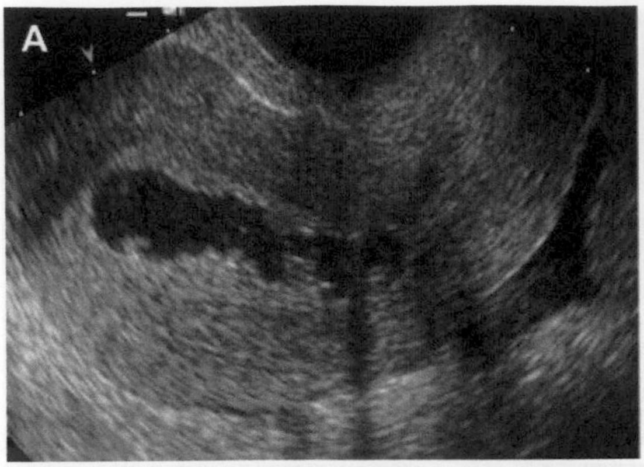

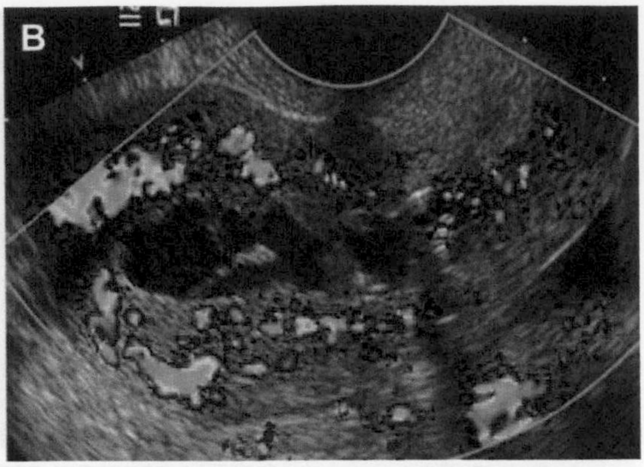

Fig. 10. (*A*) Sagittal sonohysterographic image showing diffuse irregular thickening of the endometrium without demonstrable vascular pedicle on color Doppler imaging (*B*), most consistent with diffuse endometrial hyperplasia.

hyperplasia. In cystic atrophy, there is scant identifiable intervening endometrium with multiple endometrial lucencies. This appearance is also referred to as Swiss cheese endometrium (**Fig. 12**). This appearance must be differentiated from subendometrial cysts characteristic of adenomyosis (**Fig. 13**A, B). Histopathologically, multiple dilated glands (cystic spaces) lined with atrophic endometrium are present within a dense fibrous stroma. The presence of these cysts may lead to a spuriously widened endometrial measurement, whereas the true endometrial tissue is thin.[36]

EFFECTS OF TAMOXIFEN ON THE ENDOMETRIUM

Tamoxifen citrate, widely used in the treatment of breast cancer, acts as an antiestrogenic agent in the breast. Tamoxifen has an estrogenic effect on the postmenopausal endometrium and myometrium. Long-term use has been associated with an increased incidence of endometrial proliferation, polyps, adenomyosis, leiomyomas, endometrial cystic atrophy, endometrial hyperplasia, endometrial carcinoma, and uterine sarcoma.[37–41] In a study of 238 patients on tamoxifen, the incidence of endometrial pathology was significantly higher in the symptomatic group than in the asymptomatic group (93 vs 25%).[42] A predilection for more than 1 pathologic endometrial process in patients on tamoxifen has also been established,[43] and careful consideration of multiple abnormalities is warranted (**Fig. 14**).

In asymptomatic women receiving tamoxifen, the upper limit of normal for endometrial thickness is controversial. One study referred 117 asymptomatic postmenopausal women on tamoxifen for outpatient hysteroscopy with or without

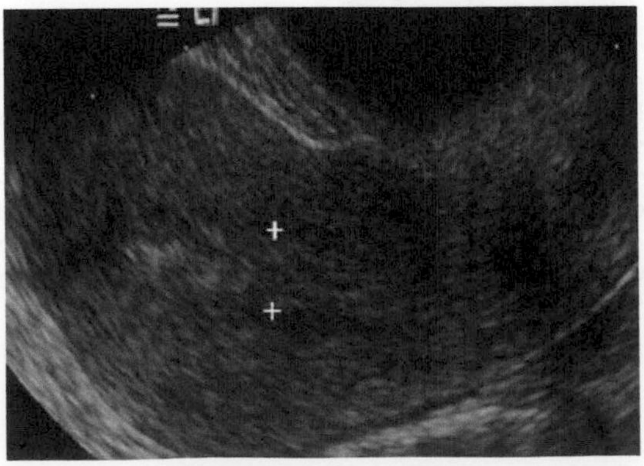

Fig. 11. Endometrial thickness measuring 6 mm in a postmenopausal woman with vaginal bleeding (*calipers*). This is the transvaginal sonogram performed before SIS in the patient shown in **Fig. 10**.

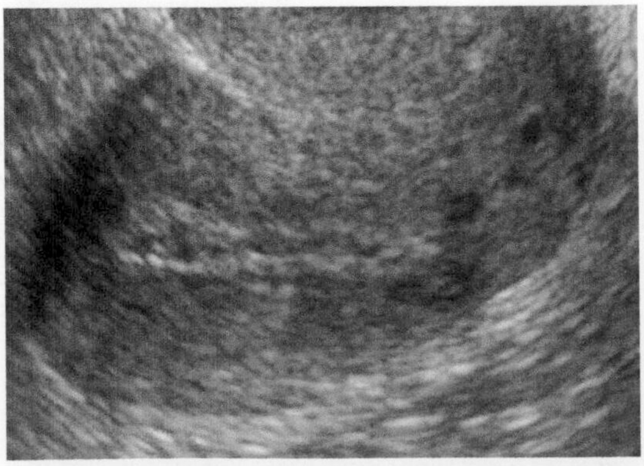

Fig. 12. Thin, cystic endometrial stripe in a postmenopausal patient with typical Swiss cheese appearance consistent with cystic atrophy. Endometrial thickness measured 4 mm. Nabothian cysts are incidentally present in the cervix.

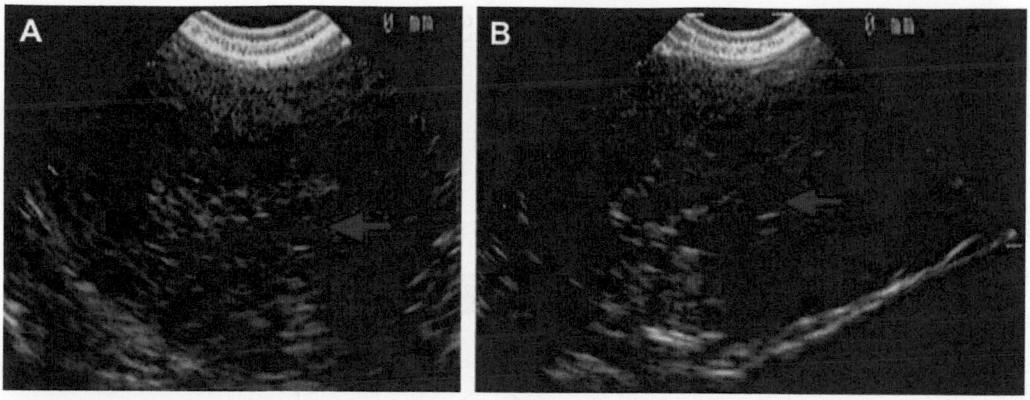

Fig. 13. (*A*) TVUS sagittal image showing multiple subendometrial cysts (*arrow*) with otherwise normal-appearing endometrial stripe. (*B*) Sagittal sonohysterographic image confirms the subendometrial location of these cysts (*arrow*). This finding is consistent with a diagnosis of adenomyosis.

directed biopsy, irrespective of endometrial thickness measurement at TVUS. Uterine abnormalities including polyps and submucosal fibroids were present in 40% of the patients, but there were no cases of endometrial hyperplasia or carcinoma. The investigators concluded the optimal endometrial thickness cutoff for detection of abnormalities was greater than 6 mm with a maximal sensitivity and specificity of 84% and 58%, respectively.[36]

However, the American College of Obstetrics and Gynecology has concluded that unless a patient on tamoxifen has been identified to be at high risk for endometrial cancer, routine endometrial surveillance in asymptomatic patients has not been effective in increasing the early detection of endometrial cancer. Such surveillance may lead to more invasive and costly diagnostic procedures

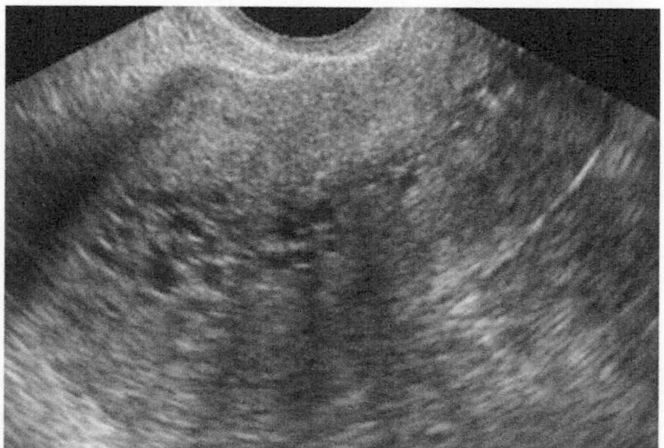

Fig. 14. Effects of tamoxifen on the endometrium in this postmenopausal patient with breast cancer and vaginal spotting manifest as diffuse thickening (10 mm) with multiple cysts seen on sagittal transvaginal sonogram. Polyps and cystic hyperplasia were revealed by undirected endometrial biopsy.

and, therefore, is not recommended. Any instance of abnormal vaginal bleeding, bloody discharge, staining, or spotting should be investigated.[44]

Endometrial polyps represent the most common endometrial pathology related to postmenopausal tamoxifen use with an estimated 2% to 10% increase in malignant degeneration compared with patients not taking tamoxifen. Further, there has been no correlation between polyp size or malignancy and duration of treatment.[45,46] Postmenopausal women taking tamoxifen have an increased risk of development of leiomyomas and adenomyosis.[38,47]

Tamoxifen therapy is associated with a statistically significantly increased risk of invasive endometrial cancer in women aged 50 years or older. The National Surgical Adjuvant Breast and Bowel Project B-14 trial reported that the cumulative rate of invasive endometrial cancer through 7 years of follow-up was 4.7 per 1000 women in the placebo group and 15.6 per 1000 women in the tamoxifen group with a relative risk of 2.2.[40,41] The risk of carcinoma increases with total duration of use and cumulative dose of tamoxifen, previous hormone replacement therapy, obesity, hypertension, and diabetes.[37]

DIFFICULTIES IN ENDOMETRIAL STRIPE MEASUREMENT

The presence of multiple myomas, unusual orientation of the uterus or patient body habitus may prohibit optimal visualization of the endometrial stripe and accurate measurement of endometrial thickness. The presence of adenomyosis or endometrial cystic atrophy may lead to misleading endometrial measurements. In these instances, if

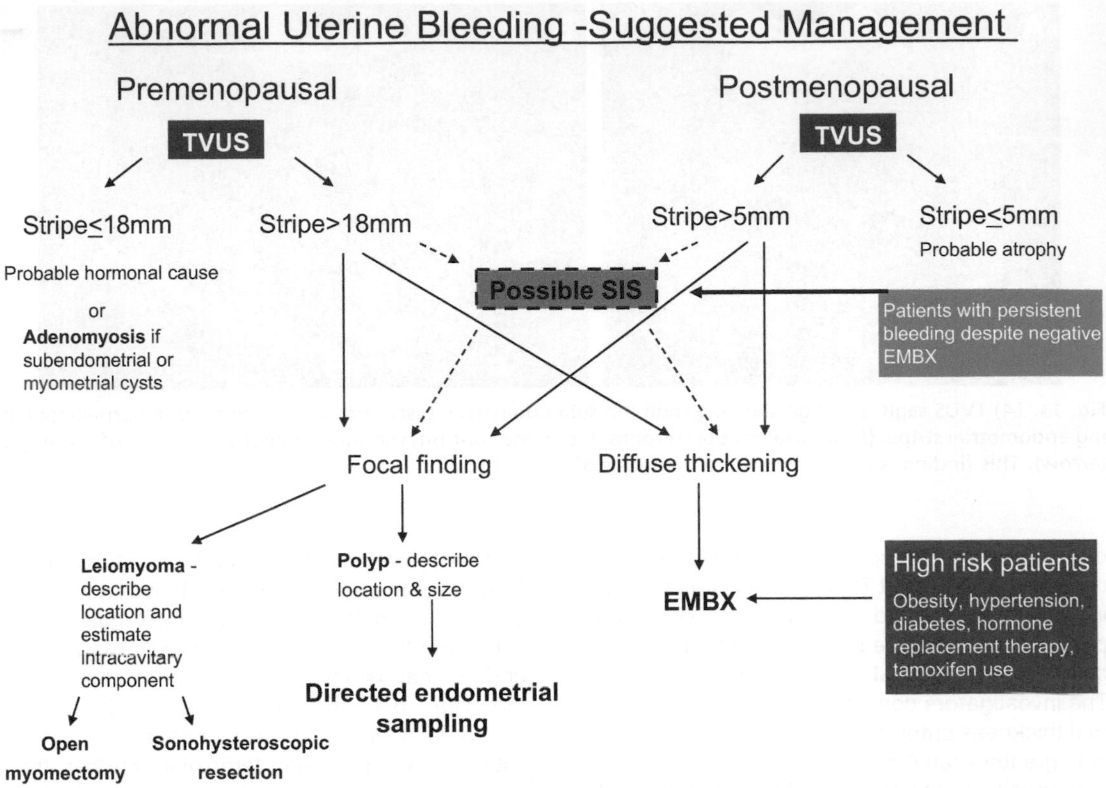

Fig. 15. Suggested algorithm for management of abnormal uterine bleeding in premenopausal, postmenopausal, and high-risk patients. In cases in which focality or diffusivity of endometrial thickening or better characterization of the endometrium is desired, SIS may be pursued after TVUS. In high-risk patients, undirected endometrial biopsy (EMBX) may be immediately undertaken. Also in patients with endometrial thickening and negative EMBX, SIS may be helpful for further assessment of possibly underlying pathology.

abnormal is bleeding present, additional workup is warranted.

SUMMARY

Appropriate triage of patients with abnormal vaginal bleeding begins with a history and physical examination. Imaging plays an integral part in the detection of endometrial disorders, and the algorithm in **Fig. 15** summarizes a suggested workup of abnormal uterine bleeding (see **Fig. 15**). A similar algorithm to that proposed in this article has recently been suggested by Shi and Lee.[48] The endometrium may be normal in thickness (≤18 mm in menstruating women and ≤5 mm in postmenopausal women), in which case the bleeding is likely hormonal or caused by atrophy in the setting of normal physical examination. However, if clinical concern persists, SIS may reveal a small, otherwise occult lesion. In cases of endometrial thickening, determination of focal or diffuse disease may be best assessed with SIS, and appropriate hysteroscopic or undirected biopsy may follow, respectively.

Alternatively, in patients who are at increased risk for endometrial cancer, such as those with morbid obesity, hypertension, diabetes, hormone replacement therapy, or tamoxifen use, endometrial thickening on routine transvaginal sonography may prompt endometrial biopsy without SIS. SIS may be useful in the setting of negative undirected biopsy and persistent bleeding.

REFERENCES

1. Awwad J, Toth T, Schiff I. Abnormal uterine bleeding in the perimenopause. Int J Fertil Menopausal Stud 1993;38(5):261–9.
2. Goldstein R, Bree R, Benson C, et al. Evaluation of the woman with postmenopausal bleeding: Society of Radiologists in Ultrasound-sponsored consensus conference statement. J Ultrasound Med 2001; 20(10):1025–36.
3. Hawwa Z, Nahhas W, Copenhaver E. Postmenopausal bleeding. Lahey Clin Found Bull 1970; 19(2):61–70.
4. Rose P. Endometrial carcinoma. N Engl J Med 1996; 335(9):640–9.

5. Guido R, Kanbour-Shakir A, Rulin M, et al. Pipelle endometrial sampling. Sensitivity in the detection of endometrial cancer. J Reprod Med 1995;40(8):553–5.
6. Goldchmit R, Katz Z, Blickstein I, et al. The accuracy of endometrial Pipelle sampling with and without sonographic measurement of endometrial thickness. Obstet Gynecol 1993;82(5):727–30.
7. Larson D, Krawisz B, Johnson K, et al. Comparison of the Z-sampler and Novak endometrial biopsy instruments for in-office diagnosis of endometrial cancer. Gynecol Oncol 1994;54(1):64–7.
8. Dijkhuizen F, Mol B, Brolmann H, et al. The accuracy of endometrial sampling in the diagnosis of patients with endometrial cancer and hyperplasia. Cancer 2000;89(8):1765–72.
9. Dubinsky T, Parvey H, Maklad N. The role of transvaginal sonography and endometrial biopsy in the evaluation of peri- and postmenopausal bleeding. AJR Am J Roentgenol 1997;169(1):145–9.
10. Smith-Bindman R, Kerlikowske K, Feldstein V, et al. Endovaginal ultrasound to exclude endometrial cancer and other endometrial abnormalities. JAMA 1998;280(17):1510–7.
11. Karlsson B, Granberg S, Wikland M, et al. Transvaginal ultrasonography of the endometrium in women with postmenopausal bleeding - a Nordic multicenter study. Am J Obstet Gynecol 1995;172(5):1488–94.
12. Ferrazzi E, Torri V, Trio D, et al. Sonographic endometrial thickness: a useful test to predict atrophy in patients with postmenopausal bleeding. An Italian multicenter study. Ultrasound Obstet Gynecol 1996;7(5):315–21.
13. Gull B, Carlsson S, Karlsson B, et al. Transvaginal ultrasonography of the endometrium in women with postmenopausal bleeding: is it always necessary to perform an endometrial biopsy? Am J Obstet Gynecol 2000;182(3):509–15.
14. Epstein E, Valentin L. Rebleeding and endometrial growth in women with postmenopausal bleeding and endometrial thickness <5 mm managed by dilation and curettage or ultrasound follow-up: a randomized controlled study. Ultrasound Obstet Gynecol 2001;18(5):499–504.
15. Gull B, Karlsson B, Milsom I, et al. Can ultrasound replace dilation and curettage? A longitudinal evaluation of postmenopausal bleeding and transvaginal sonographic measurement of the endometrium as predictors of endometrial cancer. Am J Obstet Gynecol 2003;188(2):401–8.
16. Goldstein S. The role of transvaginal ultrasound or endometrial biopsy in the evaluation of the menopausal endometrium. Am J Obstet Gynecol 2009;201(1):5–11.
17. Bredella M, Feldstein V, Filly R, et al. Measurement of endometrial thickness at US in multicentral drug trials: value of central quality assurance reading. Radiology 2000;217(2):516–20.
18. Goldstein S. Postmenopausal endometrial fluid collections revisited: look at the doughnut rather than the hole. Obstet Gynecol 1994;83(5 Pt 1):738–40.
19. Baldwin M, Dudiak K, Gorman B, et al. Focal intracavitary masses recognized with the hyperechoic line sign at endovaginal US and characterized with hysterosonography. Radiographics 1999;19(4):927–35.
20. Timmerman D, Verguts J, Konstantinovic M, et al. The pedicle artery sign based on sonography with color Doppler imaging can replace second-stage tests in women with abnormal vaginal bleeding. Ultrasound Obstet Gynecol 2003;22(2):166–71
21. Antunes A, Costa-Paiva L, Arthuso M, et al. Endometrial polyps in pre- and postmenopausal women: factors associated with malignancy. Maturitas 2007;57(4):415–21.
22. Ben-Arie A, Goldchmidt C, Laviv Y, et al. The malignant potential of endometrial polyps. Eur J Obstet Gynecol Reprod Biol 2004;115(2):206–10.
23. Elsayes K, Pandya A, Platt J, et al. Technique and diagnostic utility of saline infusion sonohysterography. Int J Gynecol Obstet 2009;105(1):5–9.
24. Breitkopf D, Frederickson R, Snyder R. Detection of benign endometrial masses by endometrial stripe measurement in premenopausal women. Obstet Gynecol 2004;104(1):120–5.
25. Farquhar C, Ekeroma A, Furness S, et al. A systematic review of transvaginal ultrasonography, sonohysterography and hysteroscopy for the investigation of abnormal uterine bleeding in premenopausal women [review]. Acta Obstet Gynecol Scand 2003;82(6):493–504.
26. Erdem M, Bilgin U, Bozkurt N, et al. Comparison of transvaginal ultrasonography and saline infusion sonohysterography in evaluating the endometrial cavity in pre- and postmenopausal women with abnormal uterine bleeding. Menopause 2007;14(5):846–52.
27. Yildizhan B, Yildizhan R, Ozkesici B, et al. Transvaginal ultrasonography and saline infusion sonohysterography for the detection of intrauterine lesions in pre- and post menopausal women with abnormal uterine bleeding. J Int Med Res 2008;36(6):1205–13.
28. Laifer-Narin S, Ragavendra N, Parmenter EK, et al. False-normal appearance of the endometrium on conventional transvaginal sonography: comparison with saline hysterosonography. AJR Am J Roentgenol 2002;178(1):129–33.
29. Dessole S, Farina M, Rubattu G, et al. Side effects and complications of sonohysterosalpingography. Fertil Steril 2003;80(3):620–4.
30. American Institute of Ultrasound in Medicine, American College of Obstetricians and Gynecologists, American College of Radiology. AIUM standard for the performance of saline infusion sonohysterography. J Ultrasound Med 2003;22:121–6.

31. Terry S, Banks E, Harris K, et al. Comparison of 3-dimensional with 2-dimensional saline infusion sonohysterograms for the evaluation of intrauterine abnormalities. J Clin Ultrasound 2009;37(5):258–62.
32. Opolskiene G, Sladkevicius P, Valentin L. Two- and three-dimensional saline contrast sonohysterography: interobserver agreement, agreement with hysteroscopy and diagnosis of endometrial malignancy. Ultrasound Obstet Gynecol 2009;33(5):574–82.
33. Benacerraf BR, Shipp TD, Bromley B. Which patients benefit from a 3D reconstructed coronal view of the uterus added to standard routine 2D pelvic sonography? AJR Am J Roentgenol 2008; 190(3):626–9.
34. Smith-Bindman R, Weiss E, Feldstein V. How thick is too thick? When endometrial thickness should prompt biopsy in postmenopausal women without vaginal bleeding. Ultrasound Obstet Gynecol 2004; 24(5):558–65.
35. Kurman R, Norris H. Endometrial hyperplasia and related cellular changes. In: Kurman RJ, editor. Blaustein's pathology of the female genital tract. New York: Springer-Verlag; 1994. p. 411–37.
36. Fong K, Kung R, Lytwyn A, et al. Endometrial evaluation with transvaginal US and hysterosonography in asymptomatic postmenopausal women with breast cancer receiving tamoxifen. Radiology 2001;220(3):765–73.
37. Berliere M, Charles A, Galant C, et al. Uterine side effects of tamoxifen: a need for systematic pretreatment screening. Obstet Gynecol 1998;91(1):40–4.
38. Cohen I, Beyth Y, Tepper R, et al. Adenomyosis in postmenopausal breast cancer patients treated with tamoxifen: a new entity? Gynecol Oncol 1995; 58(1):86–91.
39. McGonigle K, Shaw S, Vasilev S, et al. Abnormalities detected on transvaginal ultrasonography in tamoxifen-treated postmenopausal breast cancer patients may represent endometrial cystic atrophy. Am J Obstet Gynecol 1998;178(6):1145–50.
40. Fisher B, Costantino J, Redmond C, et al. Endometrial cancer in tamoxifen-treated breast cancer patients: findings from the National Surgical Adjuvant Breast and Bowel Project (NSABP) B-14. J Natl Cancer Inst 1994;86(7):527–37.
41. Fisher B, Costantino J, Wickerham D, et al. Tamoxifen for the prevention of breast cancer: current status of the National Surgical Adjuvant Breast and Bowel Project P-1 Study. J Natl Cancer Inst 2005; 97(22):1652–62.
42. Cohen I, Perel E, Flex D, et al. Endometrial pathology in postmenopausal tamoxifen treatment: comparison between gynaecologically symptomatic and asymptomatic breast cancer patients. J Clin Pathol 1999; 52(4):278–82.
43. Hulka CA, Hall DA. Endometrial abnormalities associated with tamoxifen therapy for breast cancer: sonographic and pathologic correlation. AJR Am J Roentgenol 1993; 160(4):809–12.
44. American College of Obstetricians and Gynecologists Committee on Gynecologic Practice. ACOG committee opinion. No. 336: Tamoxifen and uterine cancer. Obstet Gynecol 2006; 107(6):1475–8.
45. Mbatsogo B, Le Bouedec G, Michy T, et al. Endometrial cancers arising in polyps associated with tamoxifen use. Gynecol Obstet Fertil 2005;33(12): 975–9.
46. Schlesinger C, Kamoi S, Ascher S, et al. Endometrial polyps: a comparison study of patients receiving tamoxifen with two control groups. Int J Gynecol Pathol 1998;17(4):302–11.
47. Chalas E, Costantino J, Wickerham D, et al. Benign gynecologic conditions among participants in the Breast Cancer Prevention Trial. Am J Obstet Gynecol 2005;192(4):1230–9.
48. Shi AA, Lee SI. Radiological reasoning: algorithmic workup of abnormal vaginal bleeding with endovaginal sonography and sonohysterography. AJR Am J Roentgenol 2008;191(6 Suppl):S68–73.

The Ultrasound Workup of Adnexal Masses

Marion Brody, MD[a,*], Beverly Coleman, MD[b]

KEYWORDS

• Ultrasound • Simple • Complex • Cystic
• Adnexa • Masses

Adnexal masses, both painful and asymptomatic, are commonly encountered entities in clinical practice. Most adnexal masses are benign; however, if the examining physician determines that a palpable mass is concerning, an ultrasound is often requested to further help guide management. Ultrasound is generally the initial imaging evaluation, because it is readily available, inexpensive, and has a high negative predictive value. Depending on the clinical scenario, serum tumor marker levels may also be obtained.

Although adnexal masses may be categorized in several ways, the authors believe pattern recognition to be superior and have thus classified adnexal masses in this article as cystic, complex, or solid (**Box 1**). Commonly encountered simple masses include physiologic cysts, paratubal/paraovarian cysts, and benign cystic neoplasms. Complex masses include hemorrhagic follicular and corpus luteum cysts, peritoneal inclusion cysts, pyosalpinges or hydrosalpinges, endometriomas, teratomas, and other benign and malignant ovarian neoplasms. Solid masses include entities such as pedunculated fibroids, torsed ovaries, benign and malignant primary ovarian neoplasms, and metastases.

Ultrasound is a critical tool in precisely identifying the cause of adnexal masses, assessing the likelihood of malignancy, and helping to guide clinical and surgical management. Based on the sonographic characteristics, clinical history, and menstrual status of the patient, the sonologist may further characterize the mass as benign, indeterminant, or malignant. Sonographically benign lesions such as simple or hemorrhagic functional cysts are often managed expectantly and do not require follow-up. On the other hand, indeterminant lesions, those that cannot be categorized as benign or malignant after thorough ultrasound evaluation, may require additional imaging, such as follow-up ultrasound or magnetic resonance imaging (MRI). This classification also includes low-risk malignancies, and therefore some of these masses can be surgically removed. Diagnosis of a probable malignant neoplasm prompts the ordering physician to refer the patient for gynecologic subspecialty care and usually more complex surgery, rather than laparoscopy.

ANATOMY AND PHYSIOLOGY

The adnexa are composed of structures lateral to the uterus: the paired ovaries, fallopian tubes, broad and round ligaments, and uterine and ovarian vessels. To correctly identify adnexal pathology, the sonologist must first be able to recognize what constitutes normal adnexal morphology.

Ovaries

The ovaries are the only truly intraperitoneal structures of the adnexa and appear ovoid or almond in shape. They are supplied by both the ovarian arteries and adnexal branches of the uterine

[a] Abdominal Imaging, Department of Radiology, Hospital of the University of Pennsylvania, 3400 Spruce Street, Philadelphia, PA 19104, USA
[b] Department of Radiology, Hospital of the University of Pennsylvania, 3400 Spruce Street, Philadelphia, PA 19104, USA
* Corresponding author.
E-mail address: goodbro93@yahoo.com

Ultrasound Clin 5 (2010) 257–275
doi:10.1016/j.cult.2010.03.006

Box 1
Common sonographic appearance of adnexal masses

Cystic
- Functional cysts
- Corpus luteum (15%)
- Cystadenomas
- Paraovarian/paratubal cysts

Complex
- Hemorrhagic functional cysts
- Hemorrhagic corpus luteum
- Endometriomas
- Peritoneal inclusion cysts
- Hydrosalpinges or pyosalpinges
- Mature cystic teratomas
- Epithelial neoplasms

Solid
- Sex cord–stromal tumors (fibromas, thecomas)
- Malignant germ cell tumors
- Metastatic disease (breast, colon, stomach, appendiceal primaries)
- Brenner tumor

artery. They are covered by mesosalpinx, a fold of peritoneum that also surrounds the fallopian tubes.

Despite their numerous suspensory ligaments, the ovaries may vary considerably in position. In nulliparous women, the ovaries lie in the ovarian fossae, shallow depressions lateral to the uterus. The fossae are bordered by the external iliac vessels laterally and anteriorly and by the ureter and internal iliac vessels posteriorly. If the uterus is tilted to the right or the left, a normal anatomic variant, the ispilateral ovary may be displaced laterally. If the uterus is retroverted, the ovaries may lie on top of the uterine fundus. After pregnancy, the ovaries may remain in the superolateral position in which they were oriented to accommodate a gravid uterus. After hysterectomy, the ovaries may be found more lateral and caudad.

Ovarian size is usually discussed in terms of volume, which may be calculated by multiplying 0.5 to the product of 3 orthogonal measurements. The ovaries gradually enlarge as a girl approaches menarche. The accepted normal ovarian size in premenopausal women differs in the literature. However, reasonable maximum volumes may be considered to be 10 mL (9.8 $\pm$ 5.8) for premenopausal women and 6 mL (5.8 $\pm$ 3.6) for postmenopausal women.[1] In premenopausal women, a physiologic size discrepancy between the right and left ovary is common and typically of no clinical significance. Postmenopausal ovaries rarely show a significant size discrepancy, and therefore, ovaries that measure more than twice the volume of their contralateral counterpart are considered abnormal.

Histologically, the ovary is made up of an outer cortex, which contains follicles, and an inner medulla, which contains sex cord cells. The ovary also contains lymphatics, blood vessels, and nerves. As cortical and medullary ovarian cells are hormone sensitive, the appearance of the ovary fluctuates with each stage of the menstrual cycle. In the follicular phase (the first 14 days of a 28-day cycle), 5 to 12 thin-walled follicles of varying sizes are seen in the cortex. At ovulation, during midcycle, a dominant follicle averaging 22 mm in size releases its ovum. In the secretory phase (days 14–28), the ruptured follicle begins secreting progesterone, develops a thicker wall, and transforms into a corpus luteum. If conception does not occur, the corpus luteum gradually involutes and becomes sonographically imperceptible.

Fallopian Tubes

The fallopian tubes are paired, cylindrical, muscular structures that extend from the uterine cornu to the medial aspects of the ovaries. In contrast to the ovaries, the appearance of the fallopian tubes is generally static. They measure 8 to 12 cm in length and are supplied by tubal branches of the ovarian and uterine arteries. Anatomically, the tubes are divided into 4 segments, from proximal to distal: intramural segment, isthmus, ampulla, and infundibulum. The lateral aspects of the infundibuli contain fimbriae that open into the pelvic cavity. The tubal mucosa, or endosalpinx, is arranged in a distinctive plicae pattern, which becomes thicker toward the fimbriae. Although the mucosa is hormonally sensitive, these morphologic changes are not recognizable sonographically.

CLINICAL AND MORPHOLOGIC ANALYSIS OF ADNEXAL MASSES

A reasonable first step in evaluating an adnexal mass is to view it in the context of a patient's symptoms, age, menstrual status, and serum tumor marker levels.

Circumstances that tend to cause acute adnexal pain are acute hemorrhage into a functional or corpus luteum cyst, acute hemorrhage into an endometrioma, inflammation from pelvic infection, and ovarian torsion. Most of the remaining benign lesions either cause no symptoms and are detected by clinical examination or cause dull, chronic discomfort. Hormone-producing masses may cause virilization or vaginal bleeding. Symptoms suggestive of malignancy in any age group include refractory abdominal or pelvic pain, urinary urgency or frequency, increase in abdominal girth, and anorexia.[2]

A study by Cohen[3] outlines a demographic framework in which to contemplate adnexal masses in premenopausal women. In women in the 20s and 30s, a simple or complex adnexal mass is most likely a functional cyst, hemorrhagic corpus luteum, pelvic inflammatory process, endometrioma, mature cystic teratoma, or cystadenoma. Rarely, a mass in these patients will be a borderline malignancy or true malignancy; in which case, it is most likely a malignant germ cell or granulosa cell tumor rather than an epithelial neoplasm. In premenopausal women in their 40s, the differential diagnosis is similar; however, cystadenomas occur more commonly. In this cohort, malignant neoplasms are rare but are epithelial in origin 90% of the time.[3]

Likewise, the tendency of a woman to develop pelvic inflammatory disease or ovarian torsion decreases with age. Although postmenopausal women infrequently ovulate in the early menopause phase, years 1 to 5 after cessation of menses, they do not tend to hemorrhage into ovarian cysts nor develop corpus lutea.[4] Also, the prevalence of ovarian cancer increases with age. These statistical considerations may help narrow a differential diagnosis when faced with vexing sonographic findings.

A comprehensive review of tumor markers is beyond the scope of this discussion. However, CA 125, the most widely used tumor marker in gynecologic oncology, is worthy of mention. When combined with clinical and sonographic data, elevated CA 125 levels may help determine if a mass is more likely benign or malignant. For example, more than 80% of patients with ovarian cancer have elevated CA 125 levels, and increasing CA 125 levels correlate with disease recurrence.[5] However, only half of patients with stage I ovarian cancer have elevated CA 125 levels. Moreover, elevated levels may also be found in nonneoplastic conditions such as cirrhosis, early pregnancy, and pancreatitis.[5] Therefore, judicious interpretation of tumor marker levels is advised.

Sonographically, adnexal masses exhibit a morphologic spectrum ranging from purely cystic to completely solid. Most adnexal masses are simple unilocular cysts. In general, the differential diagnosis for these cysts is relatively limited and consists of mostly benign entities. The differential diagnosis for more complex masses is much longer. In this group, the distinction between nonneoplastic and neoplastic and between benign and malignant lesions is more challenging. In this setting, the sonographer must look for distinct or discriminating features that may implicate or eliminate specific masses.

SIMPLE CYSTIC MASSES

A simple cyst is defined as a round, unilocular structure containing anechoic fluid, demonstrating posterior acoustic enhancement, and having a smooth wall measuring less than or equal to 3 mm in maximum diameter. The differential diagnosis for an intraovarian mass with this appearance includes a follicle, a functional cyst, a corpus luteum, and a cystadenoma. As discussed earlier, the favored diagnosis varies in part depending on the age and menstrual status of the patient. If a simple cystic mass is extraovarian, it most likely represents a paraovarian or paratubal cyst; however, the differential diagnosis also includes hydrosalpinx, which is not as common.

Functional Cysts

In premenopausal women, most simple ovarian cysts measuring less than 2.5 cm in diameter are physiologic follicles.[6] If larger, they are considered functional cysts, which result from the failure of a follicle to rupture or regress (**Fig. 1**). In premenopausal women, it has been reported that 50% to

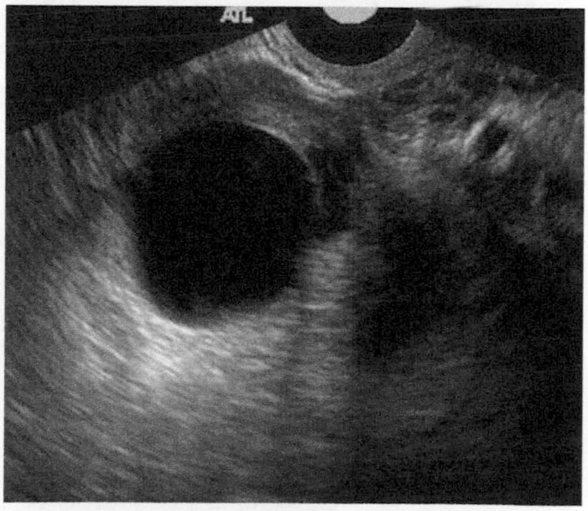

Fig. 1. Simple functional cyst. Image of the right ovary from a transvaginal ultrasound performed on a 29-year-old asymptomatic female demonstrates a simple, thin-walled, unilocular cyst with enhanced through transmission. Given the size of the cyst and the menstrual status of the patient, no additional or follow-up imaging was recommended.

60% of ovarian masses greater than 2.5 cm in diameter were functional cysts.[3] These cysts usually range in size from 2 to 8 cm but can become as large as 20 cm in maximum diameter. They can cause pelvic pain of variable intensity and usually resolve within 2 menstrual cycles.[7]

Functional cysts may develop internal hemorrhage or clot and demonstrate classic signs of debris (**Fig. 2**). On sonography, these hemorrhagic cysts are often characterized by a reticular appearance, consisting of innumerable fine, lacy echoes, which are distinct from septations by their discontinuity, delicacy, and avascularity.[7,8] The presence of these fibrin strands in a unilocular cyst has been referred to as a "fishnet, cobweb, or lacy" appearance, which makes the mass overwhelmingly more likely to be a hemorrhagic functional cyst than any other entity.[4] As the clot matures, the cyst may show clumped, avascular, hypoechoic echoes with concave margins along its wall. Conversely, mural nodules have convex margins and tend to be isoechoic to the cyst wall.[4] The characteristic appearance of retracting clot also makes the mass much more likely to be a hemorrhagic cyst (**Fig. 3**).[4,8] Hemorrhagic cysts are often indistinguishable from endometriomas but may be differentiated from the latter by their singularity and tendency to resolve over time.[7] They can have an almost solid appearance with very few cystic components.

Simple ovarian cysts are also common in postmenopausal women. In a study by Erkerhovd and colleagues,[9] ovarian cysts occurred in 3.5% to 17% of postmenopausal women. Although the

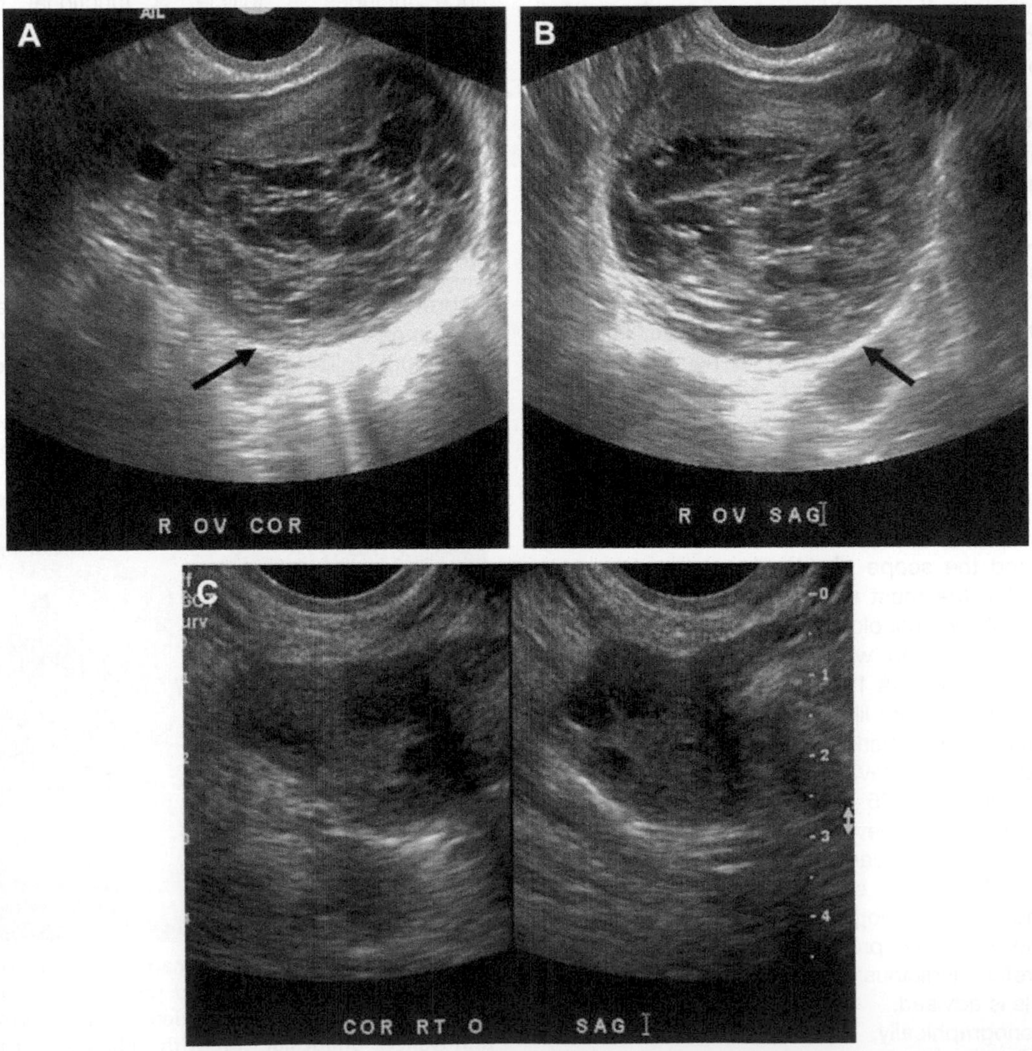

Fig. 2. Hemorrhagic functional cyst. (*A, B*) Coronal and sagittal images of the right ovary from a transvaginal ultrasound show a complex mass with reticular, lacy, discontinuous fibrin strands (*arrows*). (*C*) Transabdominal images from the same patient obtained 14 weeks later show resolution of the hemorrhagic cyst.

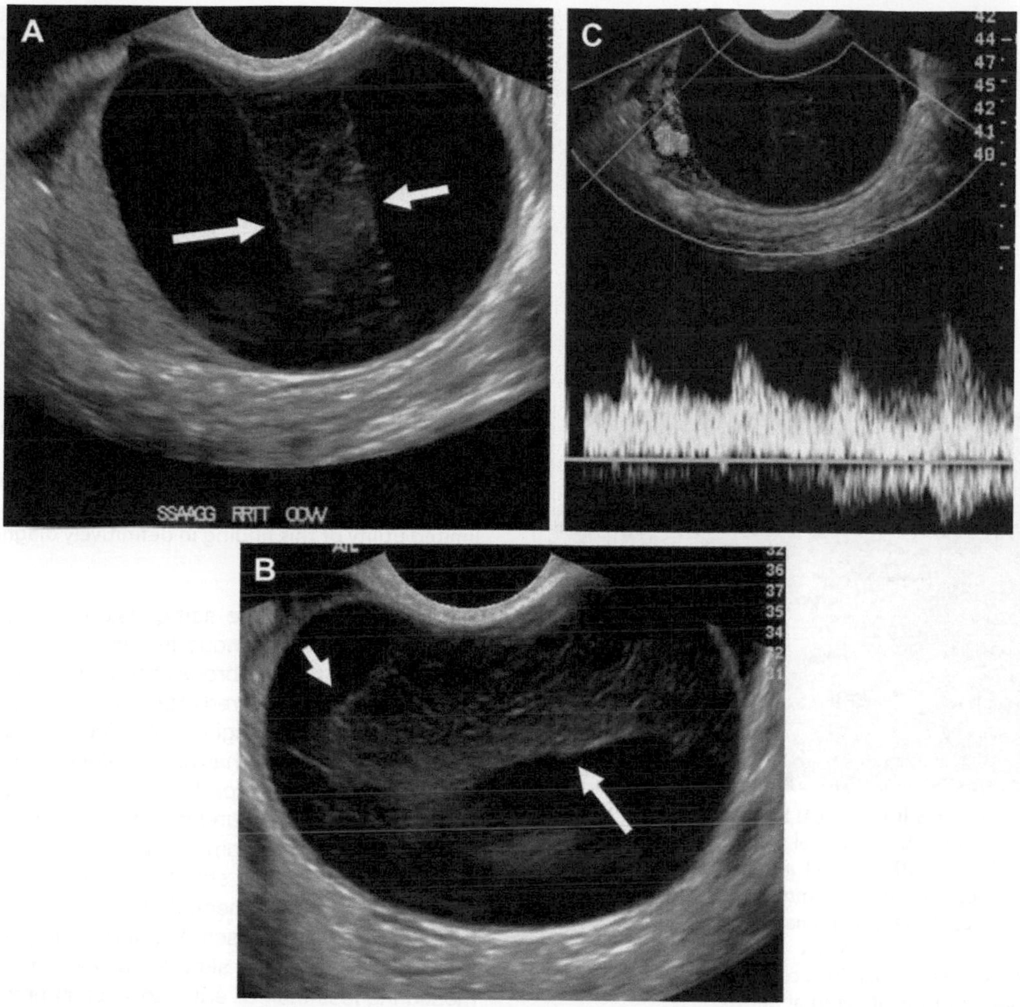

Fig. 3. Retracting clot in a hemorrhagic functional cyst. (*A, B*) Hypoechoic focus with concave margins (*arrows*), in the center of an evolving hemorrhagic functional cyst, representing retracting clot. (*C*) Note that the clot demonstrates no vascularity on color and pulsed Doppler imaging. The Doppler waveform is that of normal ovarian tissue around the cyst.

incidence of malignancy in these lesions was still low, it was double the incidence of malignancy in simple cysts seen in premenopausal women; 1.6% of the cysts were found to be malignant in postmenopausal women and 0.7% in premenopausal women.[9] All of the cases of malignancy were in cysts greater than 5 cm in diameter. Small cysts are almost certainly benign, and long-term follow-up ultrasound is helpful to assess for internal change. MRI or surgical evaluation should be considered for large or enlarging cysts because the risk of malignancy increases with size; therefore, larger masses are more concerning.

Corpus Luteum

A dominant follicle transitions to a corpus luteum cyst in premenopausal women after ovulation. About 15% of these cysts appear as thin-walled simple cysts.[9] Other appearances on sonography include thick-walled cysts with an anechoic center (27%) and cysts containing internal debris (23%).[10] They may even appear entirely solid.[6] Marked color flow in the thickened wall of the cyst with a ring of vascularity has been reported in 92% of cases,[10] which helps distinguish them as physiologic. As with hemorrhagic functional cysts, debris-containing corpus luteal cysts may be mistaken for endometriomas and can be differentiated from the latter by their resolution on follow-up scans. In the authors' practice, if a complex mass has classic features of a corpus luteum, additional imaging is not recommended (**Fig. 4**).

Cystadenoma

A unilocular simple cyst may also represent a surface epithelial neoplasm, specifically, a serous

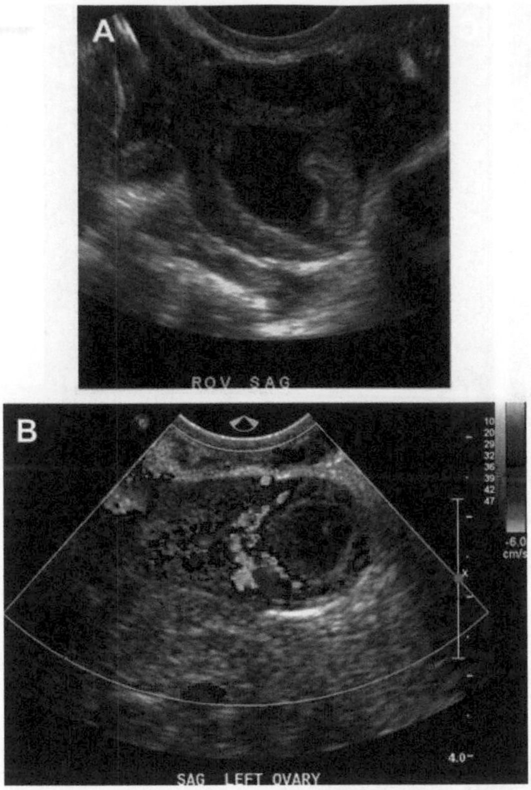

Fig. 4. Corpus luteum. (*A*) Sagittal image of the right ovary from a transvaginal ultrasound shows a thick-walled cyst with a small amount of internal debris, likely representing hemorrhage. (*B*) Transvaginal sagittal color Doppler image of the left ovary in a different patient shows a thick-walled cyst with a ring of vascularity. This corpus luteum also contains a small amount of internal debris.

or mucinous cystadenoma. Surface epithelial neoplasms, which are discussed in more depth in the subsequent section, are the most common ovarian tumors. Serous subtypes are more common than mucinous subtypes, representing 25% of all ovarian neoplasms (**Fig. 5**).[7] These tumors occur in all age groups and are bilateral in 20% of cases.[11] They are thin-walled, unilocular or bilocular, and generally do not contain solid components.[6] Sonographically, they are often indistinguishable from functional cysts except by size and their tendency to enlarge on follow-up imaging. Cystadenomas average approximately 10 cm in size but may reach up to 50 cm especially if they remain simple and unilocular.[7] These cystic neoplasms are almost always benign, even amongst postmenopausal women.[12] Mucinous subtypes may be very large and tend to be multilocular. They may also contain internal echoes because of the mucinous content or hemorrhage, in which case they may show locules of differing echogenicity within the same lesion.[5,7] Amongst both serous and mucinous tumors, the presence of solid, nonfatty, nonfibrous tissue on sonography is the most powerful predictor of malignancy.[5]

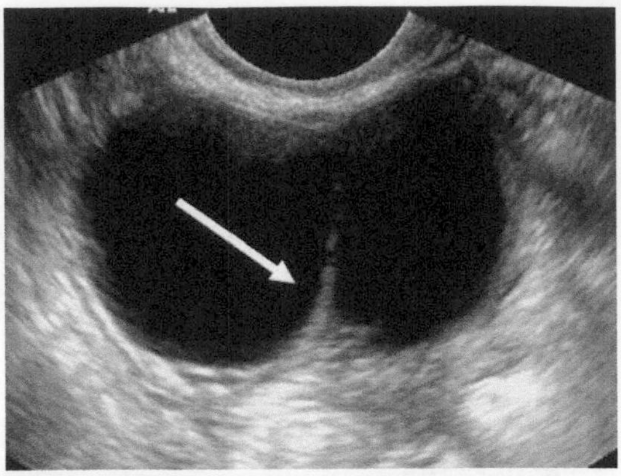

Fig. 5. Incomplete septation in a serous cystadenoma. Transvaginal image of a cystic structure in the right ovary, containing what appears to be an incomplete septation (*arrow*). This again demonstrates the limited utility of this finding in definitively diagnosing a hydrosalpinx.

The appropriate imaging follow-up protocol for cystic adnexal masses has not yet been determined and varies among departments. The Society of Radiologists in Ultrasound met in October 2009 to develop standard recommendations and will be publishing guidelines shortly for asymptomatic adnexal cyst management. At the authors' institution, the following masses do not generally require follow-up imaging: simple unilocular cysts measuring less than or equal to 4 cm in premenopausal women, complex unilocular cysts measuring less than or equal to 3 cm in premenopausal women, and simple unilocular cysts measuring less than or equal to 1 cm in postmenopausal women. In premenopausal women, larger simple or complex cystic masses usually prompt follow-up sonographic imaging in 2 menstrual cycles. In postmenopausal women, larger simple or complex cystic masses, or those associated with elevated CA 125 levels, usually prompt pelvic MRI or more short-term, serial ultrasound follow-up.

Paraovarian/Paratubal Cysts

If a simple, unilocular adnexal cyst is found to be extraovarian, it is most likely a paraovarian or paratubal cyst (**Fig. 6**). These cysts are remnants of the wolffian (mesonephric) and müllerian (paramesonephric) ducts and compose up to 20% of adnexal masses.[7] The distinction between paraovarian and paratubal cysts, which cannot be made sonographically, is clinically irrelevant.[5] These cysts can develop anywhere in the adnexa: in the broad

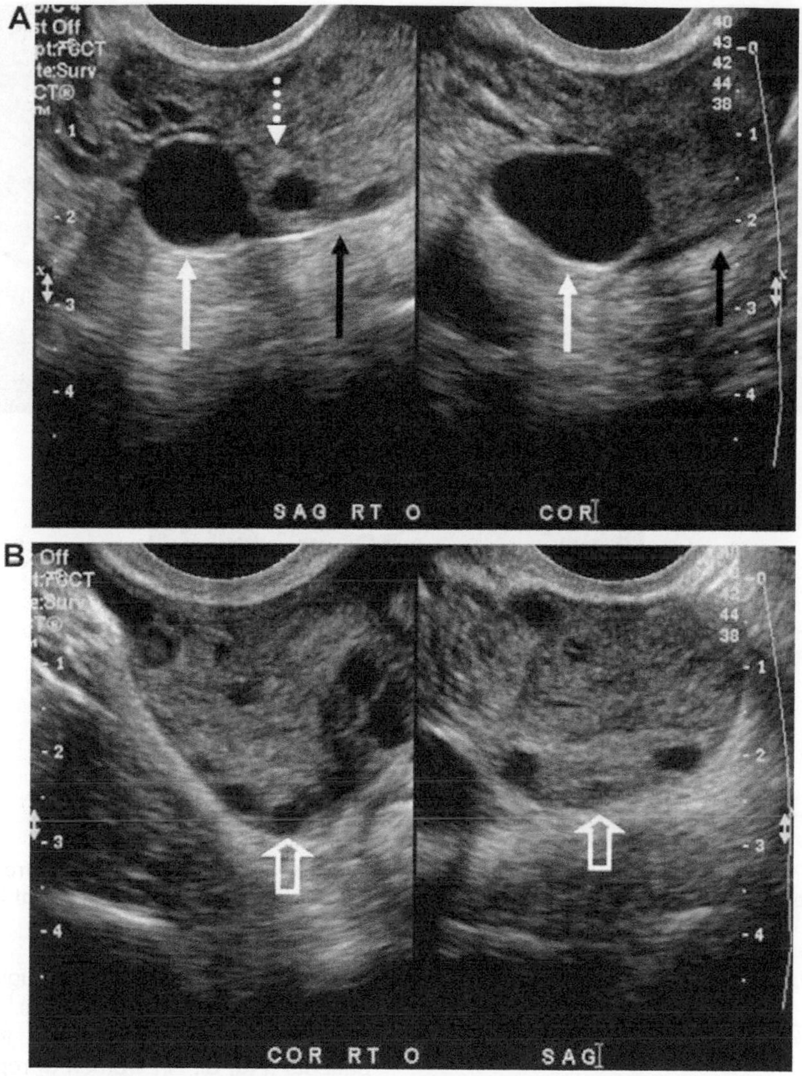

Fig. 6. Paraovarian/paratubal cyst. (*A*) Images from a transvaginal ultrasound show a unilocular, thin-walled cyst (*white arrows*) located adjacent to the right ovary (*black arrows*), which is identified by a developing follicle (*dotted white arrow*). (*B*) Additional images from the same patient demonstrate a normal-appearing ovary (*open white arrows*), separate from the cyst.

ligament, mesosalpinx, or on the ovarian surface.[7,8] The most common type of cysts are called hydatids of Morgagni, which arise from the fimbriated end of the fallopian tube.[8] These cysts are usually small but can be as large as 8 cm.[6] They are usually unilateral, unilocular, and have thin deformable walls.[7,8] Cysts that have this appearance are virtually always benign (**Fig. 7**).[13] However, up to 34% of hydatid cysts may demonstrate more complexity, such as internal hemorrhage, multilocularity, or papillary projections. The papillary projections are defined as solid projections from a cyst wall measuring greater than or equal to 3 mm.[11,13] In this circumstance, these complex cysts may actually represent cystadenofibromas, cystadenomas, or rarely, borderline or frank malignant masses.[13] In a study by Savelli and colleagues,[13] 3% of complex paratubal/paraovarian cysts were serous papillary borderline tumors, whereas all of the unilocular, simple paratubal/paraovarian cysts were found to be benign on histology.[7] Isolated case reports have described endometrioid and transitional cell carcinomas arising from paraovarian/paratubal cysts.[14,15] Typically, these cysts are asymptomatic yet infrequently may cause pain and torsion. In one study of premenarchal and young menarchal women operated for acute appendicitis, 6% of patients were found to have torsed paraovarian cysts at surgery.[16]

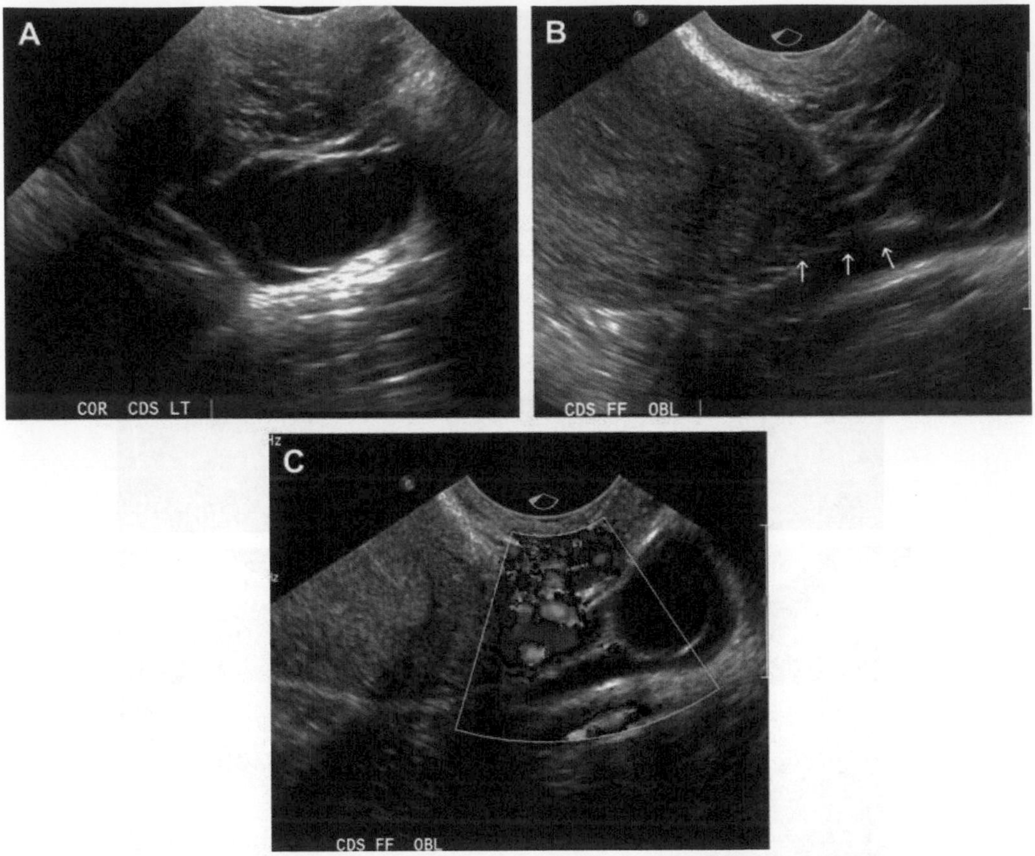

Fig. 7. Hydatid of Morgagni. Gray-scale (*A, B*) and color Doppler (*C*) images of the cul-de-sac from a transvaginal ultrasound reveal a simple, thin-walled, unilocular, avascular cyst arising from the distal end of the left fallopian tube (*arrows*).

COMPLEX MASSES

Those cystic masses that demonstrate turbid fluid, septations or calcifications, or solid components are considered complex. Hemorrhagic ovarian follicular cysts and corpus luteal cysts may be included in this classification and were discussed in the previous section. The more common adnexal masses that appear complex include endometriomas, peritoneal inclusion cysts, hydrosalpinges, and benign and malignant ovarian neoplasms. Pyosalpinges typically appear as complex adnexal masses, with increased flow in patients with systemic signs and symptoms, often presenting with pelvic pain.

Endometriosis

There are 2 types of endometriosis, diffuse and focal. Although imaging is not helpful in identifying small endometrial deposits, sonography is very useful in identifying endometriotic cysts, also known as endometriomas.[6,17] Endometriomas are islands of functional extrauterine endometrial epithelium and stroma.[7,18] They may occur anywhere in the pelvis, although the ovary is involved in 55% to 80% of cases.[5,11] Endometriomas are bilateral in one-half to one-third of patients (**Fig. 8**).[8] In women of reproductive age, endometriomas cyclically bleed and proliferate, producing discomfort, scarring, distortion of pelvic anatomy, and tubal occlusion. These lesions on sonography may appear anechoic to solid, depending on the amount and age of hemorrhage. In general, they demonstrate enhanced through transmission and contain nonvascular, diffuse low-level echoes, which have been described as "ground glass" in appearance.[6,11] They may be distinguished from hemorrhagic ovarian cysts by the homogeneity and relative immobility of the internal echoes,[6] by the tendency to be bilateral, and by persistence after 3 months of observation.[17,18] It has been estimated that 29% of endometriomas contain septations, 45% are multilocular, and 5% contain fluid-fluid levels.[6,11] The walls of endometriomas demonstrate variable thickness and 20% to 40% contain small, avascular, hyperechoic mural foci, which are thought to represent focal deposits of cholesterol left by

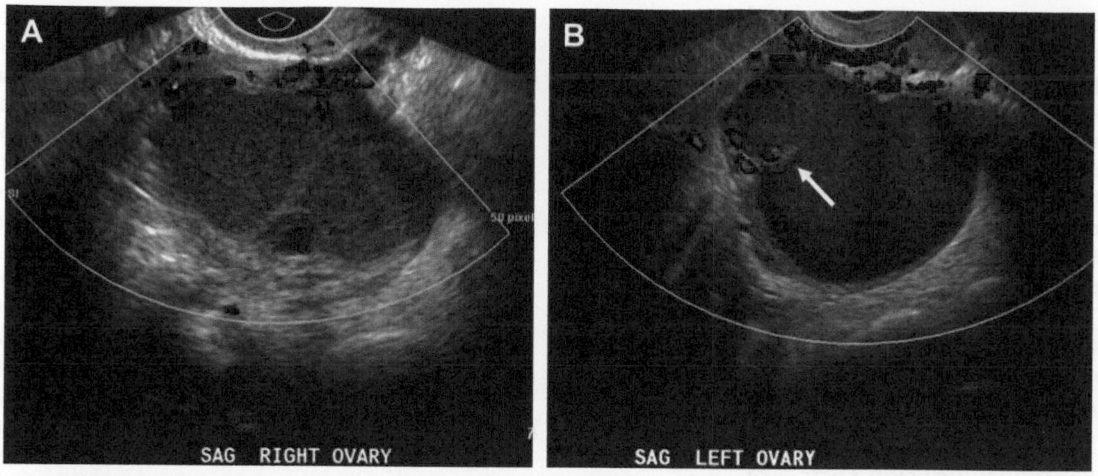

Fig. 8. Bilateral endometriomas. Transvaginal images of the ovaries demonstrate bilateral endometriomas, which may appear multilocular (*left*) or contain incomplete septations (*arrows, right*).

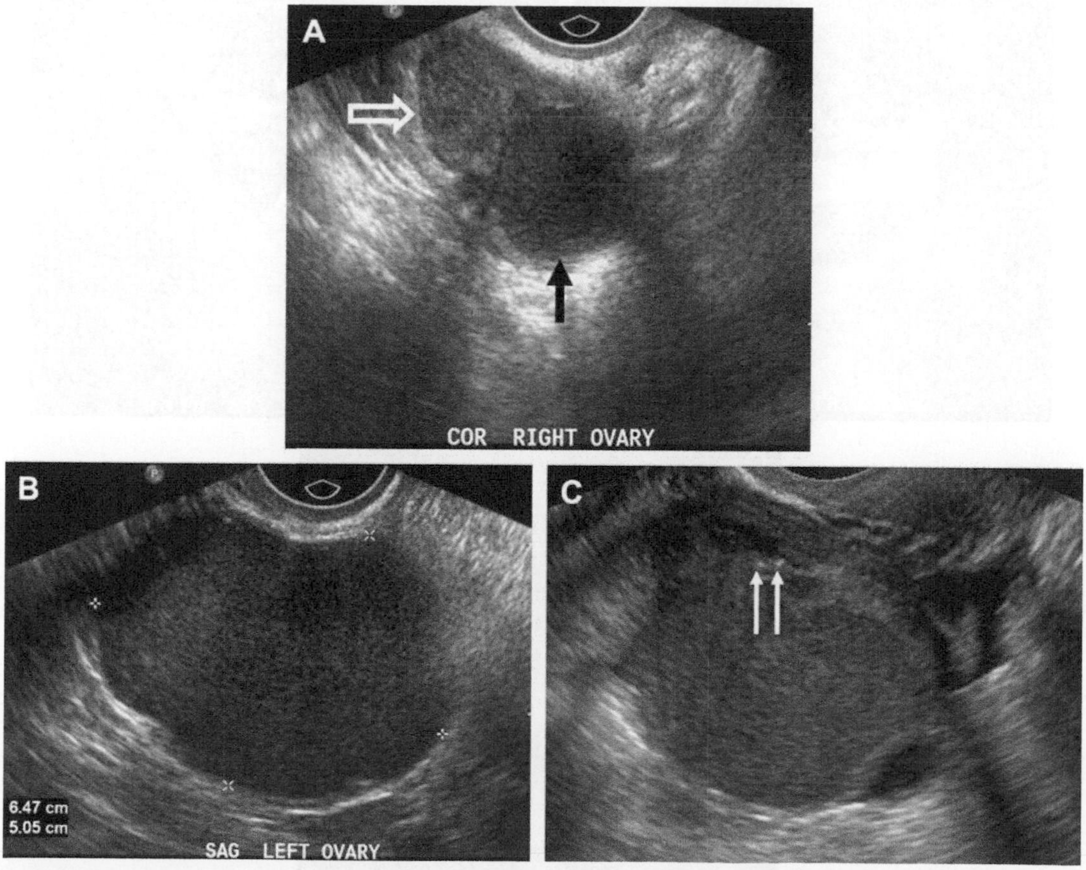

Fig. 9. Bilateral endometriomas. (*A*) Image from a transabdominal ultrasound shows a hypoechoic homogeneous mass (*solid black arrow*) with low-level echoes and enhanced through transmission, adjacent to normal ovarian tissue (*open white arrow*). (*B*) Image from a transvaginal ultrasound in the same patient demonstrates a mass with similar sonographic characteristics in the left ovary. (*C*) Transvaginal image from a different patient shows hyperechoic foci (*solid white arrows*) within the walls of an endometrioma.

degrading cell membranes.[6,8,17] A smooth-walled cyst with characteristic low-level echoes and hyperechoic mural foci is almost pathognomonic of an endometrioma (**Fig. 9**).[4] Rarely, extraovarian endometriomas may appear solid, and in such cases, they may be distinguished from neoplasms by a lack of flow on color Doppler.[6] Although endometriomas are almost always benign, malignant transformation may be suggested by polypoid projections or wall nodularity within the mass. This transformation occurs in 0.3% to 0.8% of endometriomas and most often represents metamorphosis into clear cell or endometrioid carcinomas over a long period of time.[8]

Peritoneal Inclusion Cysts

Peritoneal inclusion cysts are usually found in ovulatory patients who have had prior pelvic surgery, endometriosis, or pelvic inflammatory disease. They are formed when, as a result of prior abdominal or pelvic inflammation, physiologic ovarian fluid accumulates within nonneoplastic pelvic adhesions and entraps the ovary.[7,8,19] These masses appear as slow-growing, nongeometric shaped, thin-walled, multilocular cysts with fine internal septations that surround the ovary.[19] The ovary may be located centrally or eccentrically within the lesion (**Fig. 10**).[19,20] The septations connect to the serosal surfaces of the surrounding organs, and may distort the ovarian contour, but do not involve the ovarian parenchyma.[18,19] The walls of the mass conform to the peritoneal cavity, which is thought to be the cause of the odd shapes of these cysts.[20] The fluid is usually anechoic but may have internal echoes because of proteinaceous or hemorrhagic fluid.[6,8] The appearance of these masses has been referred to as "a spider in a web." Peritoneal inclusion cysts range in size from several millimeters to more than 20 cm.[19] These masses are protean in appearance

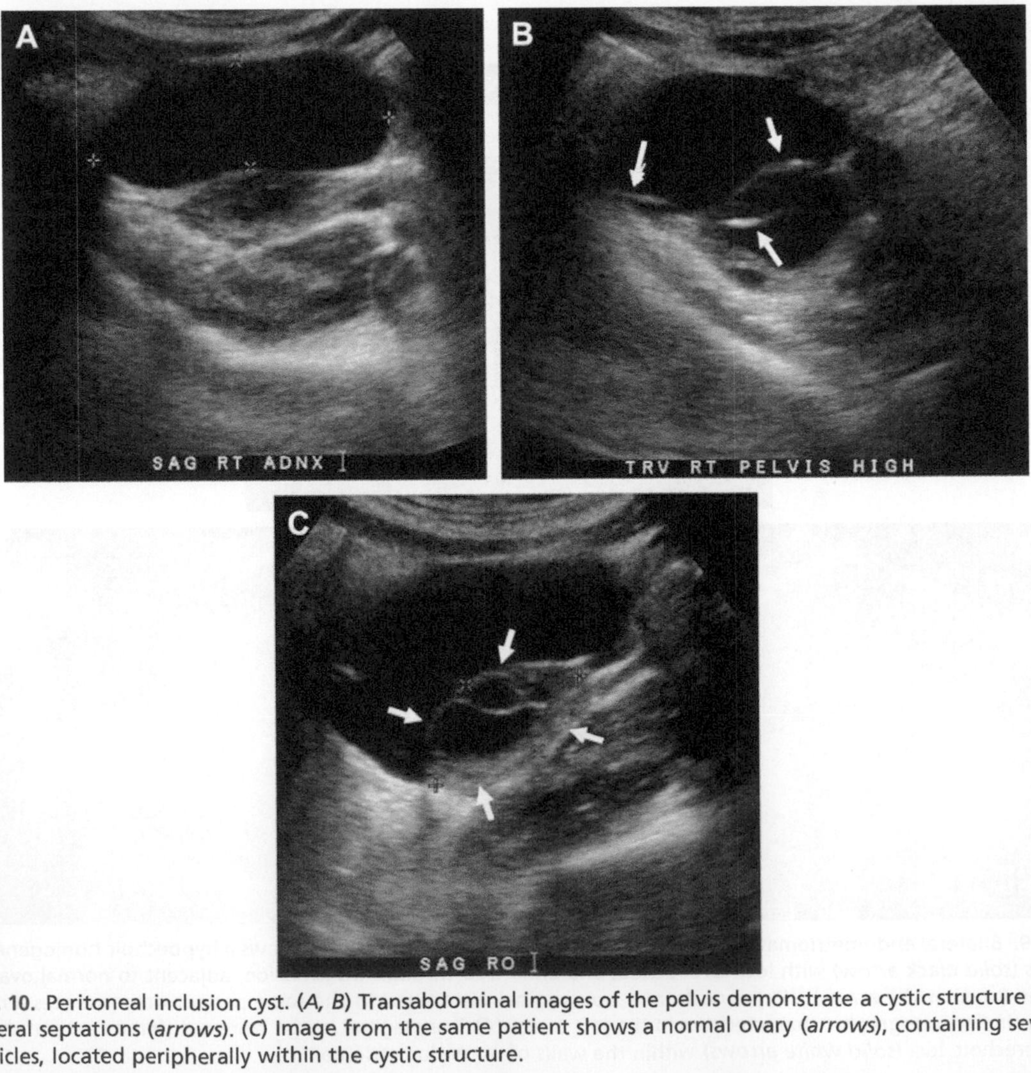

Fig. 10. Peritoneal inclusion cyst. (*A, B*) Transabdominal images of the pelvis demonstrate a cystic structure with several septations (*arrows*). (*C*) Image from the same patient shows a normal ovary (*arrows*), containing several follicles, located peripherally within the cystic structure.

and may resemble other adnexal pathology. They may contain mural nodules and incomplete septations, simulating hydrosalpinx; may appear as multiple cystic masses in the broad ligament, simulating paraovarian/paratubal cysts; and may form irregular thick septations with low-resistance flow, simulating neoplasm. In one study, the specificity of ultrasound for diagnosing peritoneal inclusion cysts was found to be as low as 67%.[19] Appropriate clinical history, stable imaging appearance on 6- to 12-month follow-up ultrasound, or MRI may help differentiate peritoneal cysts from other cystic masses.[20] Clinical management of these cysts is challenging, because their recurrence rate after surgical removal is as high as 50%.[20,21] Ultrasound-guided aspiration is an alternative form of therapy.

Hydrosalpinx

Hydrosalpinx forms when the fimbriated end of a fallopian tube is obliterated, causing the tube to distend with fluid. It occurs in up to 10% of patients with prior pelvic inflammatory disease or endometriosis.[7] Hydrosalpinx is most commonly seen as an extraovarian, tubular, fluid-filled structure. The most reliable additional ultrasound finding is a "waist sign," formed by directly opposing indentations of the tube wall.[4] Other specific features of hydrosalpinx on sonography are small round mural projections, described as "beads on a string," representing abnormal endosalpingeal folds (**Fig. 11**). In a study by Patel,[4] a combination of the previously mentioned findings in diagnosing hydrosalpinx imparted a likelihood ratio of 22:1. In the same study, helpful but less reliable features of hydrosalpinx were incomplete septations and short linear projections (mural-based linear echoes extending across less than one-third the width of the dilated tube).[4] Observing an extraovarian location may distinguish a hydrosalpinx from a cystic ovarian neoplasm. Rarely, a dilated pelvic vein may be mistaken for a hydrosalpinx, in which case the

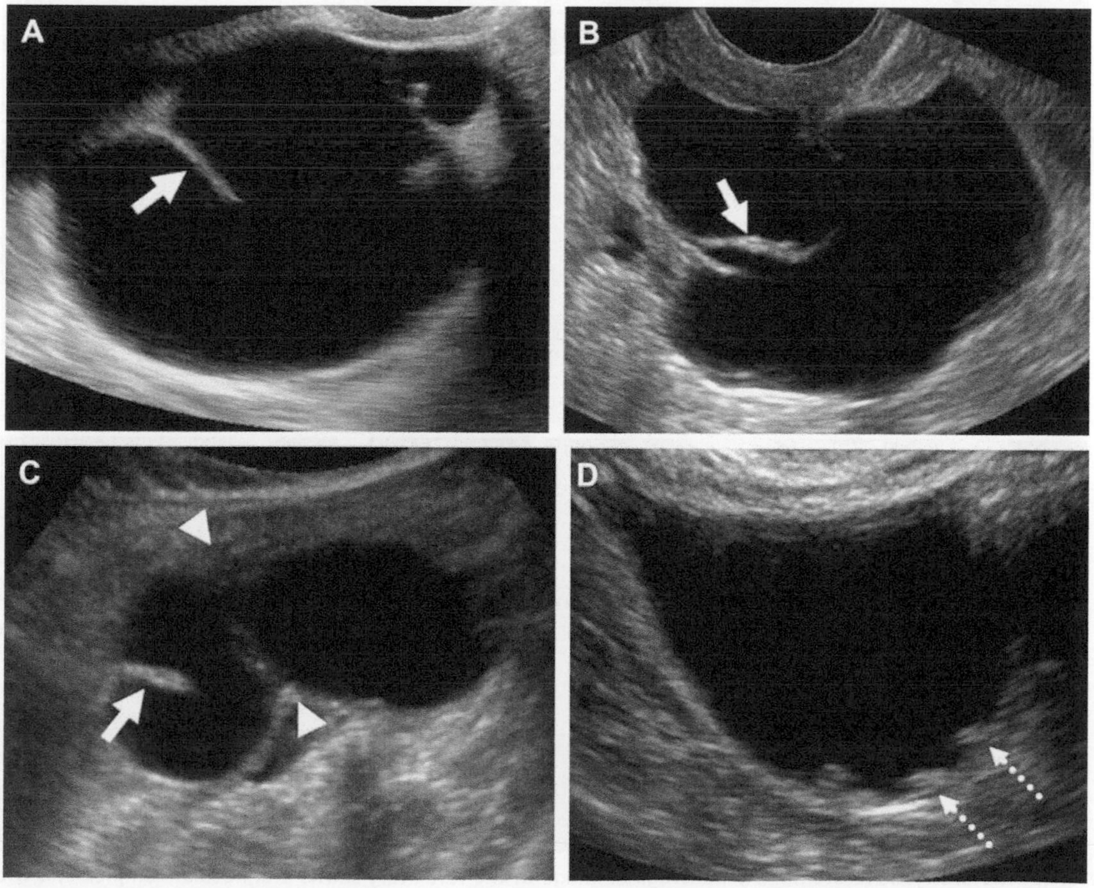

Fig. 11. Hydrosalpinx. (*A, B*) Transvaginal images of the right adnexa show an extraovarian tubular structure containing incomplete septa (*white arrows*). (*C*) Transabdominal image in a different patient shows a tubular structure containing an incomplete septation (*solid white arrow*) and a "waist sign" (*arrowheads*). (*D*) Transvaginal image from a different patient demonstrates a hydrosalpinx with small, round mural-based projections (*dotted white arrows*).

former can be easily recognized by using color Doppler, as well as by increasing gray-scale gain and looking for movement of internal echoes.[7] Statistically, paraovarian cystadenomas may usually be excluded from the differential diagnosis by their extreme rarity.

Complex Masses—Ovarian Neoplasms

Ovarian neoplasms may be categorized by cell origin: surface epithelial, germ cell, sex cord–stromal, and metastatic tumors. The most common ovarian malignancies are epithelial, which include serous, mucinous, transitional (Brenner tumor), endometrioid, and clear cell types. As previously discussed, serous and mucinous types have benign counterparts in cystadenomas, whereas endometrioid and clear cell tumors, which are also the most common subtypes arising from endometriomas, are always malignant. Germ cell tumors include teratomas, which are almost always benign, and dysgerminomas, yolk sac tumors, and embryonal carcinomas, which are virtually always malignant. Sex cord–stromal cell derivatives, which may be benign or malignant, include fibroma, thecoma, granulosa cell tumor, and Sertoli-Leydig cell tumor.

Ovarian neoplasms that almost always appear as complex masses on sonography include teratomas, epithelial neoplasms, and granulosa cell tumors. Tumors that are usually solid but may have small cystic components include certain sex cord–stromal tumors, immature germ cell tumors, and metastatic lesions, which are discussed in the subsequent section.

Mature cystic teratoma

Mature cystic teratomas are the most commonly excised ovarian tumors.[22] They occur in women

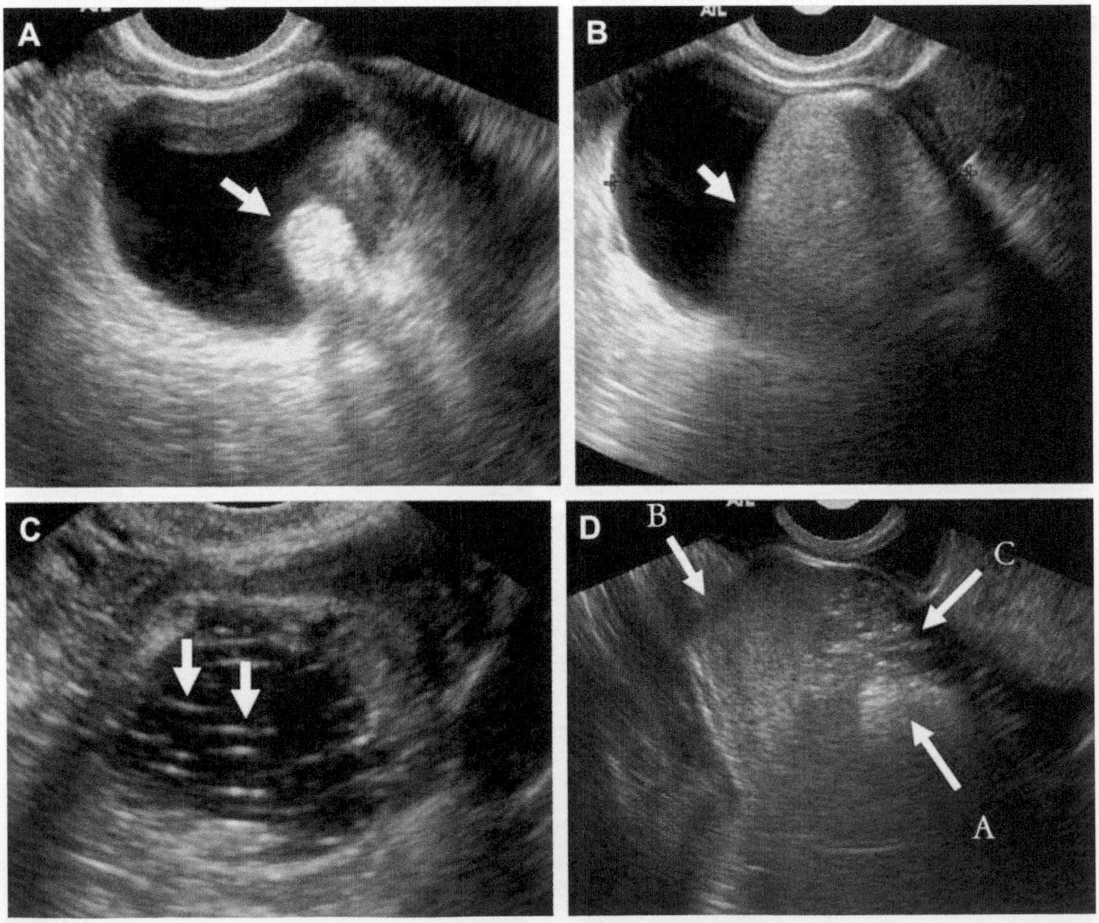

Fig. 12. Mature cystic teratoma. (*A*) Transvaginal image of the left ovary shows a unilocular complex cyst with a focal area of intraluminal bright echoes with posterior shadowing (*arrow*). (*B*) Image from the same patient shows a diffuse region of hyperechogenicity (*arrow*). (*C*) Image from the same patient shows echoes with a dot-dash configuration (*arrows*). (*D*) Transvaginal image from a different patient shows all 3 sonographic findings (*arrows*) in an ovarian mass (A, B, C).

younger than those who develop epithelial neoplasms, with a mean age of 30 years, and represent the most common ovarian mass in children. They are benign, slow-growing, congenital, cystic ovarian neoplasms derived from pluripotent cells and rarely are symptomatic.[22] Teratomas contain mature tissue often from all 3 but at least 2 germ cell layers (ectoderm, mesoderm, and endoderm), and therefore contain a variety of tissue types, including skin, brain, muscle, glandular tissue, respiratory or digestive epithelium, bone, teeth, hair, and/or fat.

Almost 90% of mature cystic teratomas are unilocular, 10% are bilateral, and almost all are hypovascular on color Doppler.[6,22] Sonographic findings that are most helpful in diagnosing mature teratomas are focal, intraluminal bright echoes that cause posterior shadowing, regional or diffuse high-amplitude echoes, and hyperechoic lines and dots.[4,22,23] Most teratomas are readily recognizable on sonography; however, a small percentage may be purely cystic, mimicking other masses. Bright, focal, shadowing echoes are seen in almost 90% of cases and are usually caused by bones, teeth, focal fat, or clumps of hair on a tubercle (also called Rokitansky nodules).[4] Some teratomas may be missed because of echogenicity similar to adjacent bowel, a finding called the "tip of the iceberg" sign. Bright, more regional, or diffuse echoes may be caused by sebum. Echoes forming lines and dots, also known as "dermoid mesh," are caused by strands of hair within nonfatty fluid. Rarely, a solitary finding may result in a false-positive diagnosis of teratoma. For example, mural foci of endometriomas, ingested material and air within bowel, and hemorrhage within a mass may produce marked focal or diffuse echogenicity. Similarly, hemorrhage within a cyst or mass may cause fibrinous linear echoes. In these instances, MRI may be helpful for superior tissue characterization. However, when several of these properties are seen together, they are virtually pathognomonic for teratoma (**Fig. 12**).[4]

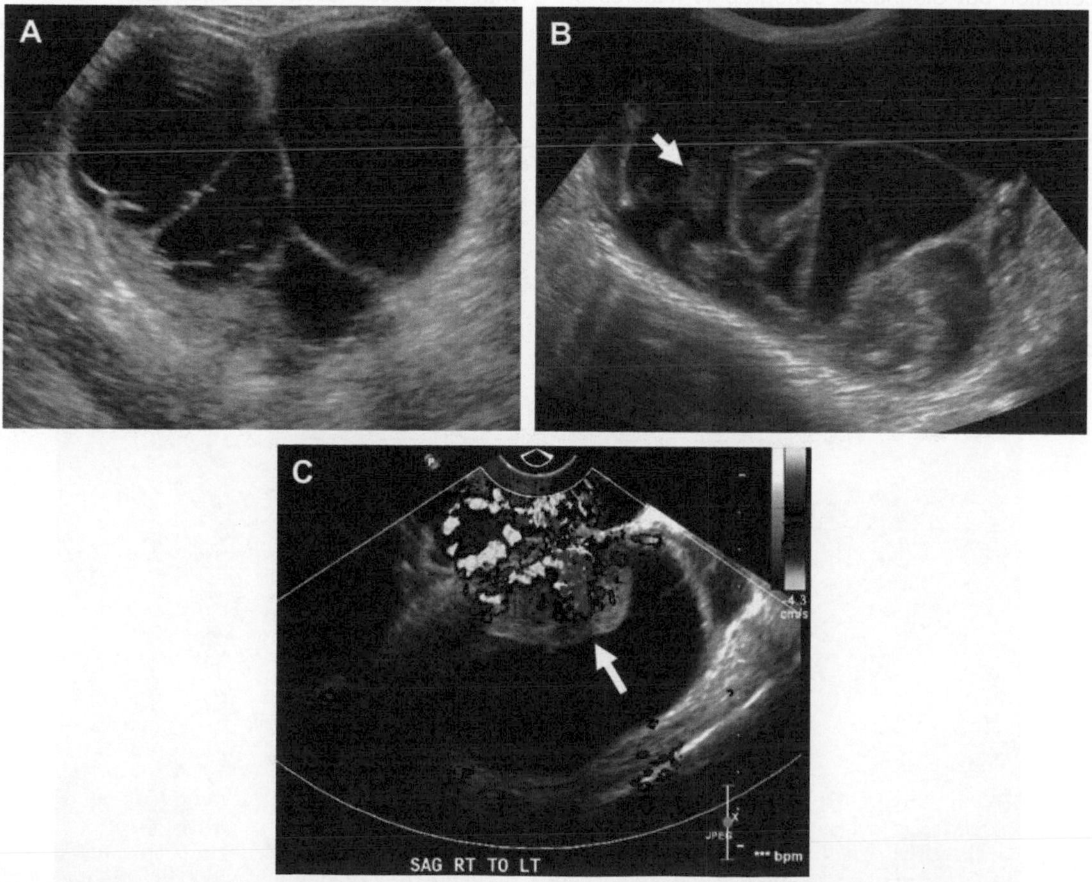

Fig. 13. Serous cystadenocarcinoma. (*A, B*) Gray-scale images of the left ovary demonstrate a complex cyst with multiple thick septations, echogenic fluid, and papillary excrescences (*arrow*). (*C*) Color Doppler image from a different patient shows a unilocular cyst containing intraluminal mural-based soft tissue with haphazardly arranged vessels (*arrow*).

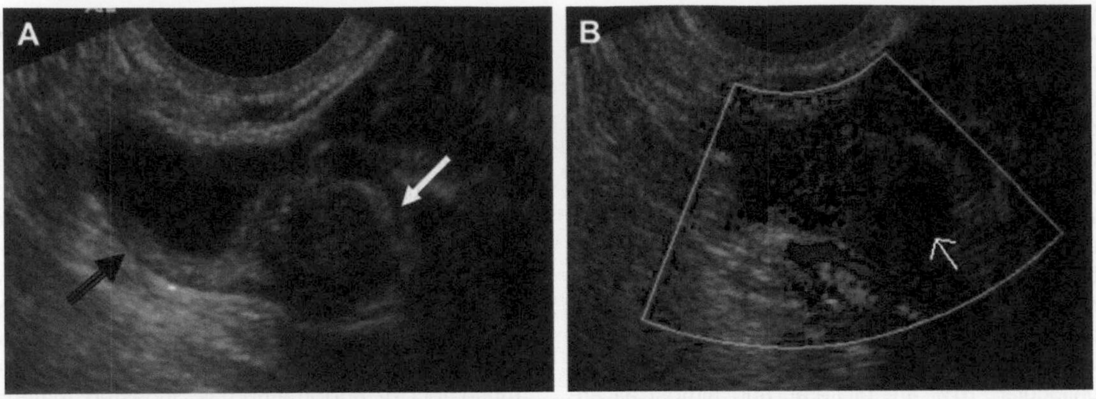

Fig. 14. Brenner tumor. (*A*) Transabdominal image shows a solid, round, well-circumscribed mass with posterior shadowing in the right ovary, which was surgically excised and found to be a Brenner tumor (*white arrow*). There is an incidental corpus luteum medial to the mass (*black arrow*). (*B*) Color Doppler image of the same lesion shows minimal vascularity within the mass.

A minority of teratomas may appear solid; however, they usually also demonstrate a prototypical finding as described earlier. Other less common but diagnostic sonographic features of teratomas include fat-fluid levels and multiple floating intracystic lipid globules. In the case of collision tumors, most often simultaneously occurring mature cystic teratomas and mucinous cystadenomas or cystadenocarcinomas, 2 adjacent septated cystic masses can be seen, 1 of which contains fat.[23]

Complications of mature cystic teratomas include torsion, rupture, autoimmune hemolytic anemia, infection, and malignant degeneration. Malignant transformation occurs in 1% to 2% of cases, usually originates from the Rokitansky nodule, and almost always forms squamous cell carcinoma.[23] Transformation generally occurs in women older than 45 years. It is often associated with elevated levels of squamous carcinoma antigen (a glycoprotein used to follow squamous cell carcinomas), CA 125, and CA 19-9.[23] By ultrasound, transmural growth of solid tissue into adjacent organs can be seen, arising from a large mass greater than 10 cm in diameter.[23] When the sonologist determines that there has been probable or frank malignant degeneration, more complex surgery supplants laparoscopic management.[23]

Epithelial neoplasms

Exactly which gray-scale and Doppler ultrasound characteristics are most helpful in determining

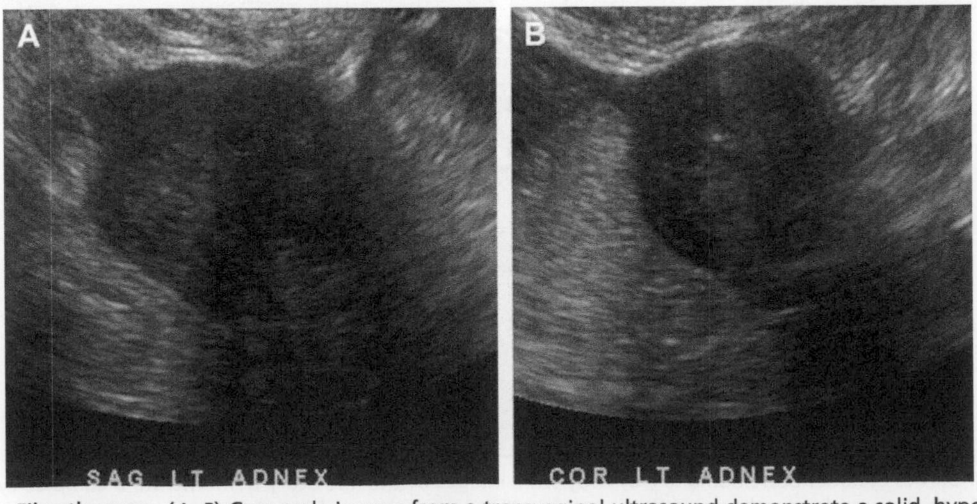

Fig. 15. Fibrothecoma. (*A, B*) Gray-scale images from a transvaginal ultrasound demonstrate a solid, hypoechoic mass with posterior shadowing in the region of the left ovary. After surgical excision, pathology confirmed that this was a fibrothecoma.

the likelihood of malignancy in adnexal masses has been the source of considerable study and debate in the radiologic and gynecologic literature. Several investigators are proponents of the use of morphologic scoring systems and mathematic models, whereas others champion the visual gestalt of an experienced sonologist. What is important is that both schools have shown reasonable diagnostic accuracy using specific sonographic findings.

As previously noted, the growth of a partially cystic mass over time and the presence of papillary projections (vascular, solid, nonfatty, nonfibrous tissue, with properties atypical of a teratoma) are most concerning for epithelial malignancy (**Fig. 13**).[5,6,24] Other concerning findings are thick septations (>2 mm), irregular, thickened walls (>3 mm), poorly defined margins, ascites and adenopathy,[4–6] stromal invasion, and haphazardly arranged vessels of changing caliber.[6] Size alone is variably regarded as predictive of malignancy. In a study by Brown,[6] almost half of the excised ovarian malignancies were less than 4 cm.

The caveat to this discussion is that, as stated earlier, many of the previously described benign masses may occasionally exhibit worrisome features that simulate malignancy. Likewise, cystadenofibromas are rare subtypes of serous epithelial tumors that, despite their low or borderline malignant potential, are likely to mimic frankly malignant masses. Cystadenofibromas occur in both premenopausal and postmenopausal women.[7,8,25] In a small study by Alcazar,[24] the most common appearance was that of a unilocular, thin-walled complex cystic mass. More than half of these masses contained papillary projections or solid nodules larger than 3 mm; and almost half

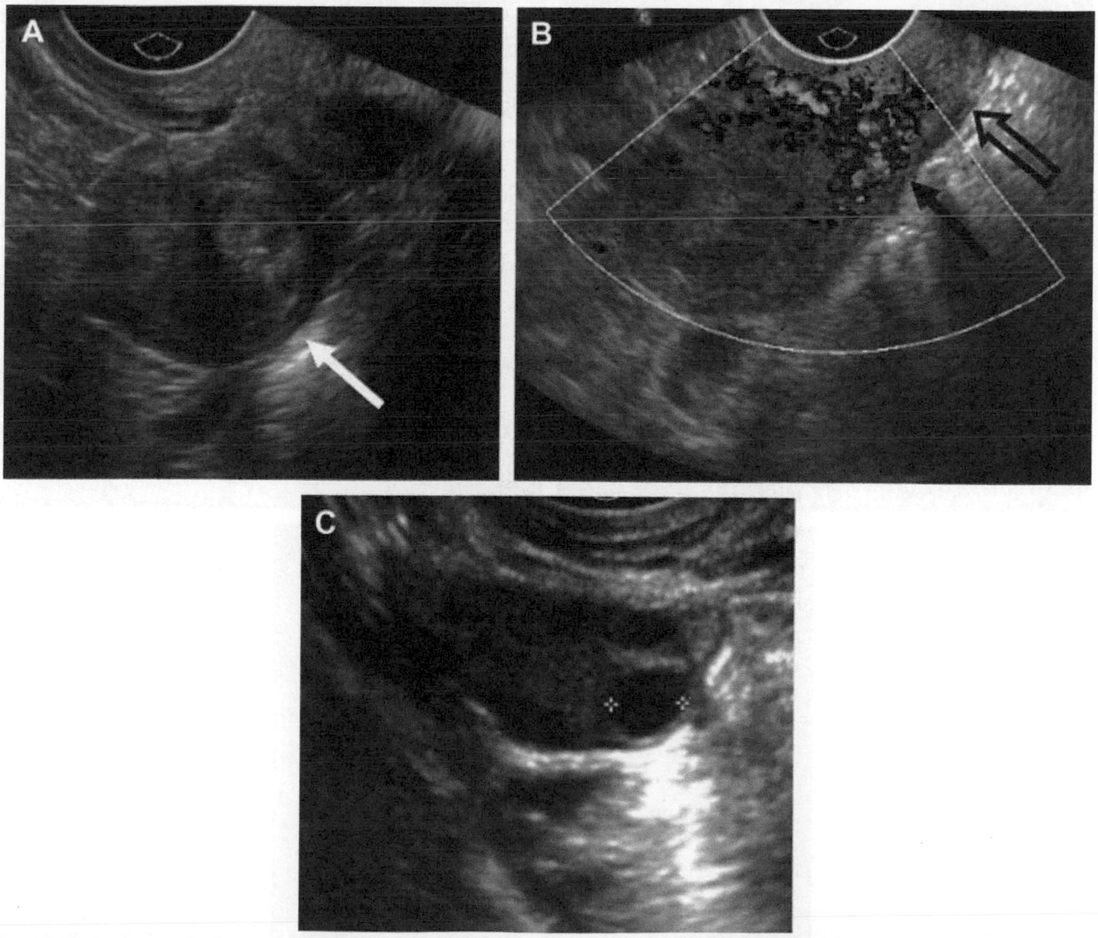

Fig. 16. Pedunculated fibroid with bridging vessels. (*A*) Gray-scale image of the right adnexa shows a mostly solid mass (*white arrow*). (*B*) Color Doppler image of the same structure shows vessels in the periphery of the mass (*solid black arrow*) connecting to the uterus (*open black arrow*). This is known as the bridging vessels sign, and indicates that the mass is a pedunculated subserosal fibroid. (*C*) A normal right ovary, containing a follicle (calipers), was visualized.

of the masses showed some vascularity, mostly within the tumor walls. One-third of these masses manifested septations or echogenic fluid. Because there is no imaging feature to confidently distinguish them from malignancy, these masses should be surgically excised.[7]

Borderline tumors or masses of low malignant potential, by definition, are true malignancies that tend to have minimal invasion on histology.[26,27] These tumors overall have a better prognosis because they affect younger women at an earlier stage than the high-grade malignancies. A study by Pascual and colleagues,[26] showed that the most predictive appearance of these masses on ultrasound has been that of unilocular cysts with intracystic papillae but without solid components or thick septa. Also in this study, borderline masses were shown to contain more echogenic fluid and demonstrate more vascularity than benign masses. Conversely, in a study by Bent and colleagues,[27] the most common appearance on MRI was that of a multiseptate cystic mass with plaquelike thickenings.

SOLID MASSES

The most common solid adnexal masses are subtypes of sex cord–stromal tumors, which arise from cells surrounding the ovarian follicles. Other adnexal masses that appear predominantly solid include metastatic disease, certain malignant germ cell tumors, and Brenner tumors (benign epithelial neoplasms) (**Fig. 14**).

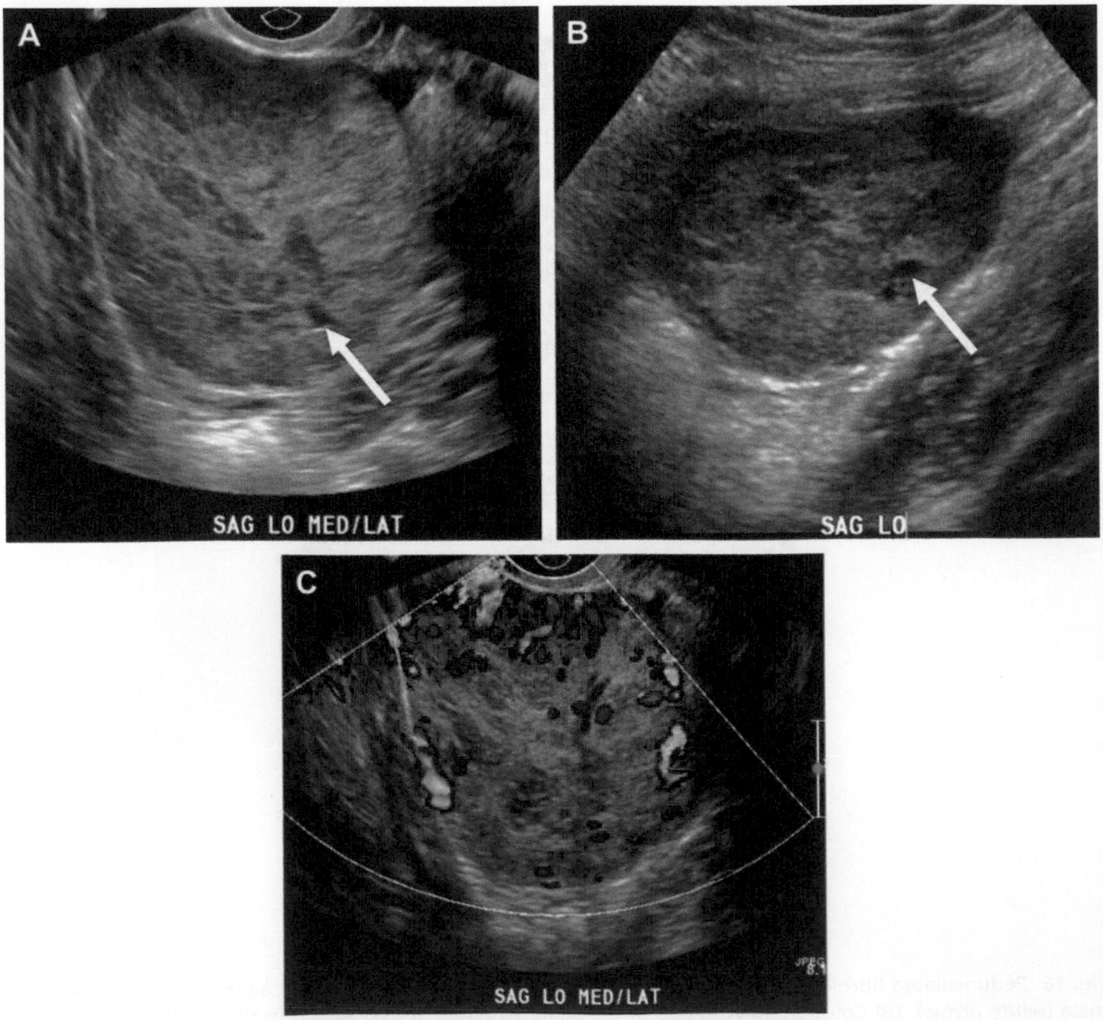

Fig. 17. Granulosa cell tumor. (*A, B*) Gray-scale images of the left ovary from a transvaginal ultrasound in a 56-year-old woman demonstrate a 4-cm, primarily solid, lobulated mass, with scattered cystic areas (*arrows*). (*C*) Color Doppler image of the same lesion demonstrates tumor vascularity.

Sex Cord–Stromal Neoplasms

Pure fibromas are benign and represent the most common sex cord–stromal tumor as well as the most common solid-appearing adnexal mass. With thecomas, they represent a spectrum of masses composed of variable amounts of estrogen-secreting cells and fibrous tissue; pure thecomas contain exclusively the former, and pure fibromas contain exclusively the latter, whereas fibrothecomas contain both (**Fig. 15**). Fibromas usually manifest as round, vascular, hypoechoic, solid masses with diffuse refractory posterior acoustic shadowing, but they may also appear hyperechoic or partially cystic.[28,29] They may be associated with Meigs syndrome, a condition in which the patient develops pleural effusions and ascites, which resolve after tumor excision. Because of the abundant fibrous tissue in fibromas, they may be mistaken for Brenner tumors (rare, benign, fibrous epithelial-derived ovarian tumors) or pedunculated fibroids. The bridging vessel sign, vessels on color Doppler extending from the uterus to the solid adnexal mass, helps to differentiate pedunculated fibroids from fibromas (**Fig. 16**).

Granulosa cell tumors, dysgerminomas, and Sertoli-Leydig cell tumors are uncommon masses that tend to present as predominantly solid masses. They are often seen in younger patients; however, granulosa cell tumor has a second peak in the postmenopausal years (**Fig. 17**). Sertoli-Leydig cell tumors are rare sex cord–stromal tumors and the most common ovarian tumor to secrete androgens. They appear as hypoechoic solid tumors and may be so small that they may be overlooked. Sertoli-Leydig cell tumor and granulosa cell

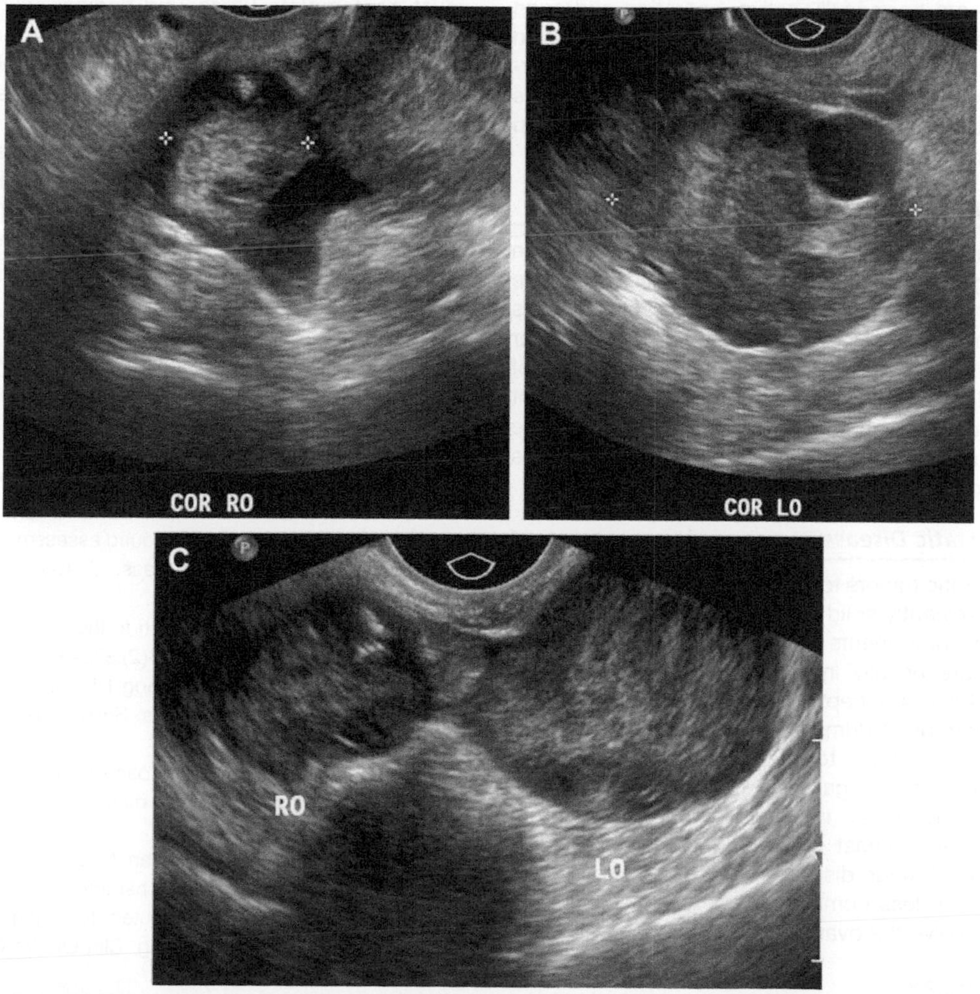

Fig. 18. Metastatic disease to the ovaries. (*A, B, C*) Transvaginal images demonstrate solid masses with tiny cystic areas on both ovaries (*cursors*) in a woman with advanced breast cancer. Metastatic disease is often not distinguishable from solid primary ovarian neoplasms except that it is more commonly bilateral.

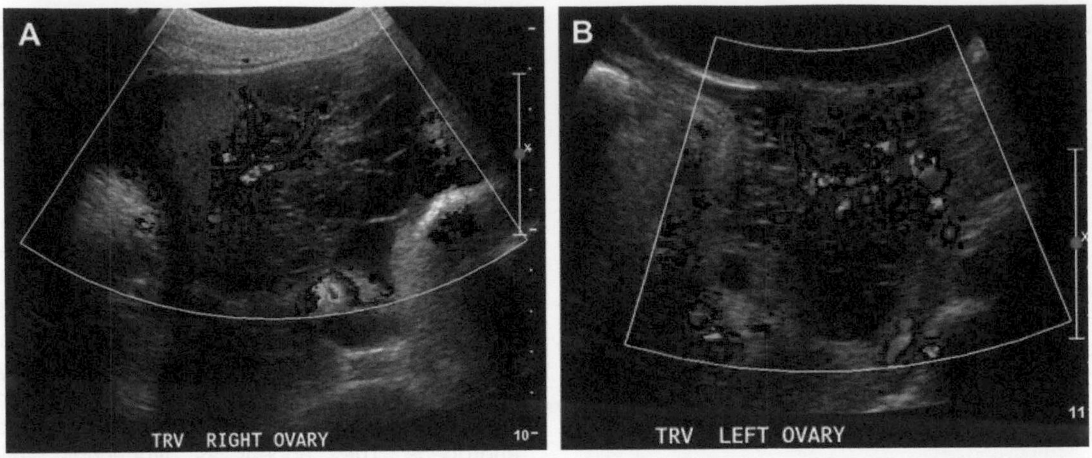

Fig. 19. Cholangiocarcinoma metastatic to the ovaries. (*A, B*) Transvaginal color Doppler images of the ovaries demonstrate vascular, mixed solid and cystic masses on both ovaries in a woman with known metastatic cholangiocarcinoma.

tumor are hormonally active, secreting androgen and estrogen, respectively. For this reason, an investigator asserts that any subtle ovarian abnormality seen in patients with virilizing symptoms should be reevaluated at least once by follow-up imaging.[4]

Malignant Germ Cell Tumors

Malignant germ cell tumors are rare and occur in younger women in their teens and 20s. These tumors are usually large, lobulated solid masses that may contain cystic areas with fibrovascular septa.[8] They may also contain speckled areas of calcification but there is generally a significant solid component.[8] Serum tumor markers may be helpful in distinguishing germ cell malignancies from other adnexal masses.

Metastatic Disease

Metastatic tumors to the ovary generally appear as predominantly solid masses but may contain tiny cystic components in a "moth-eaten" pattern.[8] They are usually indistinguishable from primary solid tumors except that they are more likely to be bilateral.[6,8] Primary neoplasms that are most often metastatic to the ovary are mammary, colonic, rectal, gastric, appendiceal, cervical, and endometrial in origin.[6] Metastases from a primary breast cancer usually occur with advanced-stage disease (**Fig. 18**).[6] Lymphomatic and other less common primary neoplasms may also involve the ovaries (**Fig. 19**).

SUMMARY

Ultrasound is usually the initial imaging modality used to assess adnexal masses. The sonologist must contemplate ultrasound findings within the clinical backdrop of patient history, demographics, and menstrual status. The goal is to identify distinguishing features of the mass and to assess its malignant potential. In some cases, follow-up ultrasound or MRI may be necessary. Familiarity with the spectrum of morphologic findings is critical, because subsequent recommendations will direct clinical and surgical management.

REFERENCES

1. Cohen HL, Tice HM, Mandel FS. Ovarian volumes measured by US: bigger than we think. Radiology 1990;177(1):189–92.
2. Le T, Giede C, Salem S, et al. Initial evaluation and referral guidelines for management of pelvis/ovarian masses. J Obstet Gynaecol Can 2009;31(7):668–80.
3. Cohen L. Transvaginal ultrasound assessment of the premenopausal ovarian mass. J Assist Reprod Genet 2007;24(11):507–12.
4. Patel MD. Practical approach to the adnexal mass. Radiol Clin North Am 2006;1(2):879–99.
5. Jeong YY, Outwater EK, Kang HK, et al. Imaging evaluation of ovarian masses. Radiographics 2000; 20(5):1445–70.
6. Brown DL. A practical approach to the ultrasound characterization of adnexal masses. Ultrasound Q 2007;23(2):87–105.
7. Heilbrun M, Olpin J, Shabaan A, et al. Imaging of benign adnexal masses: characteristic presentations on ultrasound, computed tomography, and magnetic resonance imaging. Clin Obstet Gynecol 2009;52(1):21–39.
8. Joshi M, Ganesan K, Munshi HN, et al. Ultrasound of adnexal masses. Semin Ultrasound CT MR 2008; 29(2):72–97.

9. Ekerhovd E, Wienerroith H, Staudach A, et al. Preoperative assessment of unilocular adnexal cysts by transvaginal ultrasonography: a comparison between ultrasonographic morphologic imaging and histopathologic diagnosis. Am J Obstet Gynecol 2001;184(2):48–54.
10. Durfee SM, Frates MC. Sonographic spectrum of the corpus luteum in early pregnancy: gray-scale, color, and pulsed Doppler appearance. J Clin Ultrasound 1999;27(2):55–9.
11. Shwayder JM. Pelvic pain, adnexal masses, and ultrasound. Semin Reprod Med 2008;26:252–65.
12. Modesitt SC, Pavlik EJ, Ueland FR, et al. Risk of malignancy in unilocular ovarian cystic tumors less than 10 centimeters in diameter. Obstet Gynecol 2003;102(3):594–9.
13. Savelli L, Ghi T, De Iaco P, et al. Paraovarian/paratubal cysts: comparison of transvaginal sonographic and pathological findings to establish diagnostic criteria. Ultrasound Obstet Gynecol 2006;28(3):330–4.
14. Salamon C, Tornos C, Chi DS, et al. Borderline endometrioid tumor arising in a paratubal cyst: a case report. Gynecol Oncol 2005;97(1):263–5.
15. Thomason RW, Rush W, Dave H, et al. Transitional cell carcinoma arising within a paratubal cyst: report of a case. Int J Gynecol Pathol 1995;14(3):270–3.
16. Vlhakis-Miliaras E, Miliaras D, Koutsoumis G, et al. Paratubal cysts in young females as an incidental finding in laparotomies performed for right lower quadrant abdominal pain. Pediatr Surg Int 1998;13(2–3):141–2.
17. Woodward PJ, Sohaey R, Mezzetti TP, et al. Endometriosis: radiologic-pathologic correlation. Radiographics 2001;21(1):193–216.
18. Kinkel K, Frei KA, Balleyguier C, et al. Diagnosis of endometriosis with imaging: a review. Eur Radiol 2006;16(2):285–98.
19. Guerriero S, Ajossa S, Mais V, et al. Role of transvaginal sonography in the diagnosis of peritoneal inclusion cyst. J Ultrasound Med 2004;23(9):1193–200.
20. Kiran AJ. Imaging of peritoneal inclusion cysts. AJR Am J Roentgenol 2000;174(6):1559–63.
21. Vallerie AM, Lerner JP, Wright JD, et al. Peritoneal inclusion cysts: a review. Obstet Gynecol Surv 2009;64(5):321–34.
22. Outwater EK, Siegelman ES, Hunt JL, et al. Ovarian teratomas: tumor types and imaging characteristics. Radiographics 2001;21(2):475–90.
23. Park SB, Jeong KK, Kyu-Rae K, et al. Imaging findings of complications and manifestations of ovarian teratomas. Radiographics 2008;28(4):969–83.
24. Alcazar JL, Errasti T, Minguez JA, et al. Sonographic features of ovarian cystadenofibromas. J Ultrasound Med 2001;20(8):915–9.
25. Brown DL, Kika MD, Laing FC. Adnexal masses: US characterization and reporting. Radiology 2010;252(2):342–54.
26. Pascual MA, Tressera F, Grases PJ, et al. Borderline cystic tumors of the ovary: gray-scale and color Doppler findings. J Clin Ultrasound 2002;30(2):76–82.
27. Bent CL, Sahdev A, Rockall AG, et al. MRI appearances of borderline ovarian tumors. Clin Radiol 2009;64(4):430–8.
28. Paladini D, Testa A, Van Holsbeke C, et al. Imaging in gynecological disease (5): clinical and ultrasound characteristics in fibroma and fibrothecoma of the ovary. Ultrasound Obstet Gynecol 2009;34(2):188–95.
29. Outwater EK, Wagner BJ, Mannion C, et al. Sex cord-stromal and steroid cell tumors of the ovary. Radiographics 1998;18(6):1523–46.

Sonographic Evaluation of Patients Treated with Uterine Artery Embolization

Sandra J. Allison, MD*, Darcy J. Wolfman, MD

KEYWORDS

- Ultrasound • Uterine artery embolization • UAE • UFE
- Uterine fibroid embolization • Complications
- Work-up • Follow-up

First described by Ravina and colleagues[1] in 1995, transcatheter uterine artery embolization (UAE) has become an accepted alternative to surgical and medical treatment for symptomatic fibroids.[2,3] It has been estimated that close to 100,000 procedures have been performed to date. The goal of the procedure is to produce infarction of fibroids without compromising endometrial and myometrial perfusion. Multiple postprocedural studies have demonstrated a significant decrease in uterine and fibroid volumes with associated decrease in symptoms.[4,5] When used to treat abnormal bleeding, bulk symptoms, and pain associated with fibroids, this procedure has been shown as effective and safe with minimal morbidity and mortality and clinical success in approximately 85% of patients.[6–10]

Pelvic sonography is a commonly used imaging modality pre- and post UAE. Ultrasound (US) has been used for the detection, characterization, and follow-up of fibroids. In working up a patient for embolization, US can assess for relative contraindications for embolization, such as endometriosis, malignancy, pregnancy, and pedunculated fibroids. After embolization, it can be used to monitor success by identifying regression or involution of fibroids. It can also identify complications related to the procedure.

MRI can be performed in cases where a more accurate assessment is needed or for problem solving, particularly in the pre-embolization work-up. MRI in terms of fibroid embolization has been shown to have several advantages over US. It has been shown to demonstrate higher sensitivity than transvaginal US (TVUS) in diagnosing adenomyosis.[11] Although TVUS is as effective as MRI in diagnosing and detecting fibroids, MRI has been shown to outperform US in evaluating the location, number, and size of fibroids.[12,13] Other studies have shown that MRI may be useful in predicting procedure outcome because fibroids with hemorrhagic degeneration or loss of vascular supply have been shown to have a poor response to UAE.[14,15] Furthermore, detection of persistent perfusion in a fibroid after UAE with contrast-enhanced MRI is thought to be predictive of treatment failure.[16,17]

Although MRI has been shown to have advantages over sonographic imaging to patients undergoing UAE the portability and availability of US along with its low cost make it indispensable in the evaluation of patients pre- and post UAE. With recent advances in sonography, including 3-D imaging and volume manipulation, the gap in usefulness between these 2 imaging modalities is decreasing. The focus of this article is to discuss the use of US in imaging fibroids, work-up of patients as candidates for UAE, detection of post-procedural complications, and follow-up of these patients.

Department of Radiology, Georgetown University Medical Center, 3800 Reservoir Road, NW, Washington, DC 20007, USA
* Corresponding author.
E-mail address: sa263@gunet.georgetown.edu

Ultrasound Clin 5 (2010) 277–288
doi:10.1016/j.cult.2010.03.004
1556-858X/10/$ – see front matter

PRE-EMBOLIZATION EVALUATION

Fibroid Detection and Characterization

Fibroids are benign tumors composed of smooth muscle cells, collagen, and fibrous tissue arranged in a whorl-like pattern. They are the most common pelvic tumors, occurring in up to 25% of women over age 35.

The relative amounts of smooth muscle, necrosis, calcification, and fibrous tissue within a fibroid determines its echogenicity and heterogeneity on US.[18] When the predominating tissue type is smooth muscle, the fibroid appears hypoechoic with poor sound through transmission. With degeneration, the presence of tiny cystic areas causes an increase in echogenicity and improved through transmission of sound. A fibroid may appear hypoechoic to anechoic in the setting of advanced degeneration with cystic or hemorrhagic necrosis. Dystrophic calcification presents as shadowing echogenic foci. Not all shadowing and acoustic attenuation in fibroids is associated with calcification. Radiations of sharp discrete shadowing, a defining sonographic characteristic of fibroids, are thought related to be transition zones between fibrous tissue and smooth muscle (**Fig. 1**A–D).[18]

Fibroids may be submucosal, intramural, or subserosal in location, with intramural the most common type. Sonohysterography has been shown to reliably distinguish polyps from submucosal fibroids.[19] Polyps are isoechoic to the echogenic endometrium and have preserved endometrial-myometrial interface. Fibroids are broad based, well defined, and usually hypo- to isoechoic to myometrium (**Fig. 2**A, B). Submucosal fibroids may cause disruption or displacement of the endometrial lining on TVUS.[20] Submucosal fibroids have an overlying layer of echogenic endometrium, an identifying feature that can be readily seen with sonohysterography (see **Fig. 2**B).[21] Fibroids in this location can cause metrorrhagia, which, when heavy, may result in anemia. When large enough, fibroids in other

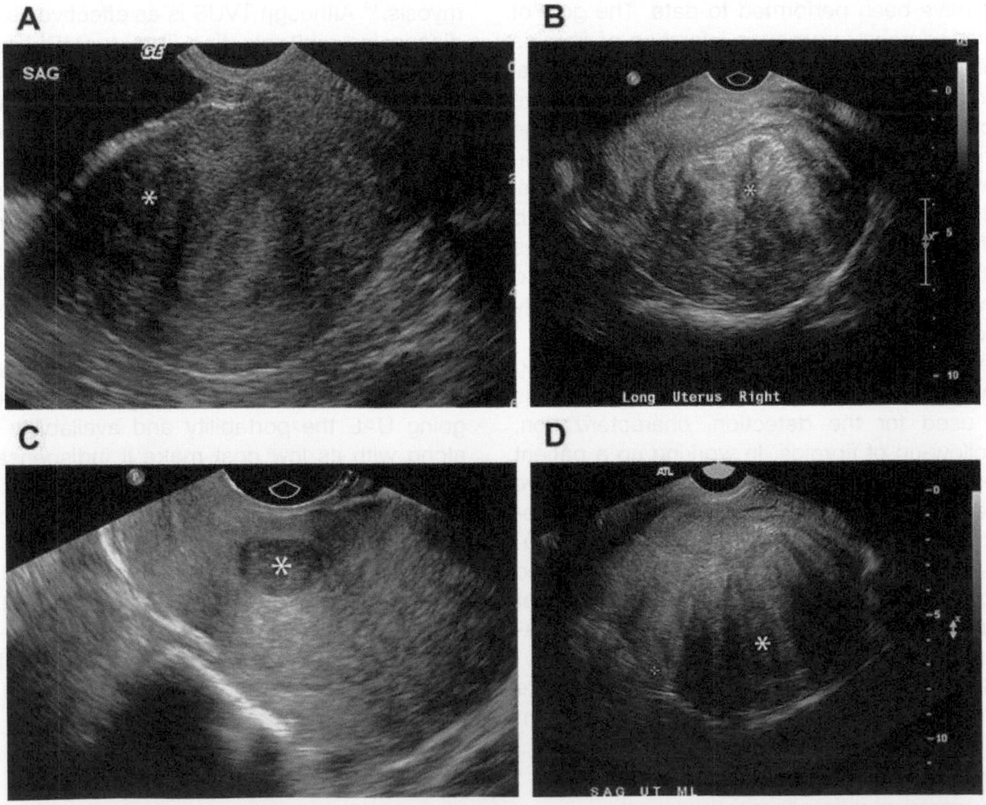

Fig. 1. Sonographic features of fibroids. (*A*) Sagittal TVUS of uterus with hypoechoic fibroid (*) with poor sound through transmission. The predominating tissue type is smooth muscle. (*B*) Increased echogenicity and improved sound transmission in this fibroid (*) is due to the presence of tiny cystic areas related to degeneration within the fibroid. (*C*) With advanced degeneration, the fibroid (*) appears hypoechoic to anechoic with improved through transmission. (*D*) Transition zones between fibroid tissue and smooth muscle are thought to cause radiations of sharp discrete shadowing within a fibroid (*).

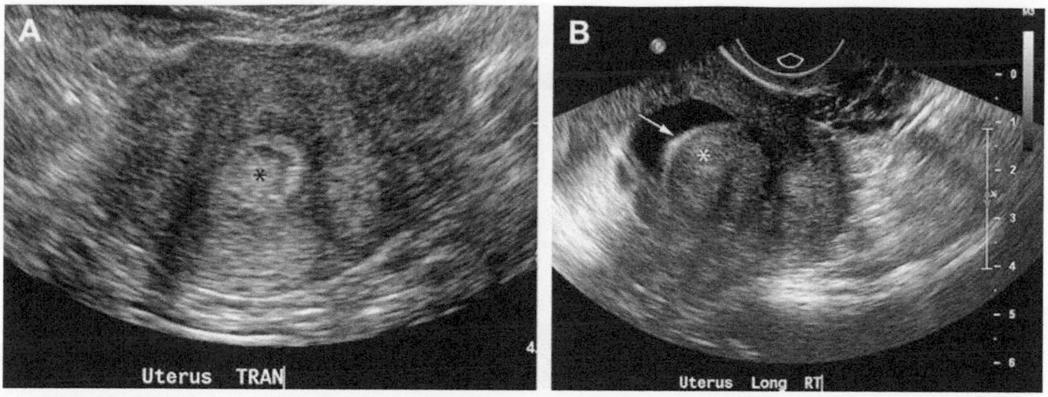

Fig. 2. Fibroid versus polyp. (*A*) Endometrial polyps (*) are typically isoechoic to endometrium whereas (*B*) fibroids (*) are isoechoic to myometrium. With sonohysterography, the echogenic endometrium (*arrow*) can be seen overlying the fibroid (*), confirming a submucosal location.

locations may cause pressure effects on adjacent organs or ligaments. Subserosal pedunculated fibroids may torse and necrose. Intramembranous fibroids (fibroids located in the broad ligament) can simulate ovarian or adnexal masses (**Fig. 3**).

When single or multiple, fibroids can cause focal or diffuse uterine enlargement, which can reach massive proportions. Depending on their location, the uterine contour may be smooth or lobulated. Although typically well defined in appearance, when a significant number of fibroids are present, they may be indistinguishable from each other. In extreme cases, the sole clue to their presence on US is an irregularly enlarged uterus with distortion or obscuration of the endometrial echo complex.[22]

Fibroids exhibit varying degrees of vascularity on color Doppler imaging. The typical Doppler pattern encountered is marked peripheral blood flow with decreased central flow or an avascular core (**Fig. 4**).[23]

Preprocedural Work-up

Gray-scale sonography can be used to assess the number and location of fibroids at baseline as well as measure the overall volume of the uterus.[24] This information is correlated with patients' presenting symptoms in the pre-embolization work-up. Sonohysterography, as discussed previously, is an indispensible tool in distinguishing submucosal fibroids from endometrial polyps in the work-up of abnormal or heavy menstrual bleeding. In addition, it can clearly depict the relationship between endometrium and underlying submucosal fibroid.[25] In contradistinction, patients presenting with symptoms of urinary frequency or urgency or constipation may attribute their symptoms to mass effect from a large intramural or subserosal fibroid encroaching on adjacent organs.[26] Gray-scale sonography may assist in predicting chances of UAE failure by assessing degree of fibroid calcification; fibroids that are advanced in degeneration

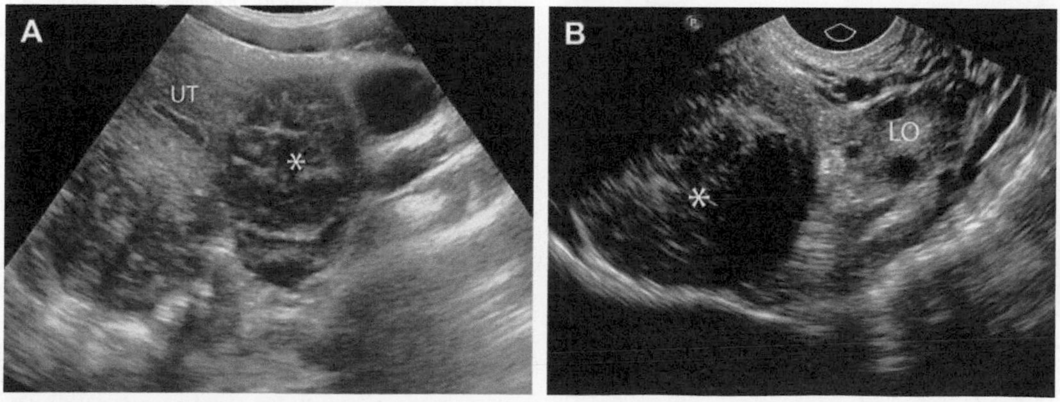

Fig. 3. Fibroid mimicking adnexal mass. (*A*) Transverse transabdominal US of a 42-year-old woman presenting with left adnexal mass. A hypoechoic mass (*) is found in the left adnexa. UT, uterus. (*B*) Sagittal TVUS of the left adnexa demonstrates hypoechoic mass (*) separate from and superior to the left ovary (LO) compatible with fibroid.

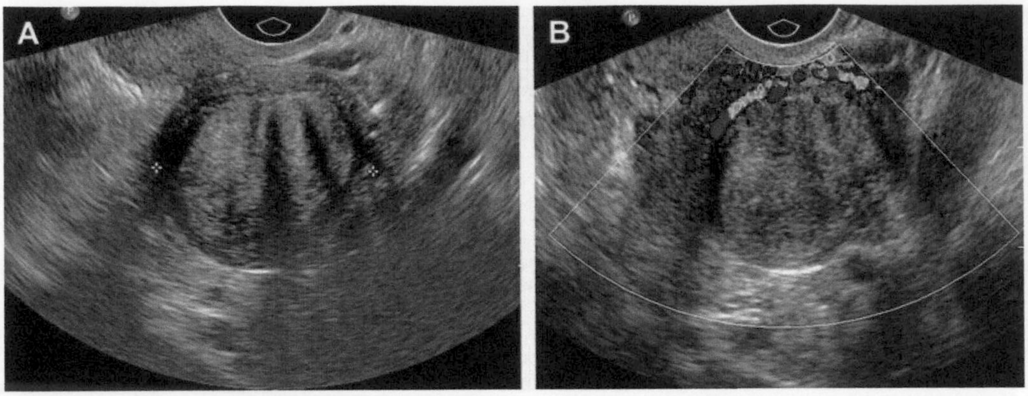

Fig. 4. Vascular pattern of fibroids. (*A*) Coronal TVUS of the uterus demonstrating fibroid with typical sharp radiating shadows. (*B*) Color Doppler US of same lesion demonstrating peripheral draping vascular pattern and absence of detectable intralesional vascularity.

are unlikely to respond to UAE.[27] The volume of a fibroid or of the entire uterus can be calculated using the formula for an ellipse, A × B × C × 0.523, designating *A*, *B*, and *C* as dimensions in the 3 orientations.[9] The largest fibroids can be measured at baseline and later followed over time. The uterine volume can also be measured and followed. This is often adequate as follow-up in the setting of multiple fibroids.[28,29] The detection and characterization of pedunculated subserosal fibroids is also important information to obtain before UAE (**Fig. 5**). The stalk of the pedunculated fibroid can be measured. If the stalk or attachment point of the fibroid measures less than 50% of its diameter, the fibroid is at risk of detachment from the uterus after complete infarction of the stalk,

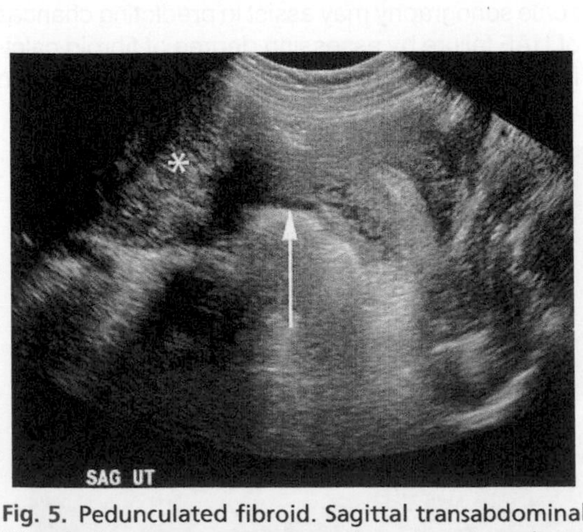

Fig. 5. Pedunculated fibroid. Sagittal transabdominal US of the uterus demonstrating a pedunculated fibroid (*) extending from the fundus. The stalk (*arrow*) can be measured to determine risk of detachment. Pedunculated fibroids in this location can be missed on TVUS as they can extend beyond the field of view.

potentially causing aseptic peritonitis.[30] In addition, it has been reported that this type of fibroid may respond less favorably to UAE due to the presence of an alternate blood supply from collateral vessels arising from the ovarian artery or from neighboring structures to which they become adherent.[31,32]

Color Doppler sonography may provide information regarding fibroid vascularity that is useful in determining which patients are best suited for UAE.[33] Fleischer and colleagues[34] suggested that a greater decrease in size after UAE can be seen with hypervascular fibroids than with hypovascular fibroids.

Color Doppler imaging may also be used to detect collateral flow not depicted on uterine artery arteriography. McLucas and colleagues[35] showed that initial uterine artery peak systolic velocity may correlate with the size and shrinkage of fibroids and uterine volume after embolization. Thus, pre-embolization Doppler may serve a role in prescreening for UAE. These investigators also found that higher peak systolic velocities were associated with a higher number of vials of particles used in embolization, as well as, the particle load used to embolize 1 L of tissue and therefore, serve as a predictor of UAE failure.

In addition to the work-up and characterization of fibroids, other abnormalities may be detected with US that may influence whether or not a patient is a candidate for UAE. One such abnormality is adenomyosis.

Adenomyosis is a condition in which ectopic endometrial glands and stroma are implanted in the myometrium. It can exist as a focal or diffuse form.[36] US has been shown to demonstrate a high degree of accuracy, sensitivity, and specificity in the diagnosis of adenomyosis.[37,38] The most common sonographic appearance of adenomyosis is myometrial heterogeneity that may be focal or diffuse, seen in approximately 75% of patients.[39] Echogenic areas within the myometrium represent heterotopic endometrial tissue whereas hypoechoic regions represent reactive smooth muscle hyperplasia.[40,41] Echogenic nodules or linear striations extending from the endometrium also represent ectopic endometrial tissue, which may lead to poor definition of the endomyometrial junction. In approximately 50% of patients, dilated cystic glands or hemorrhagic foci present as small myometrial cysts. Diffuse adenomyosis may result in asymmetric myometrial thickness or globular uterine enlargement. Focal adenomyosis, or adenomyoma, may be mistaken for a fibroid.[38–41] The lack of focal uterine contour abnormality or mass effect, elliptical shape, ill-defined margins, or increased echogenicity favor adenomyoma over fibroid.[20] Another distinguishing feature is the penetrating vascular pattern depicted with color Doppler,[42] which is different in appearance from the peripheral draping vascular pattern seen with fibroids.[43,44] An adenomyotic cyst is a rare form caused by extensive bleeding into ectopic endometrium (**Fig. 6**).[42]

Although the presence of adenomyosis was considered a cause of failed UAE in the past and a contraindication to the procedure, recent literature suggests that UAE may be a treatment option for patients with adenomyosis.[45,46]

During the work-up for UAE, US may also detect abnormalities or lesions involving the adnexa and endometrium, which can possibly explain a patient's presenting symptoms and preclude treatment with UAE. Furthermore, the presence or suspicion of uterine or adnexal malignancy is a contraindication to UAE. A discussion of adnexal

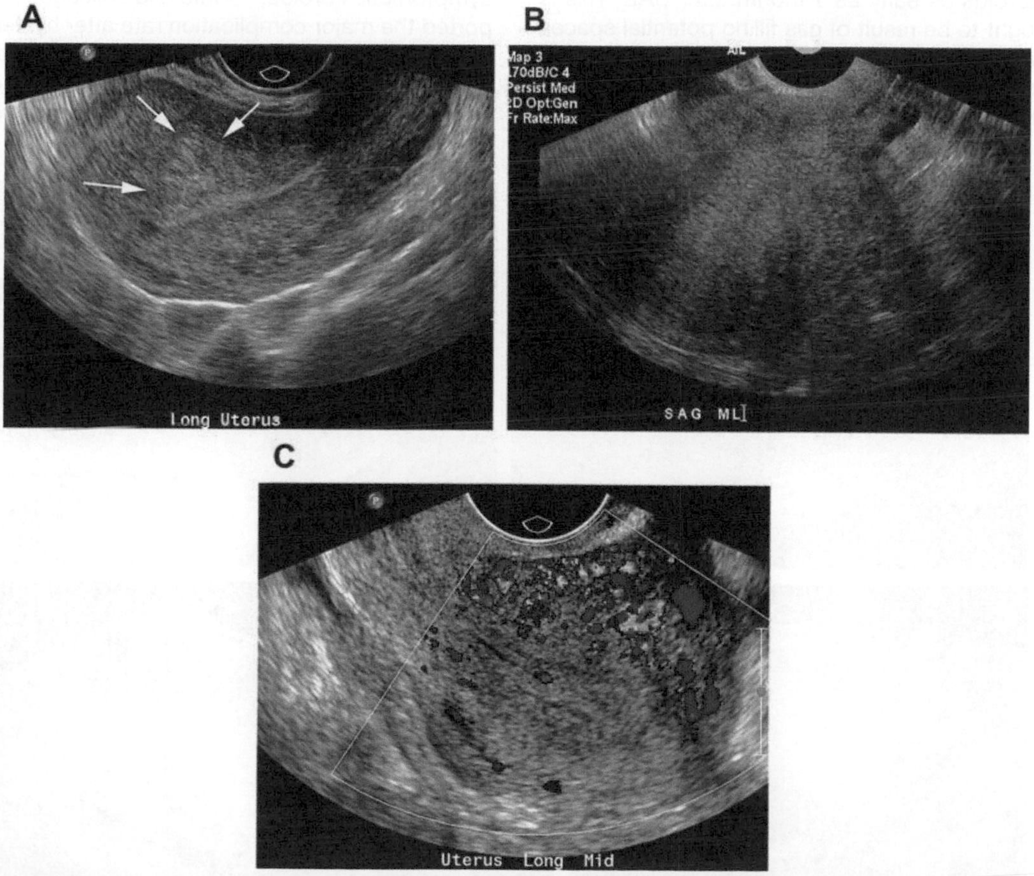

Fig. 6. Sonographic features of adenomyosis. (*A*) Sagittal TVUS of the uterus demonstrating echogenic nodules and linear striations (*arrows*) extending from the endometrium. The uterus is asymmetrically thickened anteriorly. (*B*) Sagittal TVUS of the uterus demonstrates globular enlargement and obscuration of the endometrium due to the presence of diffuse adenomyosis. (*C*) Color Doppler US demonstrates penetrating vascular pattern in the posterior myometrium in a patient with adenomyosis. This is a distinctly different vascular pattern from that seen with fibroids in **Fig. 4**B.

and other endometrial lesions is beyond the scope of this article.

POSTEMBOLIZATION IMAGING

Volume reduction of the uterus and of representative fibroids can be assessed with US. Follow-up US has shown a reduction in uterine volume of up to 40% and dominant fibroid decrease in size by up to 70%.[7,23,47] Most of the shrinkage occurs within the first 6 months after embolization followed by further reduction occurring between 6 and 12 months.[8] As with before UAE, fibroids exhibit a variety of appearances after UAE. This is thought to be due to the heterogeneous histologic composition of leiomyomas. Weintraub and colleagues[23] described a decrease in fibroid echogenicity after UAE. Others have reported heterogeneous increase in fibroid echogenicity after embolization (**Fig. 7**).[27] Air may also be detected in fibroids as early as 1 month after UAE. This is thought to be result of gas filling potential spaces created after tissue infarction and dessication.[48,49] This must not be confused with infection resulting in inappropriate management. The 2 entities may be differentiated by correlating imaging features with laboratory and clinical findings (**Fig. 8**).

Six months to 1 year after UAE, peripheral calcification may be seen formed around an increasingly hypoechoic fibroid, resulting in the fetal head sign. Natural fibroid involution and necrosis presents with a central pattern of dystrophic calcification (**Fig. 9**).[50]

On occasion, echogenic foci may be detected within uterine arteries representing polyvinyl alcohol particles that have become incorporated into blood clot forming within the uterine arteries. Color Doppler can be used to demonstrate decreased blood flow to fibroids after embolization. Flow in perifibroid vessels may persist; however, intrafibroid vascularity typically disappears.[28]

COMPLICATIONS

Major complications after UAE are rare compared with those after traditional surgical intervention for symptomatic fibroids.[51] Pinto and colleagues[52] reported the major complication rate after hysterectomy is 20% compared with 2.5% after UAE. Spies and colleagues[53] found an overall serious complication rate of 1.25%. The overall

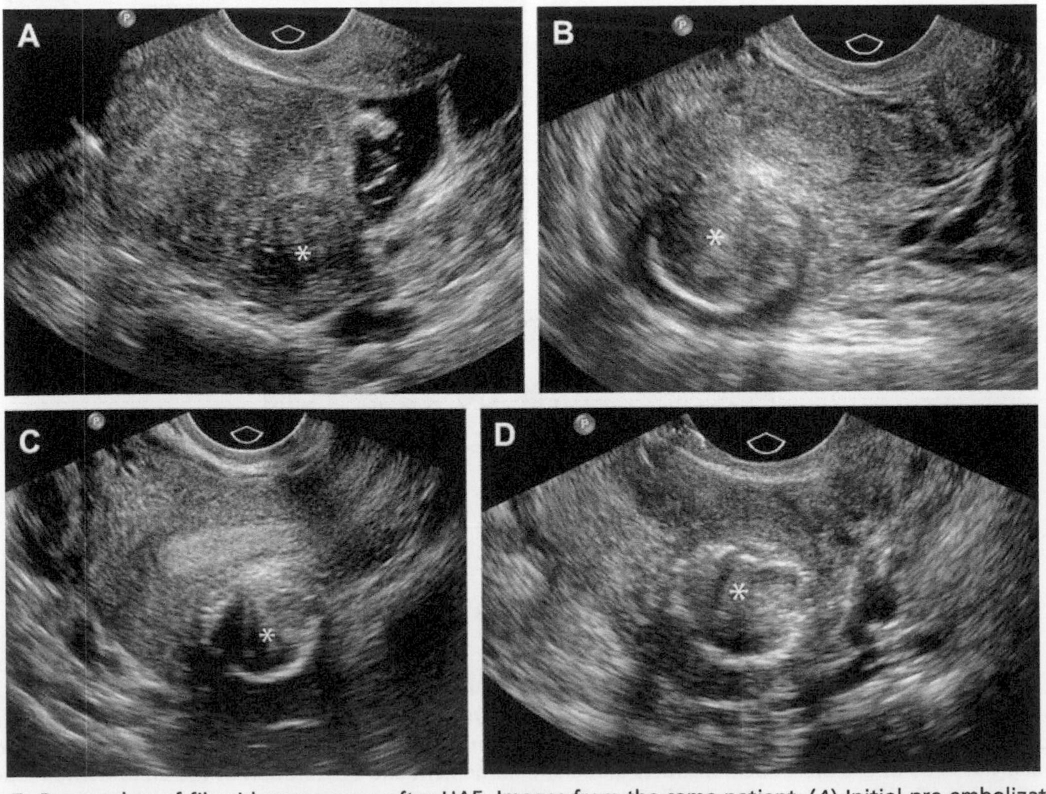

Fig. 7. Progression of fibroid appearance after UAE. Images from the same patient. (*A*) Initial pre-embolization scan. (*B*) 20 months after UAE. (*C*) 28 months after UAE. (*D*) 32 months after UAE. The fibroid (*) has changed in echogenicity and developed peripheral calcification over time.

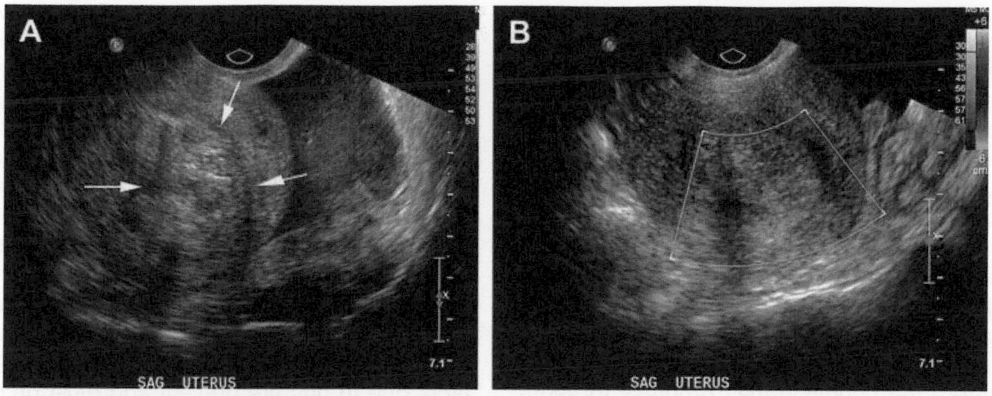

Fig. 8. Air in fibroid after UAE. A 38-year-old patient presents with pelvic pain 1 week after UAE. (*A*) Sagittal TVUS of the uterus demonstrates punctate echogenic foci within a fibroid (*arrows*) with "dirty" shadowing compatible with air. (*B*) Color Doppler demonstrates lack of significant vascularity making infection a less likely diagnosis. (*Courtesy of* Anna S. Lev-Toaff, MD, Philadelphia, PA.)

periprocedural short-term complication rate for UAE is approximately 8%. Up to 2% is related to infections.[26] Other complications are related to allergic reactions. Deaths within 30 days after UAE have been reported: 2 from uterine infection resulting in overwhelming sepsis and 1 from massive pulmonary embolism.[54–56] Recognition of complications is important because they must be treated appropriately.

Fibroid delivery or transcervical expulsion of fibroids has a reported rate of up to 3%.[57,58] At the authors' institution, this is the most common complication requiring hospitalization.[54] This occurs only with fibroids that are submucosal or intramural fibroids with at least some submucosal component. Patients experiencing fibroid expulsion may present with uterine contractions, abdominal pain, and heavy vaginal bleeding or discharge months after UAE. The presentation is not limited to the early postprocedural period and can be seen as late as 1 year after embolization.[53] These patients, in particular those with large submucosal fibroids, are also prone to infection with passage of sloughed fibroid due to necrosis acting as ideal setup for growth of bacteria transmitted from the vaginal vault.[59] In some cases, the fibroid is expelled spontaneously. In many other cases, the fibroids do not pass through the cervix spontaneously but can be identified advancing toward the cervix on serial examinations (**Fig. 10**). Those that pass into the vagina can be removed during an office visit. Those that remain firmly attached to the uterine wall may require dilatation and curettage or hysteroscopy for removal, especially if a patient is symptomatic or if the fibroid is only partially infarcted.[58,60]

Endometritis, an infection of the endometrium after UAE, has a reported prevalence of up to 1% to 2%. Afflicted patients present with pelvic pain, watery discharge, fever, and leukocytosis.

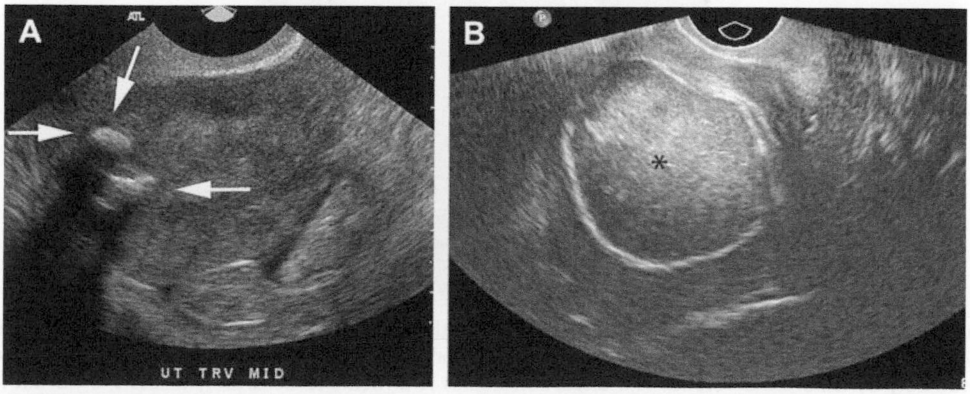

Fig. 9. Dystrophic versus post-UAE calcification. (*A*) Central pattern of dystrophic calcification (*arrows*) formed within a fibroid as a result of natural involution. (*B*) Peripheral calcification tends to form around a fibroid (*) 6 months to a year after UAE.

Endometritis may occur weeks to days after embolization. Rajan and colleagues[61] reported that all patients who developed intrauterine infections after UAE had fibroids with a submucosal component. Preprocedural antibiotic administration did not influence risk of infection. Sonographically, the uterus and endometrium may appear normal in endometritis. Other reported sonographic features include uterine enlargement, thickened heterogeneous endometrium, intracavitary fluid, and intrauterine air (**Fig. 11**A).[62] Clinical and laboratory findings should support the diagnosis. Most patients respond well to antibiotics. Untreated, the condition may progress to septicemia. Hysterectomy is the treatment in these circumstances.[53]

Pelvic inflammatory disease and tubo-ovarian abscess are rare complications of UAE but should be included in the differential diagnosis of a patient with pain accompanied by fever.[63] Patients refractory to medical treatment require drainage procedures. TVUS is the initial imaging modality of choice. Imaging features include thick-walled complex cystic adnexal masses, dilated fallopian tubes with simple or complex contents, cogwheel sign, and adnexal hyperemia detected with color Doppler imaging (see **Fig. 11**B).

Pyomyoma or suppurative leiomyoma is a rare and potentially fatal condition that has been reported after UAE. Most cases in the literature are complications of pregnancy. In both situations, the imaging findings are identical. Treatment alternatives include hysterectomy, which is favored over myomectomy with antibiotics. On US, multiple internal echoes and reverberation artifacts due to gas are present and must be distinguished from infarcting fibroids (see **Fig. 11**C).

A rare but potential complication of UAE is diffuse uterine necrosis. The reported prevalence is less than 1% and even less prevalent if the patient has intact normal pelvic collateral circulation. It is rare because occlusion of the uterine arteries is usually not complete and terminated once the fibroid blood supply is occluded. Uterine

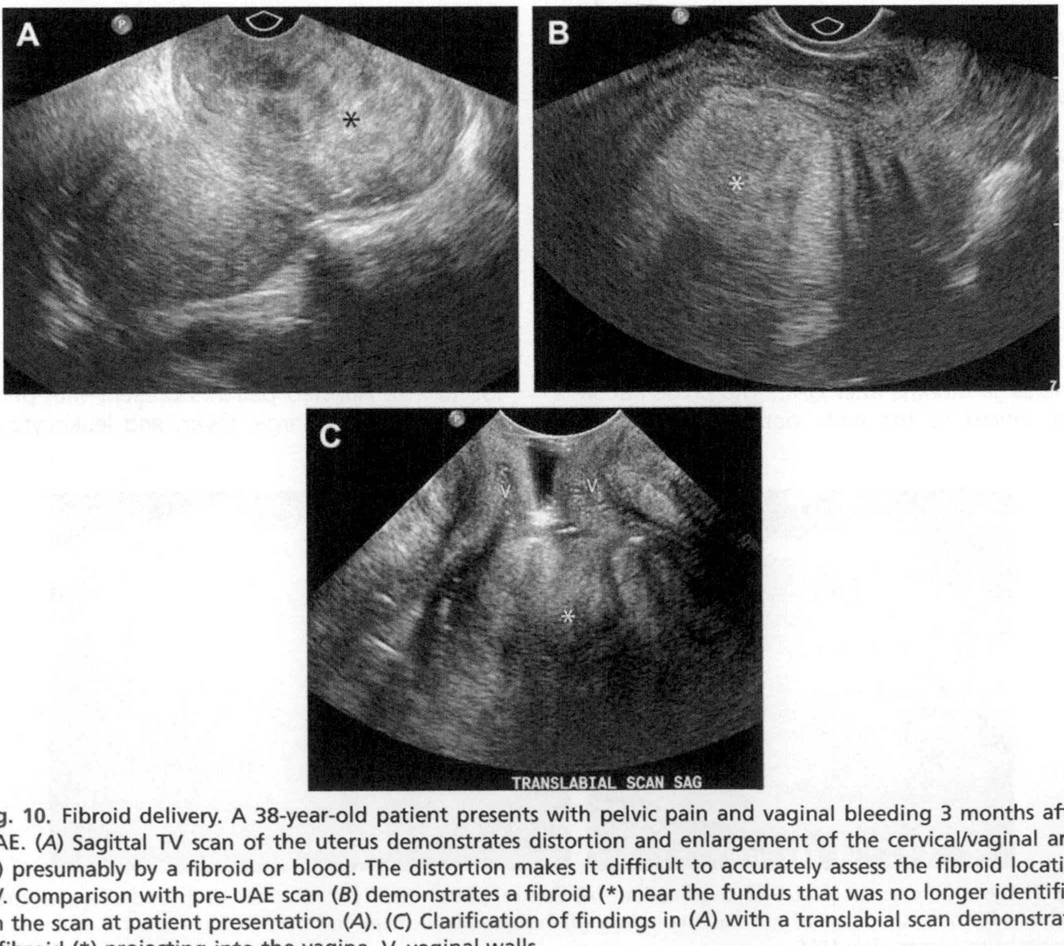

Fig. 10. Fibroid delivery. A 38-year-old patient presents with pelvic pain and vaginal bleeding 3 months after UAE. (*A*) Sagittal TV scan of the uterus demonstrates distortion and enlargement of the cervical/vaginal area (*) presumably by a fibroid or blood. The distortion makes it difficult to accurately assess the fibroid location TV. Comparison with pre-UAE scan (*B*) demonstrates a fibroid (*) near the fundus that was no longer identified on the scan at patient presentation (*A*). (*C*) Clarification of findings in (*A*) with a translabial scan demonstrates a fibroid (*) projecting into the vagina. V, vaginal walls.

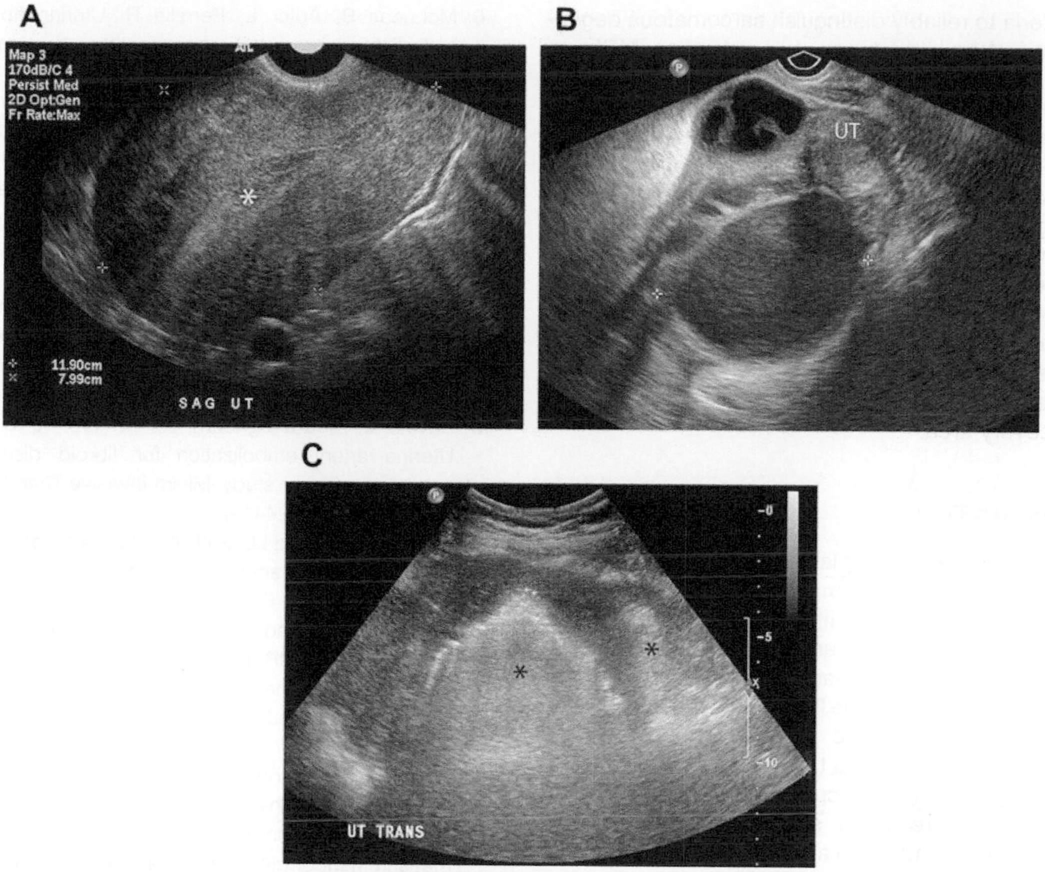

Fig. 11. Infectious complications of UAE. (*A*) Post-UAE patient with pelvic pain and discharge 1 week after UAE. Sagittal TVUS demonstrating uterine enlargement and complex fluid (*) within the uterine cavity compatible with endometritis. (*B*) TVUS of the right adnexa demonstrating a thick-walled complex cystic mass (calipers) compatible with a tubo-ovarian abscess in a patient presenting with pain and fever after UAE. UT, uterus. (*C*) Transabdominal TVUS of the uterus demonstrating diffuse increased echogenicity (*) with "dirty" shadowing due to gas within infected fibroids compatible with pyomyoma.

perfusion is also supplemented by collateral flow from ovarian, round ligament, cervical, and other pelvic vessels. Uterine necrosis has been associated with intrauterine abscess formation. Patients with abscess present with pelvic pain, vaginal discharge, fever, or leukocytosis. Hysterectomy is often required for treatment.[64] Two of the deaths reported in the first 30 days after UAE were due to uterine infection.[54,55]

Deep vein thrombosis after UAE has a reported prevalence of less than 1%.[65] This may be related to compression on large draining pelvic veins by the uterus. Resultant venous stasis leads to thrombus formation. Color Doppler sonography is the first-line modality for imaging patients with suspicion of deep vein thrombosis. The presence of thrombus within the venous lumen limits compressibility, is hypo- to hyperechoic, and may expand the vein. The spectral waveform may be dampened. Isolated reports of pulmonary embolism after UAE are in the literature with at least 1 resulting in death.[56] Both entities are treated with anticoagulation therapy.

Loss of ovarian function has been associated with UAE in up to 14 % of patients. It seems related to patient age with a higher risk in those over 45 years old.[66,67] This is thought to be related to fewer remaining oocytes at this age, which are especially vulnerable to ischemia. As embolic particles are injected into a uterine artery, the particles can migrate through anastomotic channels into the ovarian arterial vasculature, compromising ovarian perfusion.[68]

Continued growth of presumed fibroids after a technically successful embolization procedure may indicate the presence of an underlying malignancy. In this case, more definitive therapy is indicated. At least 4 cases have been reported of leiomyosarcoma discovered after UAE.[53,69–71] There are currently no published US imaging criteria to reliably distinguish sarcomatous degeneration from other types of degeneration. MRI may be helpful to distinguish fibroids from uterine sarcoma; however, there are few published data to support this.[72]

Puncture site complications are not specific to UAE because they can be associated with any angiographic procedure. These include hematoma, pseudoaneurysm, arterial dissection, and arteriovenofistula related to guide wire perforation of the arteries. These can be diagnosed sonographically. The portability of US is especially useful in this setting because patients may be imaged immediately after the procedure in the recovery area.

SUMMARY

As UAE takes its place among the treatment choices for symptomatic fibroids, radiologists need to be familiar with the pre–work-up issues, postprocedural appearance of the uterus and fibroids, and UAE-associated complications, some of which may be life threatening. Knowledge of their sonographic features should lead to prompt diagnosis and treatment.

Early studies have suggested that MRI may be helpful in predicting success of UAE. US is, however, readily available, inexpensive, and portable and should be considered as a first-line modality in the work-up of uterine fibroids for embolization. It is a cost-effective modality for repeated follow-up of patients, especially because overall volume rather than specific fibroids can be followed. US is also effective in detecting most of the commonly recognized complications that are associated with UAE.

REFERENCES

1. Ravina JH, Herbreteau D, Ciraru-Vigneron N, et al. Arterial embolization to treat uterine myomata. Lancet 1995;356:671–2.
2. Goodwin SC, Vedantham S, McLucas B, et al. Preliminary experience with uterine artery embolization for uterine fibroids. J Vasc Interv Radiol 1997;8: 517–26.
3. Spies JB, Scialli AR, Jha RC, et al. Initial results from uterine fibroid embolization for symptomatic leiomyomata. J Vasc Interv Radiol 1999;10:1149–57.
4. Messina ML, Bozzini N, Halbe HW, et al. Uterine artery embolization for the treatment of uterine leiomyomata. Int J Gynaecol Obstet 2002;79: 11–6.
5. Walker WJ, Pelage JP, Sutton C. Fibroid embolization. Clin Radiol 2002;57:325–31.
6. McLucas B, Adler L, Perrella R. Uterine fibroid embolization: nonsurgical treatment for symptomatic fibroids. J Am Coll Surg 2001;192:95–105.
7. Spies JB, Ascher SA, Roth AR, et al. Uterine artery embolization for leiomyomata. Obstet Gynecol 2001;98:29–34.
8. Walker WJ, Pelage JP. Uterine artery embolization for symptomatic fibroids: clinical results in 400 women with imaging follow-up. BJOG 2002;109: 1262–72.
9. Pron G, Bennett J, Common A, et al. The Ontario Uterine Fibroid Embolization Trial. II. Uterine fibroid reduction and symptom relief after uterine artery embolization for fibroids. Fertil Steril 2003;79:120–7.
10. Ravina J, Ciraru-Vigneron N, Aymard A, et al. Uterine artery embolization for fibroid disease: results of a 6-year study. Minim Invasive Ther Allied Technol 1999;8(6):441–7.
11. Ascher SM, Arnold LL, Patt RH, et al. Adenomyosis: prospective comparison of MR imaging and transvaginal sonography. Radiology 1994;190:803–6.
12. Omary RA, Vasireddy S, Chrisman HB, et al. The effect of pelvic MR imaging on the diagnosis and treatment of women with presumed symptomatic uterine fibroids. J Vasc Interv Radiol 2002;13: 1149–53.
13. Dueholm M, Lundorf E, Hansen ES, et al. Accuracy of magnetic resonance imaging and transvaginal ultrasonography in the diagnosis, mapping and measurement of uterine myomas. Am J Obstet Gynecol 2002;186:409–15.
14. deSouza NM, Williams AD. Uterine arterial embolization for leiomyomas: perfusion and volume changes at MR imaging and relation to clinical outcome. Radiology 2002;222:367–74.
15. Burn PR, McCall JM, Chinn RJ, et al. Uterine fibroleiomyoma: MR imaging appearances before and after embolization of uterine arteries. Radiology 2000;214:729–34.
16. Pelage JP, Guaou NG, Jha RC, et al. Uterine fibroid tumors: long-term MR imaging outcome after embolization. Radiology 2004;230:803–9.
17. Katsumori T, Nakajima K, Tokuhiro M. Gadolinium-enhanced MR imaging in the evaluation of uterine fibroids treated with uterine artery embolization. AJR Am J Roentgenol 2001;177:303–7.
18. Kliewer MA, Hertzberg BS, George PY. Acoustic shadowing from uterine leiomyomas: sonographic-pathologic correlation. Radiology 1995; 196:99–102.
19. Davis PC, O'Neill MJ, Yoder IC, et al. Sonohysterographic findings of endometrial and subendometrial conditions. Radiographics 2002;22:803–16.
20. Lev-Toaff AS, Toaff ME, Liu JB, et al. Value of sonohysterography in the diagnosis and management of abnormal uterine bleeding. Radiology 1996;201: 179–84.

21. Becker E Jr, Lev-Toaff AS, Kaufman EP, et al. The added value of transvaginal sonohysterography over transvaginal sonography alone in women with known or suspected leiomyoma. J Ultrasound Med 2002;21:237–47.
22. Gross BH, Silver TM, Jaffe MH. Sonographic features of uterine leiomyomas: analysis of 41 proven cases. J Ultrasound Med 1983;2:401–6.
23. Weintraub JL, Romano WJ, Kirsch MJ, et al. Uterine artery embolization: sonographic imaging findings. J Ultrasound Med 2002;21:633–7.
24. Bree RL, Bowerman RA, Bohm-Velez M, et al. US evaluation of the uterus in patients with postmenopausal bleeding: a positive effect on diagnostic decision-making. Radiology 2000;216: 260–4.
25. Dueholm M, Forman A, Jensen ML, et al. Transvaginal sonography combined with saline contrast sonohysterography in evaluating the uterine cavity in premenopausal patients with abnormal uterine bleeding. Ultrasound Obstet Gynecol 2001;18: 54–61.
26. Hovsepian DM, Siskin GP, Bonn J, et al. Quality improvement guidelines for uterine artery embolization for symptomatic leiomyomata. J Vasc Interv Radiol 2001;12:1011–20.
27. Ghai S, Rajan DK, Benjamin MS, et al. Uterine artery embolization for leiomyomas: pre-and postprocedural evaluation with US. Radiographics 2005;25: 1159–76.
28. Tranquart F, Brunereau L, Cottier JP, et al. Prospective sonographic assessment of uterine artery embolization for the treatment of fibroids. Ultrasound Obstet Gynecol 2002;19:81–7.
29. Goodwin SC, Bonilla SM, Sack D, et al. Reporting standards for uterine artery embolization for the treatment of uterine leiomyomata. J Vasc Interv Radiol 2001;12:1011–20.
30. Goodwin SC, Wong GC. Uterine artery embolization for uterine fibroids: a radiologist's perspective. Clin Obstet Gynecol 2001;44:412–24.
31. Nikolic B, Spies JB, Abbara S, et al. Ovarian artery supply of uterine fibroids as a cause of treatment failure after uterine artery embolization: a case report. J Vasc Interv Radiol 1999;10:1167–70.
32. Katsumuri T, Akazawa K, Mihara T. Uterine artery embolization for pedunculated subserosal fibroids. AJR Am J Roentgenol 2005;184:399–402.
33. Muniz CJ, Fleischer AC, Donnelly AF, et al. Three-dimensional color Doppler sonography and uterine artery arteriography of fibroids: assessment of changes in vascularity before and after embolization. J Ultrasound Med 2002;21:129–33.
34. Fleischer AC, Donnelly EF, Campbell MG, et al. Three-dimensional color Doppler sonography before and after fibroid embolization. J Ultrasound Med 2000;19:701–5.
35. McLucas B, Perrella R, Goodwin S, et al. Role of uterine artery Doppler flow in fibroid embolization. J Ultrasound Med 2002;21:113–20.
36. Outwater EK, Siegelman ES, Van Deerlin V. Adenomyosis: current concepts and imaging considerations. Am J Roentgenol 1998;170:437–41.
37. Reinhold C, Atri M, Mehio A, et al. Diffuse uterine adenomyosis: morphologic criteria and diagnostic accuracy of endovaginal sonography. Radiology 1995;197:609–14.
38. Reinhold C, Tafazoli F, Mehio A, et al. Uterine adenomyosis: endovaginal US and MR imaging features with histopathologic correlation. Radiographics 1999;19(Spec No):S147–160.
39. Fedele L, Bianchi S, Dorta M, et al. Transvaginal ultrasonography in the diagnosis of diffuse adenomyosis. Fertil Steril 1992;58:94–7.
40. Atri M, Reinhold C, Mehio AR, et al. Adenomyosis: US features with histologic correlation in an in-vitro study. Radiology 2000;215:783–90.
41. Kuligowska E, Deeds L III, Lu K III. Pelvic pain: overlooked and underdiagnosed gynecologic conditions. Radiographics 2005;25:3–20.
42. Lyons EA. Ultrasound evaluation of bleeding in the non-pregnant patient. Presented at the 102nd Annual Meeting of the American Roentgen Ray Society. Atlanta (GA), April 28–May 3, 2002.
43. Chiang CH, Chang MY, Hsu JJ, et al. Tumor vascular pattern and blood flow impedance in the differential diagnosis of leiomyoma and adenomyosis by color Doppler sonography. J Assist Reprod Genet 1999; 16:268–75.
44. Botsis D, Kassanos D, Antoniou G, et al. Adenomyoma and leiomyoma: differential diagnosis with transvaginal sonography. J Clin Ultrasound 1998;26: 21–5.
45. Siskin GP, Tublin ME, Stainken BF, et al. Uterine artery embolization for the treatment of adenomyosis: clinical response and evaluation with MR imaging. AJR Am J Roentgenol 2001;177:297–302.
46. Jha RC, Takahama J, Imaoka I, et al. Adenomyosis: MRI of the uterus treated with uterine artery embolization. AJR Am J Roentgenol 2003;181:851–6.
47. Worthington-Kirsch RL, Popky GL, Hutchins FL Jr. Uterine arterial embolization for the management of leiomyomas: quality-of-life assessment and clinical response. Radiology 1998;208:625–9.
48. Vott S, Bonilla SM, Goodwin SC, et al. CT findings after uterine artery embolization. J Comput Assist Tomogr 2000;24:846–8.
49. Stein LA, Valenti D. Soft- tissue case 36: ischemic necrosis of a large uterine fibroid after embolization. Can J Surg 2000;43:410 467.
50. Nicholson TA, Pelage JP, Ettles DF. Fibroid calcification after uterine artery embolization: ultrasonographic appearance and pathology. J Vasc Interv Radiol 2001;12:443–6.

51. Nott V, Reidy J, Forman R, et al. Complications of fibroid embolization. Minim Invasive Ther Allied Technol 1999;8:421–4.
52. Pinto I, Chimeno P, Romo A, et al. Uterine fibroids: uterine artery embolization versus abdominal hysterectomy for treatment – a prospective, randomized, and controlled clinical trial. Radiology 2003;226:425–31.
53. Spies JB, Spector A, Roth AR, et al. Complications after uterine artery embolization for leiomyomas. Obstet Gynecol 2002;100:873–80.
54. Vashist A, Studd J, Carey A, et al. Fatal septicemia after fibroid embolization. Lancet 1999;354:307–8.
55. De Blok S, de Vries C, Prinssen HM, et al. Fatal sepsis after uterine artery embolization with microspheres. J Vasc Interv Radiol 2003;14:779–83.
56. Lanocita R, Frigerio LF, Patelli G, et al. A fatal complication of percutaneous transcatheter embolization for treatment of uterine fibroids [abstract]. Presented at the 11th Annual Meeting of the Society for Minimally Invasive Therapy. Boston (MA), September 16–18,1999.
57. Laverge F, D'Angelo A, Davies NJ, et al. Spontaneous expulsion of three large fibroids after uterine artery embolization. Fertil Steril 2003;80:450–2.
58. Abbara S, Spies JB, Scialli AR, et al. Transcervical expulsion of a fibroid as a result of uterine artery embolization for leiomyomata. J Vasc Interv Radiol 1999;10:409–11.
59. Brunereou L, Herbreteau D, Gallas S, et al. Uterine artery embolization in the primary treatment of uterine leiomyomas: technical features and prospective follow-up with clinical and sonographic examinations in 58 patients. AJR Am J Roentgenol 2000;175:1267–72.
60. Braude P, Reidy J, Nott V, et al. Embolization of uterine leiomyomata: current concepts in management. Hum Reprod Update 2000;6:603–8.
61. Rajan DK, Beecroft JR, Clark TW, et al. Risk of intrauterine infectious complications after uterine artery embolization. J Vasc Interv Radiol 2004;15:1415–21.
62. Nalaboff KM, Pellerito JS, Ben-Levi E. Imaging the endometrium: disease and normal variants. Radiographics 2001;21:1409–24.
63. Nikolic B, Nguyen K, Martin LG, et al. Pyosalpinx developing from a preexisting hydrosalpinx after uterine artery embolization. J Vasc Interv Radiol 2004;15:297–301.
64. Godfrey CD, Zbella EA. Uterine necrosis after uterine artery embolization for leiomyoma. Obstet Gynecol 2001;98:950–2.
65. Kitamura Y, Ascher SM, Cooper CJ, et al. Imaging manifestations of complications associated with uterine artery embolization. Radiographics 2005;25:S119–132.
66. Payne JF, Robboy SJ, Haney AF. Embolic microspheres within ovarian arterial vasculature after uterine artery embolization. Obstet Gynecol 2002;100:883–6.
67. Chrisman HB, Saker MB, Ryu RK, et al. The impact of uterine fibroid embolization on resumption of menses and ovarian function. J Vasc Interv Radiol 2000;11:699–703.
68. Razavi MK, Wolanske KA, Hwang GL, et al. Angiographic classification of ovarian artery-to-uterine artery anastomosis: initial observations in uterine fibroid embolization. Radiology 2002;224:707–12.
69. Marret H, Alonso AM, Cottier JP, et al. Leiomyoma recurrence after uterine artery embolization. J Vasc Interv Radiol 2003;14:1395–9.
70. Joyce A, Hessami S, Heller D. Leiomyosarcoma after uterine artery embolization: a case report. J Reprod Med 2001;46:278–80.
71. D'Angelo A, Amso NN, Wood A. Uterine leiomyosarcoma discovered after uterine artery embolization. J Obstet Gynaecol 2003;23:686–7.
72. Wolfman DJ, Kishimoto K, Sala E, et al. Distinguishing uterine sarcoma from leiomyoma on magnetic resonance imaging [abstract]. Presented at the RSNA 95th Scientific Assembly and Annual Meeting. Chicago (IL), November 29–December 4, 2009.

Applications of Ultrasound in Gynecologic Oncology

Darcy J. Wolfman, MD*, Sandra J. Allison, MD

KEYWORDS

- Gynecologic oncology • Ultrasound
- Gynecologic imaging • Gynecologic malignancy

In patients with gynecologic malignancy, ultrasound (US) has many established applications, including the diagnosis and staging of ovarian cancer, endometrial cancer, and gestational trophoblastic disease (GTD); detection of recurrent and/or metastatic disease, including ovarian and cervical cancer and GTD; and diagnosis and guidance for treatment of postoperative complications.

DIAGNOSIS AND STAGING OF GYNECOLOGIC MALIGNANCY

Ovarian Cancer

US is considered the initial imaging modality of choice to help distinguish a benign ovarian lesion from a malignant one. Although a likely benign lesion can be followed or removed by a general gynecologist, suspicion of a malignant ovarian mass should initiate referral to a gynecologic oncologist who can better perform the more complex therapeutic and staging surgery for ovarian carcinoma. Morphologic features remain the primary US criteria for differentiating benign from malignant ovarian masses. Hence, transvaginal ultrasound (TVS) is the critical US imaging approach because of the improved spatial and soft tissue resolution afforded by the higher frequency endovaginal probe. Nonetheless, transabdominal US remains an important, complementary component of this US examination when a larger field of view is required. For example, if a lesion is displaced out of the pelvis or is so large that it is incompletely visualized by TVS. In addition, transabdominal imaging is required for evaluation of secondary findings in ovarian cancer, such as ascites, peritoneal implants, and hydronephrosis. These secondary findings are important not only because they can confirm the suspicion of a malignant ovarian mass, but these findings are also necessary for staging a malignant ovarian mass.

Numerous studies have reported that when strict US criteria and a pattern recognition approach for identification of benign ovarian masses are used, US has a nearly 95% to 99% negative predictive value in excluding malignancy.[1–7] US features consistent with benign etiology include smooth, thin walls; few, thin septations; and absence of solid components or mural nodularity. Besides specific US features that suggest a benign etiology, several benign etiologies are diagnosed by pattern recognition. Simple cysts will be anechoic with a smooth, thin wall and posterior acoustic enhancement. Endometriomas often contain uniform low-level echoes but should still demonstrate a smooth, thin wall, increased through transmission, and no internal vascularity. Hemorrhagic cysts may have characteristic lace-like internal echoes. The internal echogenicity of

Department of Radiology, Georgetown University Hospital, 3800 Reservoir Road, NW, Washington, DC 20007, USA
* Corresponding author. Department of Radiology, Georgetown University Hospital, 3800 Reservoir Road, NW, Washington, DC 20007.
E-mail address: darcywolfman@yahoo.com

Ultrasound Clin 5 (2010) 289–298
doi:10.1016/j.cult.2010.03.003
1556-858X/10/$ – see front matter

hemorrhagic cysts may be quite complex and even irregular; however, the appearance of the internal echoes will change over time and internal vascularity should never be noted. Several US patterns associated with dermoid cysts have been described including uniform increased echogenicity with posterior acoustic attenuation, echogenic shadowing mural nodules, and layering with or without floating debris.

Conversely, mural nodules, mural thickening or irregularity, solid components, and thick septations (>3 mm) suggest malignancy (**Fig. 1**). Although these morphologic features have a high sensitivity for malignancy, the specificity is low.[1–7] The low specificity reflects overlap in the imaging appearance of benign and malignant lesions. For example, benign lesions such as hemorrhagic cysts, cystadenomas, or cystadenofibromas may have thick septations and apparent mural nodules and Brenner's tumors, fibromas, and fibrothecomas are solid but benign. Furthermore, pedunculated fibroids, dermoids, and endometriomas can masquerade as solid ovarian lesions. Even with the low specificity of these morphologic features, if US findings suggestive of a malignant ovarian mass are seen, further evaluation is mandatory.

The use of color and pulse Doppler in the evaluation of ovarian masses is controversial. Some investigators consider blood flow characteristics to be merely confirmatory whereas others consider the Doppler examination to be a helpful discriminator.[8–11] Increased number of often tortuous vessels with arteriovenous shunts is characteristic of tumor neovascularity. Malignant neovascularity lacks the normal amount of smooth muscle cells in the vessel walls. Researchers had hoped that Doppler evaluation, which could potentially assess vascular compliance or resistance as well as vessel morphology, density, and distribution, would be helpful in characterizing ovarian masses. Malignant lesions more often demonstrate increased vessel density and tortuosity than benign lesions, but significant overlap exists. Malignant ovarian lesions also tend to demonstrate higher peak systolic velocities and lower resistive indices than benign masses, but again, considerable overlap exists and no discriminatory cutoff values are accepted.[8–11]

Three-dimensional (3D) US is a new imaging technique that may improve characterization of adnexal masses. Several studies have shown that 3D power Doppler US improved specificity and positive predictive value compared with conventional 2D US[12,13]; however, other studies have shown no added value with 3D power Doppler US compared with conventional 2D US.[14] Further research is needed with this technique to better define its role in the characterization of adnexal masses.

Scoring systems have been proposed to standardize evaluation of ovarian masses in an attempt to improve specificity.[15–17] Brown and colleagues[17] used a stepwise logistic regression analysis to determine the most discriminating gray-scale and Doppler sonographic features of malignancy. They reported that a multiparameter approach, which assessed for nonhyperechoic solid components, central blood flow on color Doppler, ascites, and thick septations, had a 93% sensitivity and specificity for malignancy. To achieve 100% sensitivity, specificity dropped to 86% in this study.[17] However, Timmerman and colleagues[18] reported similar sensitivity and specificity and interobserver variability when readers used subjective criteria for evaluating ovarian masses rather than a standardized approach.

US has a limited role in the staging of ovarian cancer; however, US can be used to detect the presence of ascites, peritoneal implants, and

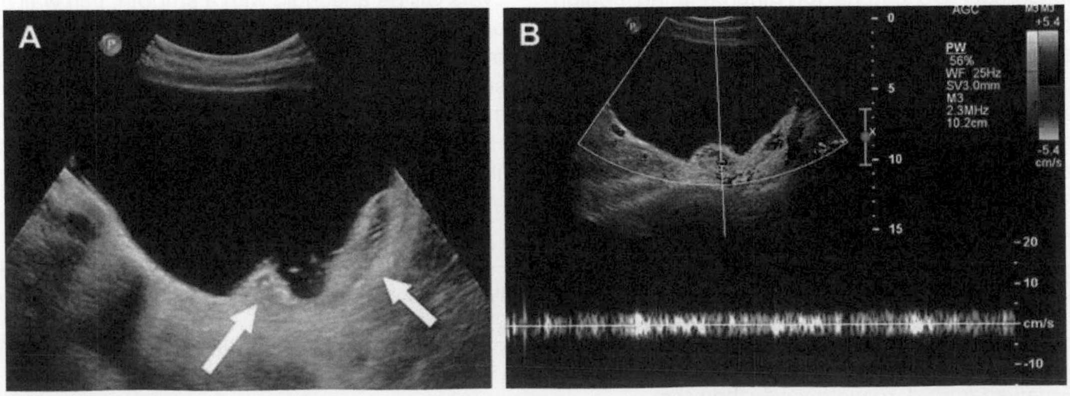

Fig. 1. Ovarian cancer. Transvaginal gray-scale (*A*) and color Doppler (*B*) images demonstrating a cystic lesion with mural nodularity (*white arrow* in *A*) with color flow (*B*).

hydronephrosis. These findings are not only useful for the staging of ovarian cancer, they can be used to confirm the malignant nature of an indeterminate adnexal mass. Transabdominal US is an excellent modality for identifying ascites (**Fig. 2**A) and hydronephrosis and can be used to guide biopsy, paracentesis, or renal collecting system stent placement; however, detection of peritoneal disease by transabdominal US is limited (see **Fig. 2**B). Although the specificity of US in documenting peritoneal spread of disease is slightly higher than CT or MR, the sensitivity for the detection of implants smaller than 2 cm is low.[19,20] If an indeterminate adnexal mass is found, it is worthwhile to evaluate for peritoneal spread of disease with US because a positive finding will limit the need for further imaging and initiate referral to a gynecologic oncologist. A negative result, however, should not be taken as proof that peritoneal implants are not present.

Endometrial Cancer

Endometrial biopsy and/or dilation and curettage has traditionally been the gold standard for histologic diagnosis of endometrial pathology. However, if routine endometrial sampling were performed in all women with postmenopausal bleeding, only 1 of every 10 samples would be expected to be positive. In addition, significant sampling error has been reported with false-negative rates ranging from 2% to 6%.[21–26] To decrease unnecessary endometrial biopsies, screening patients with postmenopausal bleeding with TVS and/or sono-hysterography (SHG) has been advocated.[27–33]

Double-layer endometrial thickness greater than 4 or 5 mm on TVS is used as the sole US criterion for determining whether endometrial sampling is warranted in postmenopausal patients (**Fig. 3**).[27,28] This endometrial thickness is based on numerous trials that looked to establish a threshold endometrial thickness in postmenopausal patients below which endometrial pathology is unlikely. However, the specificity of this criterion is low, ranging from 59% to 63%.[28,34]

When endometrial thickness is greater then 5 mm, endometrial sampling is suggested not only because of increased posttest probability of endometrial carcinoma but also because of the inability of TVS and/or SHG to differentiate accurately between benign and malignant causes of endometrial thickening.[29,35–38] In a meta-analysis of 35 articles including 5892 women, Smith-Bindman and colleagues[28] reported that when using a cutoff of 5 mm for endometrial thickness, 96% of women with endometrial cancer had an abnormal TVS. In this series, a woman with a 10% pretest probability of endometrial carcinoma and a negative TVS had a posttest probability of endometrial carcinoma of only 1%. They concluded that TVS is highly accurate in identifying a subgroup of patients at extremely low risk, obviating the need for endometrial sampling in these patients.

In women taking hormone replacement therapy (HRT), the specificity of the 5-mm cutoff is even lower, as HRT increases endometrial thickness. However, because the pretest probability of endometrial carcinoma is also likely increased in these patients, the same cutoff value of 4 or 5 mm is generally used. In women on sequential HRT regimens, scanning should be performed after the progesterone part of the cycle when the endometrium is expected to be at its thinnest.

Investigators have attempted to correlate the morphology of the endometrium on US with

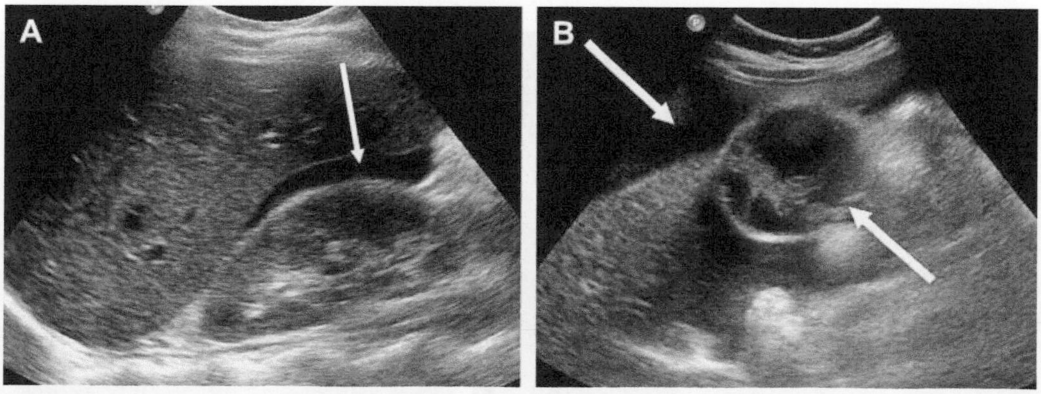

Fig. 2. Ascites and peritoneal implant secondary to ovarian cancer. Transabdominal gray-scale images demonstrating ascites (*white arrows* in *A* and *B*) and peritoneal implant (*white arrows* in *B*) in a patient with an indeterminate adnexal mass.

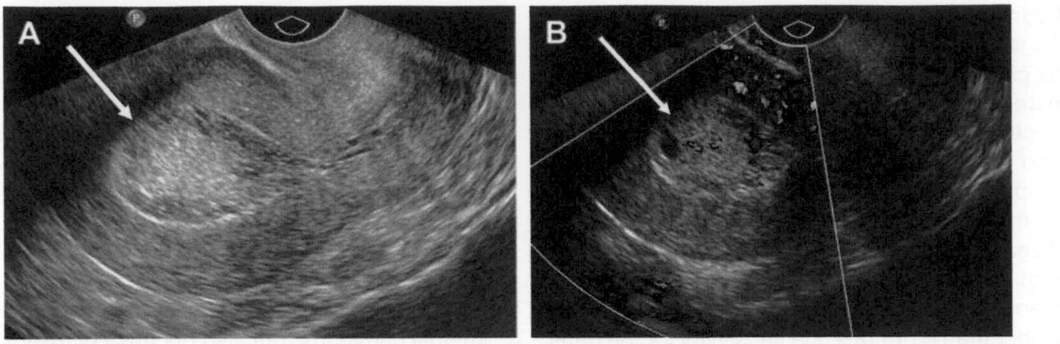

Fig. 3. Thickened endometrium. Transvaginal gray-scale (*A*) and color Doppler (*B*) images of a thickened endometrium (*white arrows*).

histology to increase specificity. Endometrial cancer tends to be an irregular, heterogeneous mass, whereas endometrial hyperplasia tends to be more homogeneous and echogenic. Cystic areas within the endometrium are more often associated with polyps, cystic endometrial hyperplasia, or tamoxifen use,[39–41] rather than with endometrial carcinoma. Still, considerable overlap exists between these morphologic features. The most specific, and only reliable, US finding for endometrial carcinoma is invasion of the myometrium or disruption of the subendometrial halo by an endometrial mass (**Fig. 4**).

On SHG, endometrial carcinoma is most commonly depicted as a broad-based, irregular mass.[37] Difficulty in distending the endometrial cavity has also been described.[42] Three-dimensional SHG has been reported to be more accurate than either TVS or 2D SHG for the diagnosis of endometrial carcinoma. Endometrial volume and thickness are reported to be higher in patients with postmenopausal bleeding and endometrial carcinoma than in patients without endometrial carcinoma[43]; however, no specific thresholds have been established.

Doppler US has not been shown to be useful in distinguishing benign from malignant endometrial pathology as a wide range of peak systolic velocities and resistive indices have been reported for benign and malignant endometrial pathology.[44] Benign endometrial polyps are more likely to have a single feeding vessel, whereas cancers more often have numerous feeding vessels and generalized increased vascularity.[45]

Depth of myometrial invasion is an important aspect of staging endometrial cancer. Further, depth of myometrial invasion is often used by gynecologic oncologists to decide whether to perform pelvic lymph node dissection in patients with known endometrial cancer; as depth of myometrial invasion is one of the most important factors associated with lymph node metastasis.[46] Unfortunately, evaluation of depth of myometrial invasion with 2D TVS has yielded varying results compared with MR, which is considered the gold standard. A recent article, however, showed that

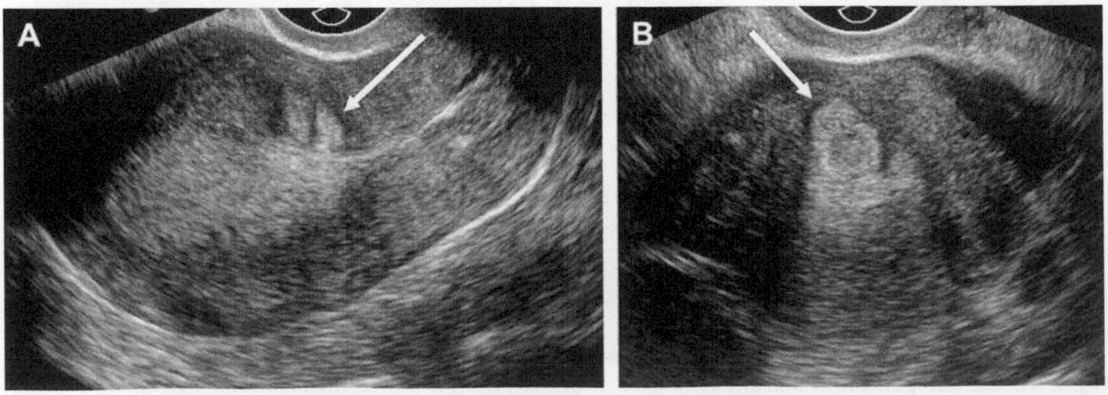

Fig. 4. Endometrial cancer. Long (*A*) and coronal (*B*) transvaginal gray-scale images demonstrating a thickened endometrium with myometrial invasion (*white arrows*) diagnostic of endometrial cancer.

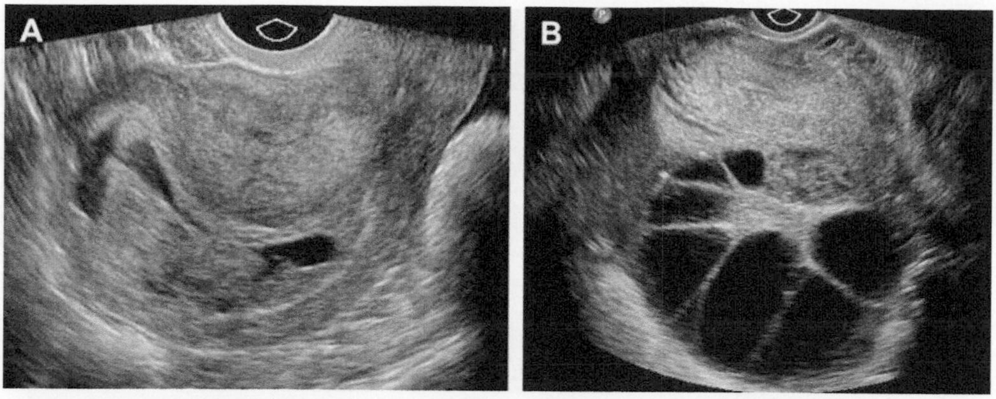

Fig. 5. Gestational trophoblastic disease. Transvaginal gray-scale image (*A*) demonstrates an echogenic mass expanding the endometrial canal in a patient with a positive beta-hcg. Transvaginal gray-scale image of the right ovary (*B*) in the same patient with multiple enlarged cysts, compatible with theca-leutin cysts.

3D TVS improved the accuracy in predicting depth of myometrial invasion compared with conventional 2D US.[47] Although more research in this area is needed, 3D TVS looks promising to evaluate for depth of myometrial invasion before surgery.

Gestational Trophoblastic Disease

TVS is considered the study of choice in the evaluation of suspected GTD. In patients with GTD, TVS examination most commonly demonstrates an echogenic, heterogeneous mass with cystic spaces distending the endometrial cavity (**Fig. 5**A).[48–53] In the case of complete hydatidiform mole, the cystic spaces correspond to the hydropic villi.[48,49] GTD is usually extremely vascular, demonstrating increased vessel density and an abnormal uterine arterial waveform characterized by high peak systolic velocity and high diastolic blood flow (low RI) compared with the normal uterine arterial waveform.[50–53] Irregularity of the border of the mass or asymmetric extension of the mass into the myometrium suggests myometrial invasion.

With GTD, the ovaries may become enlarged with numerous theca lutein cysts (**Fig. 5**B). This ovarian enlargement can result in symptomatic ovarian torsion or hemorrhage.[54,55] However, theca lutein cysts may not be detected in the early stages of the disease.[50,52]

DETECTION OF RECURRENT OR METASTATIC DISEASE

Ovarian Cancer

US plays a limited role in the detection of recurrent ovarian cancer, with the greatest sensitivity in detecting recurrent tumor in the pelvis or around the liver and right hemidiaphragm in the setting of ascites.[56] The sensitivity of US in detecting microscopic disease, miliary peritoneal seeding, and macroscopic disease smaller than 2 cm of the peritoneum and/or omentum is poor.[56,57]

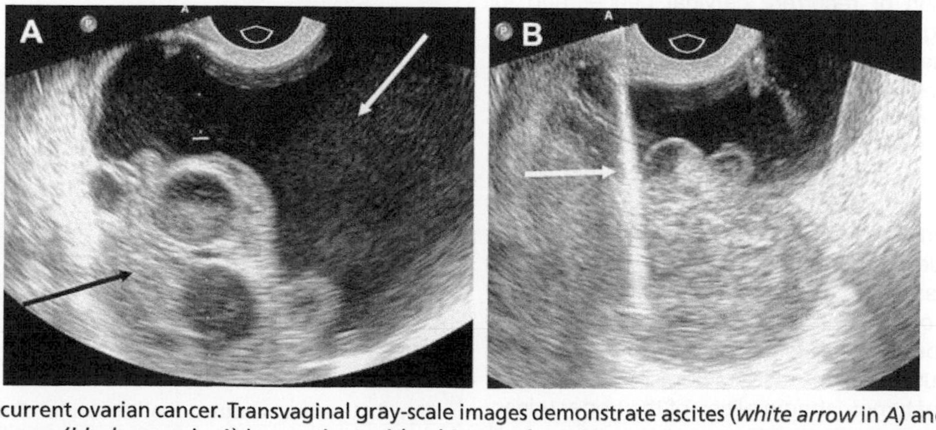

Fig. 6. Recurrent ovarian cancer. Transvaginal gray-scale images demonstrate ascites (*white arrow* in *A*) and a solid and cystic mass (*black arrow* in *A*) in a patient with a history of ovarian cancer. Transvaginal biopsy of the lesion was performed (*white arrow* in *B*).

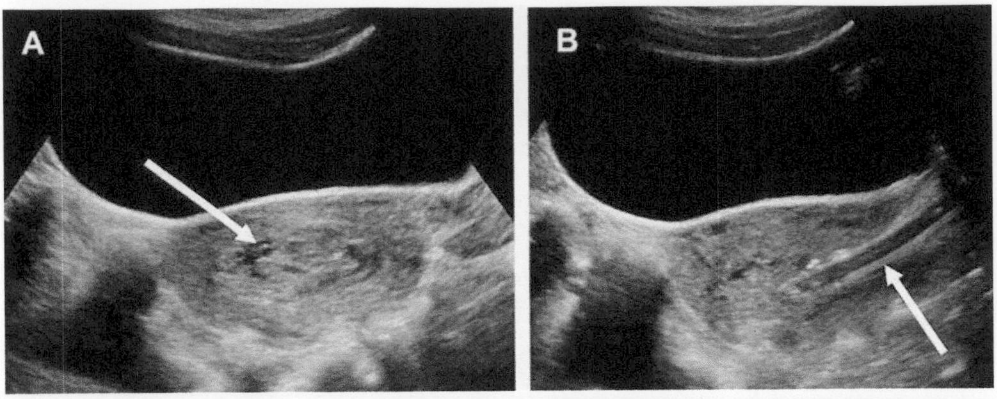

Fig. 7. Recurrent GTD. Transabdominal gray-scale image showing an echogenic mass in a patient with a history of GTD (*arrow* in *A*). Transabdominal US was used to help guide methotrexate injection (*arrow* in *B*).

Additionally, small, plaquelike lesions on the pelvic peritoneum or lesions high in the false pelvis are often missed on US.[57] Therefore, US is not sufficient to replace second-look laparotomy (which is still performed in some centers) or CT in making patient-management decisions.[56] Despite these limitations, US is more accurate than clinical examination[56,57] and can be used to confirm a clinical suspicion of gross recurrent disease (**Fig. 6**A). US can also be used to guide biopsy areas of suspected recurrence (**Fig. 6**B).

New-onset ascites in a patient with a history of ovarian cancer is a worrisome finding and one that is easily diagnosed with US. Further, US can be used to guide paracentesis.

Cervical Cancer

Cervical cancer is diagnosed by physical examination and pap smear and, therefore, US has a limited role in the evaluation of cervical cancer. Transrectal ultrasound (TRUS) has a role, albeit small, in the evaluation of recurrent cervical cancer and for biopsy guidance in selected patients.[58,59] Reports from one study indicate that in approximately 25% of cases, TRUS provides information that is complementary to that obtained from CT. TRUS is most likely to be helpful in patients with small-volume recurrence in areas of previous irradiation.[58] Unfortunately, differentiation between radiation fibrosis and recurrent disease cannot be made on the basis of sonographic soft tissue appearance or Doppler vascularity. TRUS-guided biopsy of these areas can be performed. Furthermore, because of its limited field of view, TRUS is not useful in the assessment of the cephalic extent of tumor, abnormalities of the upper urinary tract, or the presence of extrapelvic metastases.[58] Transabdominal imaging can serve to screen for hydronephrosis and guide ureteral stent placement.

Gestational Trophoblastic Disease

US can be used to assess for persistent or recurrent GTD by documenting an endometrial mass. Persistent GTD can be treated with US-guided direct injection of methotrexate (**Fig. 7**).[60]

GTD is the most common cause of uterine vascular malformations. These vascular malformations usually present after treatment is complete and can be easily diagnosed with US (**Fig. 8**). Recently, it has been shown that these vascular malformations can be treated with uterine artery embolization.[61]

DIAGNOSIS OF POSTTREATMENT COMPLICATIONS

Following radiation therapy or surgery, patients with gynecologic malignancy may present with complications. US can be useful for the diagnosis of multiple complications, but also for treatment guidance.

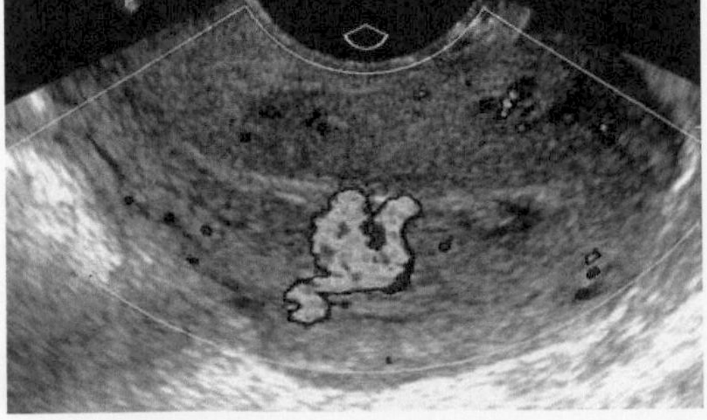

Fig. 8. Uterine vascular malformation. Transvaginal color Doppler image demonstrating a vascular malformation in a patient with a history of GTD.

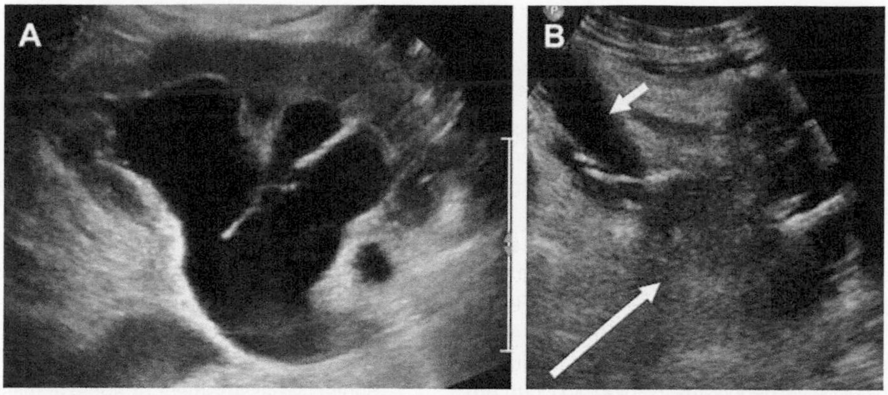

Fig. 9. Hydronephrosis and hydroureter. Gray-scale images demonstrate hydronephrosis in a patient with a history of ovarian cancer (*A*) and dilated ureter (*short white arrow* in *B*) with obstruction by a soft tissue mass in the pelvis (*long arrow* in *B*), proven to be recurrent ovarian cancer.

In the gastrointestinal tract, abscesses may develop following radiation therapy or surgery secondary to bowel leak. Although CT is considered the first-line imaging modality, US can be used to diagnose focal fluid collections in the setting of suspected bowel leak. Once a collection has been identified, US can be used to guide placement of a percutaneous drainage catheter in the collection, which is considered the treatment of choice.[62]

Multiple complications of the urinary system can be diagnosed with US (**Fig. 9**). Ureteral stricture following radiation therapy is diagnosed by US as hydronephrosis and hydroureter. It is important to keep in mind that if a ureteral stricture secondary to radiation therapy is suspected in US, recurrent disease must be included in the differential diagnosis and excluded before intervention.[63] US can be used both to biopsy sites of possible recurrence and to guide placement of a ureteral stent.

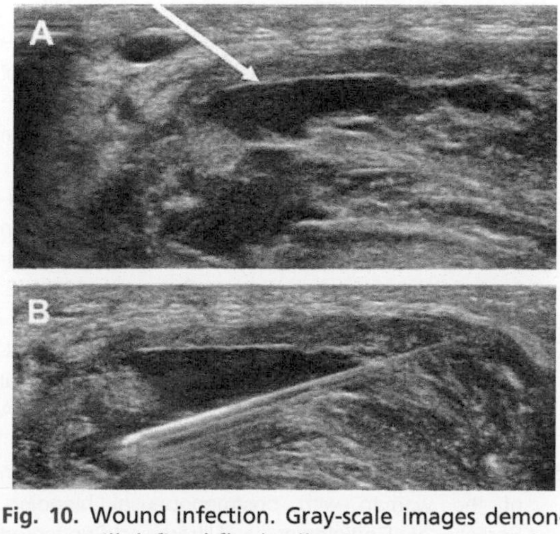

Fig. 10. Wound infection. Gray-scale images demonstrate an ill-defined fluid collection (*arrow* in *A*) that was underlying an abdominal incision. Collection was drained with US guidance (*B*).

Bladder contraction following radiation therapy can be diagnosed on US with pre- and postvoid bladder imaging. A contracted bladder demonstrates decreased filling on prevoid images and little change in bladder configuration between pre- and postvoid images. A thickened bladder wall is also often present.

Clinically significant urinary leak occurs in 5% of patients and can lead to abscess or urinoma.[64,65] Ultrasound is useful not only in the diagnosis of abscess or urinoma but in guidance for placement of percutaneous drains and ureteral stents.

Wound infections occur in 4% of patients undergoing a surgical procedure. Many of these infections do not require imaging, however US is the modality of choice to diagnose underlying fluid collection and to guide drainage of a subcutaneous collection (**Fig. 10**).

SUMMARY

Ultrasound is useful for the diagnosis, staging, and detection of suspected recurrence or metastatic disease in multiple gynecologic malignancies. Further, US can be useful for paracentesis guidance, biopsy of suspected disease recurrence or metastatic disease, and evaluation of postoperative complications.

REFERENCES

1. Brown DL, Frates MC, Laing FC, et al. Ovarian masses: can benign and malignant lesions be

differentiated with color and pulsed Doppler US? Radiology 1994;190:333–6.
2. Buy JN, Ghossain MA, Hugol D, et al. Characterization of adnexal masses: combination of color Doppler and conventional sonography compared with spectral Doppler analysis alone and conventional sonography alone. AJR Am J Roentgenol 1996;166:385–93.
3. DiSantis DJ, Scatarige JC, Kemp G, et al. A prospective evaluation of transvaginal sonography for detection of ovarian disease. AJR Am J Roentgenol 1993;161:91–4.
4. Mendelson EB, Bohm-Velez M. Transvaginal ultrasonography of pelvic neoplasms. Radiol Clin North Am 1992;230:703–34.
5. Jain KA. Prospective evaluation of adnexal masses with endovaginal gray-scale and duplex and color Doppler US: correlation with pathologic findings. Radiology 1994;191:63–7.
6. Stein SM, Laifer-Narin S, Johnson MB, et al. Differentiation of benign and malignant adnexal masses: relative value of gray-scale, color Doppler, and spectral Doppler sonography. AJR Am J Roentgenol 1995;164:381–6.
7. Timor-Tritsch IE, Lerner JP, Monteagudo A, et al. Transvaginal ultrasonographic characterization of ovarian masses by means of color flow-directed Doppler measurements and a morphologic scoring system. Am J Obstet Gynecol 1993;168:909–13.
8. Hamper UM, Sheth S, Abbas FM, et al. Transvaginal color Doppler sonography of adnexal masses: differences in blood flow impedance in benign and malignant lesions. AJR Am J Roentgenol 1993;160:1225–8.
9. Kurjak A, Predanic M, Kupesic-Urek S, et al. Transvaginal color and pulsed Doppler assessment of adnexal tumor vascularity. Gynecol Oncol 1993;50:3–9.
10. Levine D, Feldstein VA, Babcock CJ, et al. Sonography of ovarian masses: poor sensitivity of resistive index for identifying malignant lesions. AJR Am J Roentgenol 1994;162:1355–9.
11. Fleischer AC, Brader KR. Sonographic depiction of ovarian vascularity and flow: current improvements and future applications. J Ultrasound Med 2001;20:241–50.
12. Cohen LS, Escobar PF, Scharm C, et al. Three-dimensional power Doppler ultrasound improves the diagnostic accuracy for ovarian cancer prediction. Gynecol Oncol 2001;82(1):40–8.
13. Geomini PM, Coppus SF, Kluivers KB, et al. Is three-dimensional ultrasonography of additional value in the assessment of adnexal masses? Gynecol Oncol 2007;106(1):153–9.
14. Jokubkiene L, Sladkevicius P, Valentin L. Does three-dimensional power Doppler ultrasound help in discrimination between benign and malignant ovarian masses? Ultrasound Obstet Gynecol 2007;29(2):215–25.
15. DePriest PD, Varner E, Powell J, et al. The efficacy of a sonographic morphology index in identifying ovarian cancer: a multi-institutional investigation. Gynecol Oncol 1994;55:174–8.
16. Kurjak A, Predanic M. New scoring system for prediction of ovarian malignancy based on transvaginal color Doppler sonography. J Ultrasound Med 1992;11:631–8.
17. Brown DL, Doubilet PM, Miller FH, et al. Benign and malignant ovarian masses: selection of the most discriminating gray-scale and Doppler sonographic features. Radiology 1998;208:103–10.
18. Timmerman D, Schwarzler P, Collins WP, et al. Subjective assessment of adnexal masses with the use of ultrasonography: an analysis of interobserver variability and experience. Ultrasound Obstet Gynecol 1999;13:8–10.
19. Kurtz AB, Tsimikas JV, Tempany CMC, et al. Diagnosis and staging of ovarian cancer: comparative values of Doppler and conventional US, CT, and MR imaging correlated with surgery and histopathologic analysis—report of the Radiology Diagnostic Oncology Group. Radiology 1999;212:19–27.
20. Tempany CM, Zou KH, Silverman SG, et al. Staging of advanced ovarian cancer: comparison of imaging modalities—report from the Radiological Diagnostic Oncology Group. Radiology 2000;215:761–7.
21. Word B, Gravlee LC, Widerman GL. The fallacy of simple uterine curettage. Obstet Gynecol 1958;12:642–8.
22. Grimes DA. Diagnostic dilatation and curettage: a reappraisal. Am J Obstet Gynecol 1982;142:1–6.
23. Koonings PP, Moyer DI, Grimes DA. A randomized clinical trial comparing Pipelle and Tis-U-Trap for endometrial biopsy. Obstet Gynecol 1990;75:293–5.
24. Stock RJ, Kanbour A. Prehysterectomy curettage. Obstet Gynecol 1975;45:537–41.
25. Guido RS, Kanbour-Shakir A, Rulin MC, et al. Pipelle endometrial sampling. Sensitivity in the detection of endometrial cancer. J Reprod Med 1995;40:553–5.
26. Hofmeister FJ. Endometrial biopsy: another look. Am J Obstet Gynecol 1974;118:773–7.
27. Karlsson B, Granberg S, Wikland M, et al. Transvaginal ultrasonography of the endometrium in women with postmenopausal bleeding—a Nordic multicenter study. Am J Obstet Gynecol 1995;172:1488–94.
28. Smith-Bindman R, Kerlikowske K, Feldstein VA, et al. Endovaginal ultrasound to exclude endometrial cancer and other endometrial abnormalities. JAMA 1998;280:1510–7.
29. Goldstein RB, Bree RL, Benson CB, et al. Evaluation of the woman with postmenopausal bleeding. Society of Radiologist in Ultrasound-Sponsored Consensus Conference Statement. J Ultrasound Med 2001;20:1025–36.

30. Medverd JR, Dubinsky TJ. Cost analysis model: US versus endometrial biopsy in evaluation of peri- and postmenopausal abnormal vaginal bleeding. Radiology 2002;222:619–27.
31. Dubinsky TJ, Parvey HR, Maklad N. The role of transvaginal sonography and endometrial biopsy in the evaluation of peri- and postmenopausal bleeding. AJR Am J Roentgenol 1997;169:145–9.
32. Lev-Toaff AS, Toaff ME, Liu JB, et al. Value of sonohysterography in the diagnosis and management of abnormal uterine bleeding. Radiology 1996;201:179–84.
33. Laifer-Narin S, Ragavendra N, Parmenter EK, et al. False-normal appearance of the endometrium on conventional transvaginal sonography: comparison with saline hysterosonography. AJR Am J Roentgenol 2002;178:129–33.
34. Langer RD, Pierce JJ, O'Hanlan KA, et al. Transvaginal ultrasonography compared with endometrial biopsy for the detection of endometrial disease. N Engl J Med 1997;337:1792–8.
35. Atri M, Nazarnia S, Aldis AE, et al. Transvaginal US appearance of endometrial abnormalities. Radiographics 1994;14:483–92.
36. Laifer-Narin SL, Ragavendra N, Lu DS, et al. Transvaginal saline hysterosonography: characteristics distinguishing malignant and various benign conditions. AJR Am J Roentgenol 1999;172:1513–20.
37. Dubinsky TJ, Stroehlein K, Abu-Ghazzeh Y, et al. Prediction of benign and malignant endometrial disease: hysterosonographic-pathologic correlation. Radiology 1999;210:393–7.
38. Williams PL, Laifer-Narin SL, Ragavendra N. US of abnormal uterine bleeding. Radiographics 2003;23:703–18.
39. Sheth S, Hamper UM, Kurman RJ. Thickened endometrium in the postmenopausal woman: sonographic-pathologic correlation. Radiology 1993;187:135–9.
40. Hann LE, Giess CS, Bach AM, et al. Endometrial thickness in tamoxifen-treated patients: correlation with clinical and pathological findings. AJR Am J Roentgenol 1997;168:657–61.
41. Hulka CA, Hall DA. Endometrial abnormalities associated with tamoxifen therapy for breast cancer: sonographic and pathologic correlation. AJR Am J Roentgenol 1993;160:809–12.
42. Affinito P, Palomba S, Pellicano M, et al. Ultrasonographic measurement of endometrial thickness during hormonal replacement therapy in postmenopausal women. Ultrasound Obstet Gynecol 1998;11:343–6.
43. Bonilla-Musoles F, Raga R, Osborne NG, et al. Three dimensional hysterosonography for the study of endometrial tumors: comparison with conventional transvaginal sonography, hysterosalpingography, and hysteroscopy. Gynecol Oncol 1997;65:245–52.
44. Sheth S, Hamper UM, McCollum ME, et al. Endometrial blood flow analysis in postmenopausal women: can it help differentiate benign from malignant causes of endometrial thickening? Radiology 1995;195:661–5.
45. Sladkevicius P, Valentin L, Marsal K. Endometrial thickness and Doppler velocimetry of the uterine arteries as discriminators of endometrial status in women with postmenopausal bleeding: a comparative study. Am J Obstet Gynecol 1994;171:722–8.
46. Creasman WT, Morrow CP, Bundy BN, et al. Surgical pathologic spread patterns of endometrial cancer: a Gynecologic Oncology Group Study. Cancer 1987;60:2035–40.
47. Alcazar JL, Galvan R, Albela S, et al. Assessing myometrial infiltration by endometrial cancer: uterine virtual navigation with three-dimensional US. Radiology 2009;250(3):776–83.
48. Green CL, Angtuaco TL, Shah HR, et al. Gestational trophoblastic disease: a spectrum of radiologic diagnosis. Radiographics 1996;16:1371–84.
49. Wagner BJ, Woodward PJ, Dickey GE. From the archives of the AFIP. Gestational trophoblastic disease: radiologic-pathologic correlation. Radiographics 1996;16:131–48.
50. Lazarus E, Hulka C, Siewert B, et al. Sonographic appearance of early complete molar pregnancies. J Ultrasound Med 1999;18:589–94.
51. Benson CB, Enest DR, Bernstein MR, et al. Sonographic appearance of first trimester complete hydatidiform moles. Ultrasound Obstet Gynecol 2000;16:188–91.
52. Dobkin GR, Berkowitz RS, Goldstein DP, et al. Duplex ultrasonography for persistent gestational trophoblastic tumor. J Reprod Med 1991;36:14–6.
53. Taylor KJ, Schwartz PE, Kohorn EI. Gestational trophoblastic neoplasia: diagnosis with Doppler US. Radiology 1987;165:445–8.
54. Miyasaka M, Hachiya J, Furuya Y, et al. CT evaluation of invasive trophoblastic disease. J Comput Assist Tomogr 1984;9:459–62.
55. Sanders C, Rubin E. Malignant gestational trophoblastic disease: CT findings. AJR Am J Roentgenol 1987;148:165–8.
56. Murolo C, Constantini S, Foglia G, et al. Ultrasound examination in ovarian cancer patients. A comparison with second look laparotomy. J Ultrasound Med 1989;8:441–3.
57. Khan O, Cosgrove DO, Fried AM, et al. Ovarian carcinoma follow-up: US versus laparotomy. Radiology 1986;159:111–3.
58. Meanwell CA, Rolfe EB, Blackledge G, et al. Recurrent female pelvic cancer: assessment with transrectal ultrasonography. Radiology 1987;162:278–81.
59. Squillaci E, Salzini MC, Grandinetti ML, et al. Recurrence of ovarian and uterine neoplasms: diagnosis with transrectal US. Radiology 1988;169:355–8.

60. Su WH, Wang PH, Chang SP. Successful treatment of a persistent mole with myometrial invasion by direct injection of methotrexate. Eur J Gynaecol Oncol 2001;22:283–6.
61. Lim AK, Agarwal R, Seckl MJ, et al. Embolization of bleeding residual uterine vascular malformations in patients with treated gestational trophoblastic tumors. Radiology 2002;222:640–4.
62. Castro JR, Issa P, Fletcher GH. Carcinoma of the cervix treated by external beam irradiation alone. Radiology 1970;95:163.
63. McIntyre JF, Eifel PJ, Levenback C, et al. Ureteral stricture as a late complication of radiotherapy for stage 1B carcinoma of the uterine cervix. Cancer 1995;75:836.
64. Hancock KC, Copeland RJ, Gershenson DM, et al. Urinary conduits in gynecologic oncology. Obstet Gynecol 1986;67:680.
65. Regan JB, Barrett DM. Stented versus nonstented ureteroileal anastomoses: is there a difference with regard to leak and stricture? J Urol 1985;134:1101.

Three-Dimensional Gynecologic Ultrasound

Ashley Corbett Bragg, MD*, Teresita L. Angtuaco, MD

KEYWORDS

• Three-dimensional • Ultrasound • Pelvis • Uterus • Adnexa

OVERVIEW

Three-dimensional (3D) ultrasound has gained popularity in obstetric imaging because of its ability to render lifelike images of the fetus. This ability has increased patient appreciation of the prenatal sonogram and has led expectant mothers to request such images on routine prenatal examinations. Although the application of 3D ultrasound in gynecology is a much later development, its diagnostic potential has been recognized especially in the diagnosis of uterine pathology. The surface-rendered image allows visualization of a more anatomically relatable image, which is particularly helpful for both patients and clinicians. Counseling of patients is improved with more easily recognizable images on 3D ultrasound because patients and clinicians can better relate to what the sonographer and sonologist are seeing.

In gynecologic imaging, 3D ultrasound should be viewed as a supplement to, rather than a replacement of, the conventional 2D technique. Although 3D probes may be used with both transabdominal and transvaginal techniques, it is the transvaginal application that has proved most useful. Conventional transabdominal transverse and longitudinal images translate to axial and sagittal planes using the transvaginal approach. In addition, 3D imaging has added the unique dimension of coronal images, which were not possible with 2D ultrasound because of limitations of the bony pelvis. In addition, because of anteflexion or retroflexion of the uterus, the coronal plane can be more accurately aligned with the uterine body. The addition of the coronal plane proves particularly useful in the assessment of external uterine contour, leading to more precise assessment of congenital uterine anomalies when all 3 scan planes are displayed simultaneously (**Fig. 1**).[1,2]

TECHNICAL ASPECTS

The 3D ultrasound technique is technically easier in gynecologic imaging than in obstetrics due to less complex and nonmoving subjects, as compared with fetal imaging. These technical aspects lead to a less steep learning curve as one converts from traditional 2D ultrasound to 3D imaging. Data for 3D ultrasound may be acquired in 2 different ways. In an off-line freehand system, traditional 2D probes are used to obtain 3D images using traditional 2D ultrasound machines. More commonly today, the automated technique is used in which dedicated 3D probes are used along with internal integrated 3D systems software built into the state-of-the-art ultrasound system.[3] Although 3D ultrasound does not replace conventional 2D imaging, it is dependent on obtaining high-quality 2D images. Using the automated 3D technique, data can be processed within the ultrasound machine or in an off-line workstation. Because the automated technique is more commonly used today, the remainder of this discussion focuses on automated technique.

The 3D automated technique stores complete sets of volume data in a computer memory so

Department of Radiology, University of Arkansas for Medical Sciences, #556, 4301 West Markham, Little Rock, AR 72205, USA
* Corresponding author.
E-mail address: ACBragg@uams.edu

Ultrasound Clin 5 (2010) 299–311
doi:10.1016/j.cult.2010.03.001
1556-858X/10/$ – see front matter

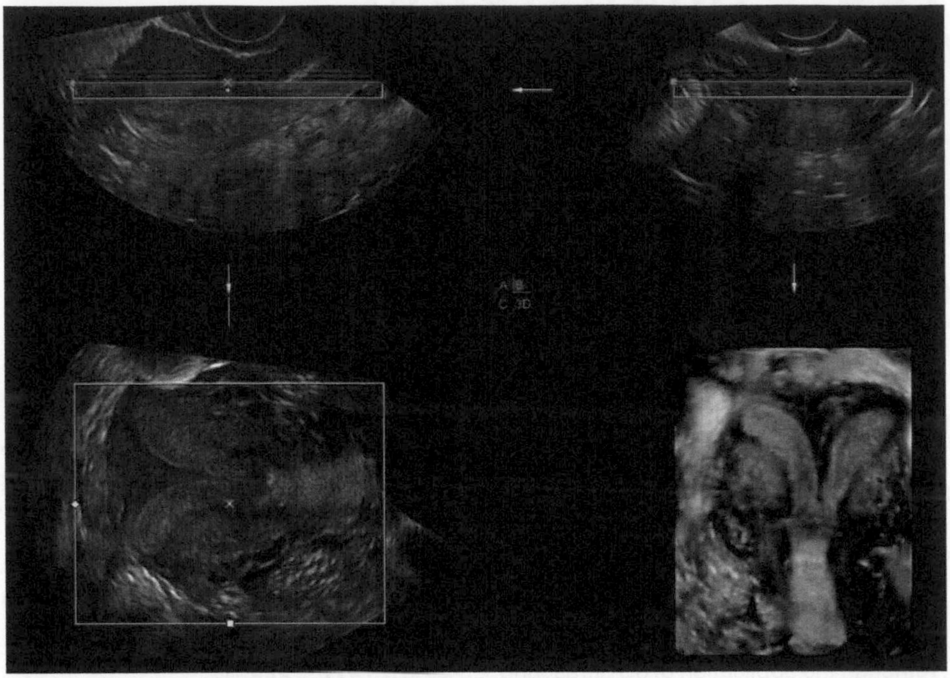

Fig. 1. Three-dimensional manipulation of the volume data allows simultaneous display of sagittal, axial, and coronal images. A point of reference on each image is moved, resulting in corresponding changes in the images displayed on all planes. A surface-rendered image in the fourth frame is a projection of the coronal image in the correct anatomic plane. (*Courtesy of* Beryl Benacerraf, MD, Boston, MA, USA.)

that it can be accessed for reconstruction in any desired image plane. Four steps are necessary to accomplish this: data acquisition, 3D visualization, volume processing of images, and storage of images. In this way, data can also be displayed as 3D volume–rendered images. Specialized 3D transducers perform volume acquisition with the touch of a button. Instead of individual slices, obtained in 2D ultrasound, 3D volumes of data are obtained. A single sweep of the transducer at a specified angle is used to acquire the entire volume set. The acquired data are then stored digitally in an electronic volume memory. The acquired data can then be retrieved from the memory to be displayed as multiplanar sections. Typically, the axial, sagittal, and coronal planes are displayed on a monitor simultaneously. As 1 plane is manipulated, the other planes are automatically rotated or shifted to display the focus in 3 planes simultaneously. This capability allows precise anatomic location of any area of interest, which is not possible with 2D ultrasound.

The ability to view all 3 planes simultaneously is advantageous in many ways. Using the 3D technique, the distinction between artifactual and true findings becomes more apparent as all 3 orthogonal planes are displayed simultaneously. This distinction proves to be advantageous over 2D ultrasound, where it is often difficult to separate true from artifactual findings. Storage and retrieval of complete volumes of data as well as multiplanar display and surface rendering are allowed by 3D ultrasound. The ability to store data has huge implications in terms of decreased scan times and evaluation of data after the patient leaves, and tremendously increases patient throughput in a busy service. An endovaginal 3D ultrasound examination can be performed in less than 10 seconds,[1] increasing convenience for the patient and the physician. The data may then be manipulated at a later time. In addition, discussion with peers and referring physicians can take place at more convenient times without the physical presence of the patient. If needed, retrospective analysis may be performed years later.

Volume calculation using 3D ultrasound is becoming a popular application of this technique. Recent work on 3D ultrasound with 3D power Doppler allows calculation of 3 objective indices of vascularity with high intraobserver reproducibility.[4] The vascularization index (VI) is the ratio of power Doppler information within the total dataset to both color and gray information. The flow index (FI) represents the mean power Doppler signal intensity. The vascularization flow index is a combination of the other 2 indices. All of these show potential for future applications of 3D imaging.

CLINICAL APPLICATIONS

Uterine Abnormalities

Congenital anomalies

Uterine congenital anomalies have been traditionally evaluated with contrast hysterosalpingography (HSG), which is considered the gold standard test in evaluating uterine anomalies. HSG is an invasive test requiring the presence of a physician in radiology or gynecology and requiring radiation exposure. HSG is limited in its evaluation of the external uterine contour but accurately depicts the internal uterine cavity. In recent years, the use of saline infusion sonohysterography (SIS) using 2D ultrasound has become a viable alternative to contrast HSG. SIS involves infusing saline into the uterine cavity before ultrasound examination to characterize the uterine cavity better. However, SIS is also limited in assessing uterine anomalies by its inability to assess the uterus in the coronal plane. The 3D ultrasound technique has added to our understanding of uterine anomalies, allowing characterization of both the internal and external uterine contour of the uterus.[2,3] With a reported 100% sensitivity and specificity for detection of an anomalous uterus, 3D ultrasound is proving to be an accurate alternative to HSG and supplement to 2D ultrasound for the detection and characterization of uterine anomalies.[5] Accurate diagnosis of uterine anomalies is essential in fertility patients who have recurrent spontaneous abortions. As many as 24% of women with recurrent pregnancy loss may have uterine anomalies.[6] Women with septate uteri have a significantly higher proportion of first-trimester loss. Women with an arcuate uterus have a significantly greater proportion of second-trimester loss and preterm labor compared with women with a normal uterus.[7] These patients have good outcomes after surgical intervention, making accurate diagnosis essential.[8] **Figs. 2–5** demonstrate several uterine anomalies using 3D ultrasound.

There have been reports of the added benefit of combining 3D ultrasound and SIS. Lev-Toaff and colleagues[9] determined that 3D SIS added valuable information in 69% of cases compared with 2D SIS and in 92% of cases compared with HSG. An additional benefit of combining 3D ultrasound and SIS is the ability to analyze data after scanning the patient. This procedure shortens examination time and time that the uterine cavity is distended, thus reducing patient discomfort, which is particularly helpful when uterine distension is difficult to achieve because of restricted capacity or free passage of saline into the open fallopian tubes, thus preventing optimum visualization of the endometrial cavity.

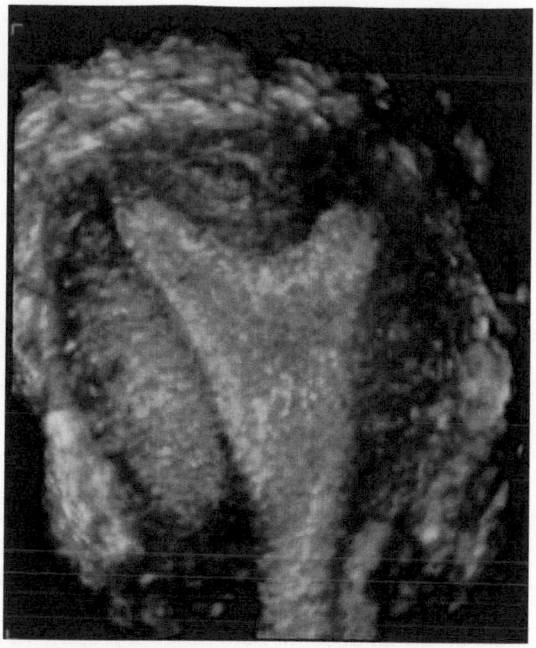

Fig. 2. Arcuate uterus. There is a shallow indentation of the superior border of the endometrial cavity. The fundal myometrium is smooth. (*Courtesy of* Beryl Benacerraf, MD, Boston, MA, USA.)

Myomas

The distinction between intramural and submucosal myomas can be difficult with 2D sonography, which becomes critical in women contemplating whether to undergo surgical resection or local ablation of submucosal myomas to preserve fertility (**Fig. 6**). The 3D ultrasound

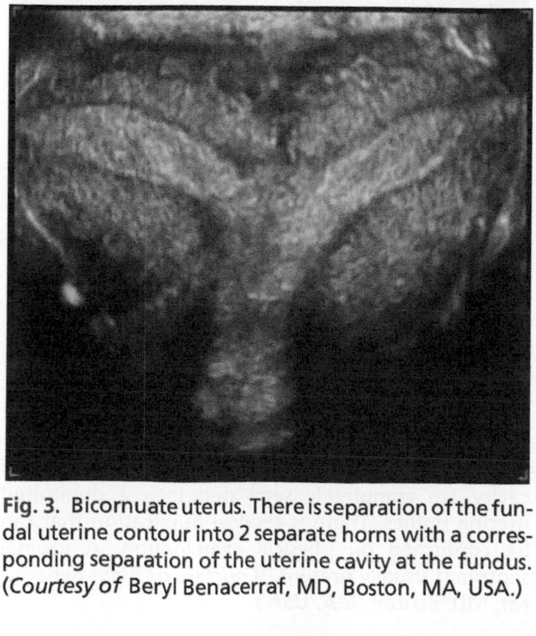

Fig. 3. Bicornuate uterus. There is separation of the fundal uterine contour into 2 separate horns with a corresponding separation of the uterine cavity at the fundus. (*Courtesy of* Beryl Benacerraf, MD, Boston, MA, USA.)

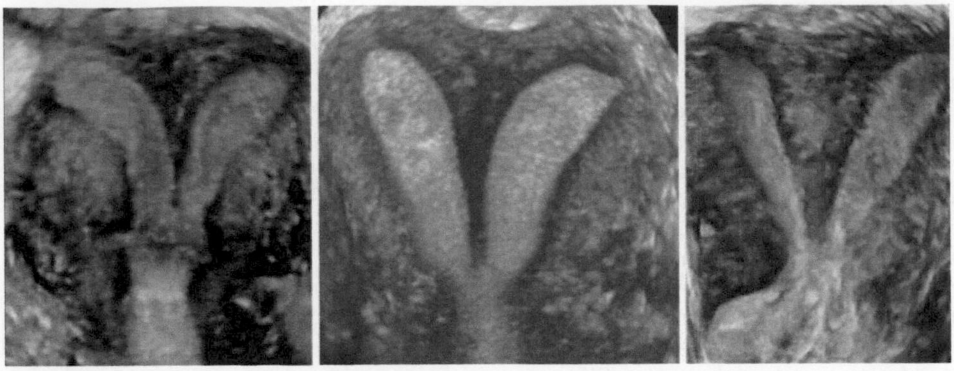

Fig. 4. Septate uterus. Varying degrees of uterine septation are demonstrated. Note that the uterine contour remains continuous at the fundus. (*Courtesy of* Beryl Benacerraf, MD, Boston, MA, USA.)

technique is useful in the evaluation of myomas and can provide precise anatomic location of the abnormality (**Fig. 7**).[3] The simultaneous display of 3 imaging planes also allows better visualization of subtle myomas that can be confused with artifacts on 2D ultrasound. Both 2D sonography with SIS and 3D ultrasound improve diagnostic accuracy in these cases.[10] Therefore, the examination can be chosen based on preference and availability.

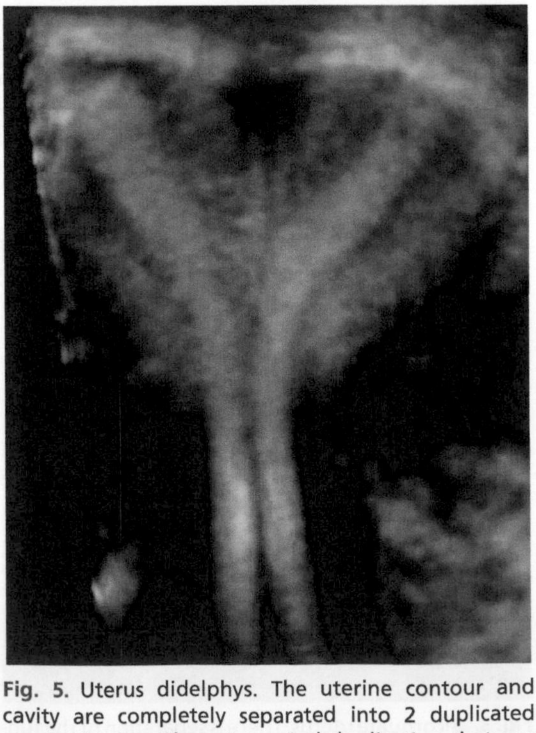

Fig. 5. Uterus didelphys. The uterine contour and cavity are completely separated into 2 duplicated uterine bodies. There is cervical duplication that can be confirmed on physical examination. A vaginal septum is usually present. (*Courtesy of* Beryl Benacerraf, MD, Boston, MA, USA.)

In patients with symptomatic uterine myomas who are considering uterine embolization, 3D ultrasound with Doppler may play an important role in evaluating the uterine vascularity before and after embolization.[11] The presence of collateral vessels on preembolization examination negatively influences the outcome of embolization and is better assessed using 3D ultrasound compared with 2D. The 3D ultrasound technique allows more accurate assessment of the changes in vascularity and volume before and after embolization, an important prognostic indicator.[12]

Dysmenorrhea

Pelvic pain can be caused by numerous pelvic conditions. Patients with defined masses or inflammatory conditions on ultrasound comprise only a minority of those who present with recurrent or chronic pelvic pain. Some studies have been performed to assess myometrial vascularization in patients with dysmenorrhea. Initial studies by Royo and Alcazar[13] suggest that in patients with severe dysmenorrhea, there is increased myometrial vascularization in the early menstrual phase. Improved visualization and characterization of uterine vascularity using 3D ultrasound and 3D power Doppler may in the future play an increasingly important role in evaluating patients with severe dysmenorrhea.

Endometrial pathology

Conventionally, transvaginal 2D sonography has been used to evaluate the endometrium and measure endometrial thickness. This evaluation is sufficient in most instances when the patient's menstrual history corroborates with endometrial thickness and morphology. However, in patients with menorrhagia or menometrorrhagia, further evaluation is usually warranted. This evaluation is especially important in women with postmenopausal bleeding and thickened endometrium

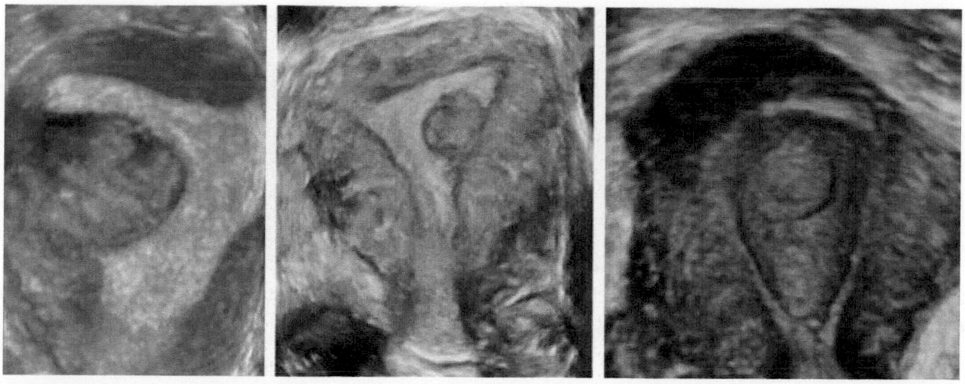

Fig. 6. Submucous myomas. The uterine cavity is indented by myomas that arise from the submucosal myometrium. This examination is adequate to confirm any suspicion raised by the 2D images. Further evaluation with sonohysterography is avoided. (*Courtesy of* Beryl Benacerraf, MD, Boston, MA, USA.)

greater than 5 mm. SIS improves diagnostic accuracy in 2D ultrasound evaluation of the endometrium and detects subtle polyps that may be invisible on conventional 2D ultrasound. However, although its acceptance is increasing, it is not widely available in many ultrasound clinics because of the extra time involved in the process and the skill required to perform the procedure. SIS is a cost-effective way to accurately evaluate the endometrium but can be time consuming in centers where it is not performed regularly. Evaluation of the endometrium with 3D ultrasound has proved particularly useful in patients with endometrial lesions and in determining intrauterine device (IUD) placement.

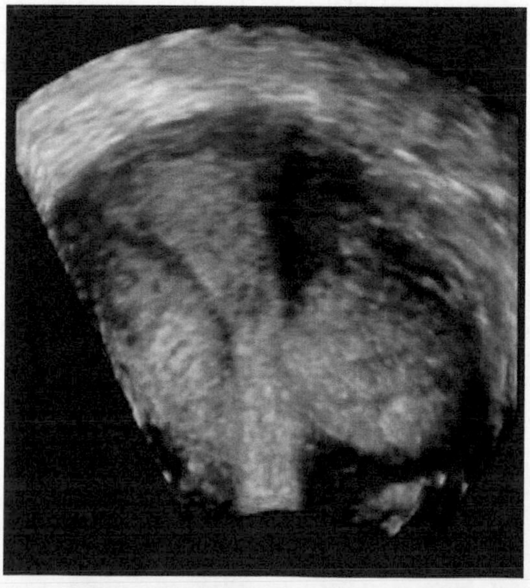

Fig. 7. Transmural myoma. The uterine mass spans the whole uterine wall and indents both the endometrial and serosal surfaces. Myomectomy will have to be performed transabdominally rather than through an endometrial approach.

Endometrial carcinoma Most patients with known endometrial carcinoma are not evaluated by sonography. Other studies such as magnetic resonance imaging or computed tomography are preferred for the important preoperative staging information they can provide. However, because endometrial cancer is always a differential diagnosis in older women with postmenopausal bleeding, this diagnosis may first be suspected on initial ultrasound. Accurate and reliable calculation of endometrial volume can be performed in 3D ultrasound, which is more accurate than measurement of uterine thickness for evaluation for endometrial carcinoma.[5] Using an endometrial volume of 13 mL, there is 100% sensitivity and 98% specificity for diagnosing endometrial carcinoma in 3D ultrasound, which is much more accurate than the measurement of 1.5 cm endometrial thickness conventionally used with 2D ultrasound.[3] Volume calculation of the endometrium has a low interexaminer variability as well. The 3D ultrasound technique also improves diagnostic accuracy in assessing myometrial or cervical invasion by endometrial cancer as compared with 2D ultrasound.[14]

Endometrial polyps La Torre and colleagues[15] investigated the evaluation of endometrial polyps with 2D and 3D ultrasound in a group of patients who later underwent hysteroscopy, confirming the presence of endometrial polyps. A poor specificity of 69%, suggesting polyps in 23 patients, was demonstrated by 2D ultrasound. Specificity improved to 94.1% when combined with SIS. Polyps were diagnosed by 3D ultrasound in 18 patients with a specificity of 88.8%. When combined with saline infusion, all polyps were

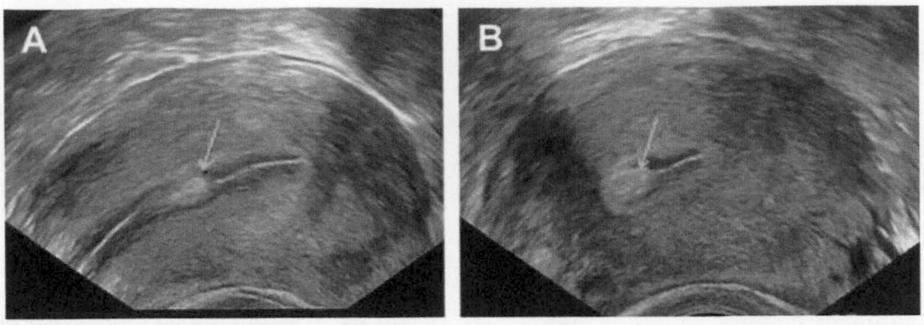

Fig. 8. Endometrial polyp. Endovaginal sagittal (*A*) and coronal (*B*) images of the uterine cavity show a focal area of echogenicity highly suspicious for a polyp (*arrow*).

correctly identified, demonstrating a clear role for 3D ultrasound with and without saline infusion in evaluating endometrial lesions. Other studies, including one by Sylvester and colleagues,[10] do not show marked improvement in accuracy when comparing 2D ultrasound with SIS to 3D ultrasound with or without SIS. Therefore, the sonographic examination may be chosen based on availability and individual preference. As more experience is gained with this technique, there is increasing popularity for the notion that 3D sonography may decrease the need for SIS because of its enhanced definition of endometrial pathology (**Figs. 8** and **9**).

IUD placement Display of 3 orthogonal planes has proved invaluable in IUD detection and location, which can be problematic with 2D ultrasound (**Figs. 10** and **11**).[3] In the past, IUD visualization was not as problematic with ultrasound because of the echogenic signature of most devices. Nowadays, however, some IUDs may be difficult to separate from the endometrium and create some difficulty in detection and display (**Fig. 12**). The 3D ultrasound technique increases the conspicuity of these devices and accurately depicts their location and orientation relative to the endometrial canal (**Fig. 13**). An added advantage is the ability of 3D to depict not just the central echo of the device but also the negative shadow image that may be seen posterior to the IUD (**Fig. 14**). It also becomes important to demonstrate penetration of parts of the IUD into the myometrial wall in those patients who desire removal of the device (**Fig. 15**). This capability is a distinct advantage over conventional 2D sonography.

ADNEXAL MASSES

The application of 3D ultrasound in the adnexa is not as well established as its role in uterine abnormalities. However, various studies have shown 3D ultrasound to be more sensitive and specific than

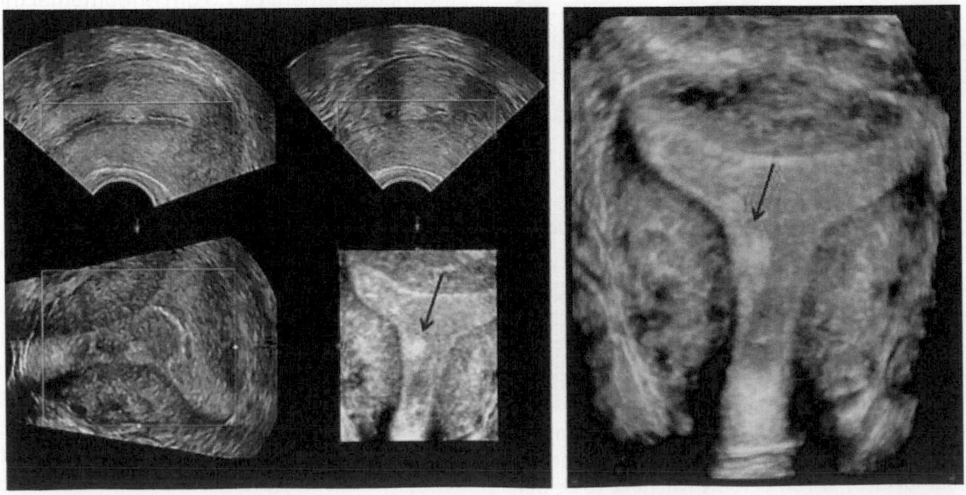

Fig. 9. Three-dimensional rendering of the endometrial cavity confirms the presence of the polyp that arises predominantly from the lateral uterine wall (*arrow*).

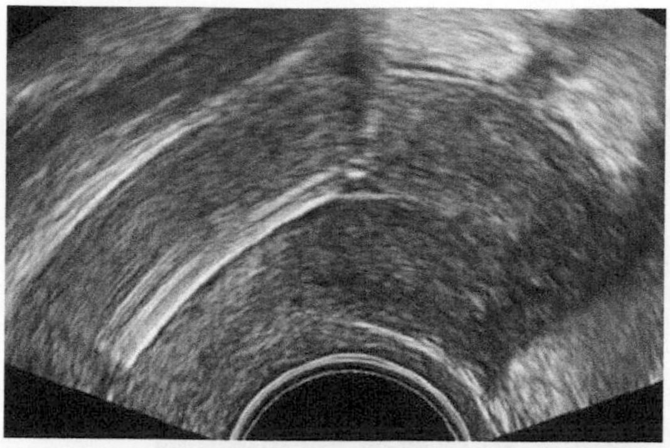

Fig. 10. Intrauterine device (IUD). A very echogenic stem of the IUD is easily seen on this sagittal view. (*Courtesy of* Beryl Benacerraf, MD, Boston, MA, USA.)

2D ultrasound in the evaluation of adnexal pathology. Volume calculation of irregularly shaped structures such as the ovaries is more accurate than measurements in 3 planes using 2D ultrasound, and is especially helpful in patients with polycystic ovarian syndrome (PCOS) in which volume calculations may be critical. Volume calculations also play a significant role in follicle size determination in patients with infertility. In 2D ultrasound, evaluation of the adnexa is limited by the limited motion of the transvaginal probe. This limitation is overcome using 3D ultrasound.[2]

In addition, 3D ultrasound with 3D power Doppler has proved useful in the evaluation of indeterminate adnexal masses. Using 2D ultrasound, masses are characterized as benign or malignant based on tumor diameter or volume, presence of septations and papillary projections, subjective estimate of echogenicity, and the presence of free fluid. Lower resistance blood flow is typically seen in malignant lesions. The 3D ultrasound technique allows visualization of masses in 3 orthogonal planes, allowing more accurate understanding of mass characterization and relation to adjacent structures. Early studies performed to evaluate 3D power Doppler suggest that masses are more likely malignant if there is central vascular flow, vascular flow in excrescences, flow in septations, or chaotic or complex architecture of vasculature. In a study by Geomini and colleagues[16] evaluating adnexal masses, all patients scheduled for resection of adnexal masses underwent preoperative 2D with power Doppler and 3D ultrasound with power Doppler. This study demonstrated important parameters for distinguishing benign from malignant lesions using 3D ultrasound with 3D power Doppler. Key parameters identified in this study were central location of vessels, mean gray index, and flow index. In 3D ultrasound, mean gray index and flow index are objective quantitative parameters based on the number of gray-scale color voxels. In 2D ultrasound these parameters are not measurable, and echogenicity is subjectively assessed by the examiner. Location of vessels is more accurately assessed with 3D ultrasound and 3D power Doppler, and allows better spatial awareness of vascularity. Multiple studies have shown improved diagnostic accuracy using 3D ultrasound and 3D power Doppler compared with 2D ultrasound. In 50 patients evaluated in a study by Laban and colleagues,[17] 3D ultrasound with 3D power Doppler identified all 31 cases of malignancy with a sensitivity of 100%, specificity of 84%, positive predictive value of 91%, and accuracy of 94%, demonstrating clear improvement over 2D ultrasound. Preoperative evaluation of borderline adnexal masses with 3D ultrasound may introduce laparoscopic surgery as an option to patients, decreasing surgical morbidity and mortality.[18]

POLYCYSTIC OVARIAN SYNDROME

Ultrasound plays an important role in patients with PCOS. In fact, the presence of polycystic ovaries is commonly detected by ultrasound. Ultrasound criteria used for diagnosis of PCOS include 10 to 12 follicles or more measuring 2 to 9 mm in any plane as well as increased ovarian volume of one or both ovaries measuring 10 cm^3 or more. A study by Allemand and colleagues[19] has shown that 2D ultrasound may underestimate the absolute

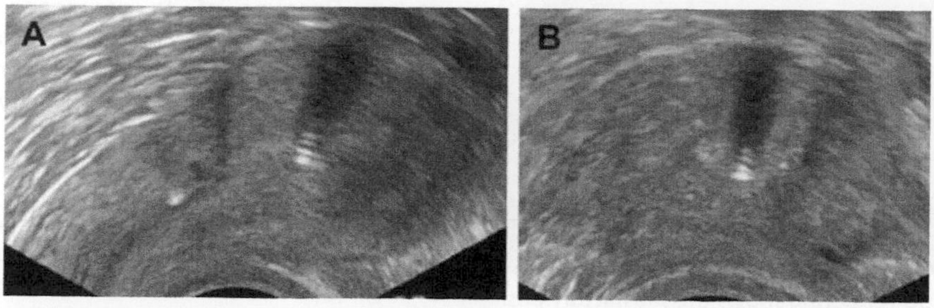

Fig. 11. IUD. Endovaginal sagittal (*A*) and coronal (*B*) images of the uterus show partial visualization of the IUD but its position relative to the uterine cavity is not clear.

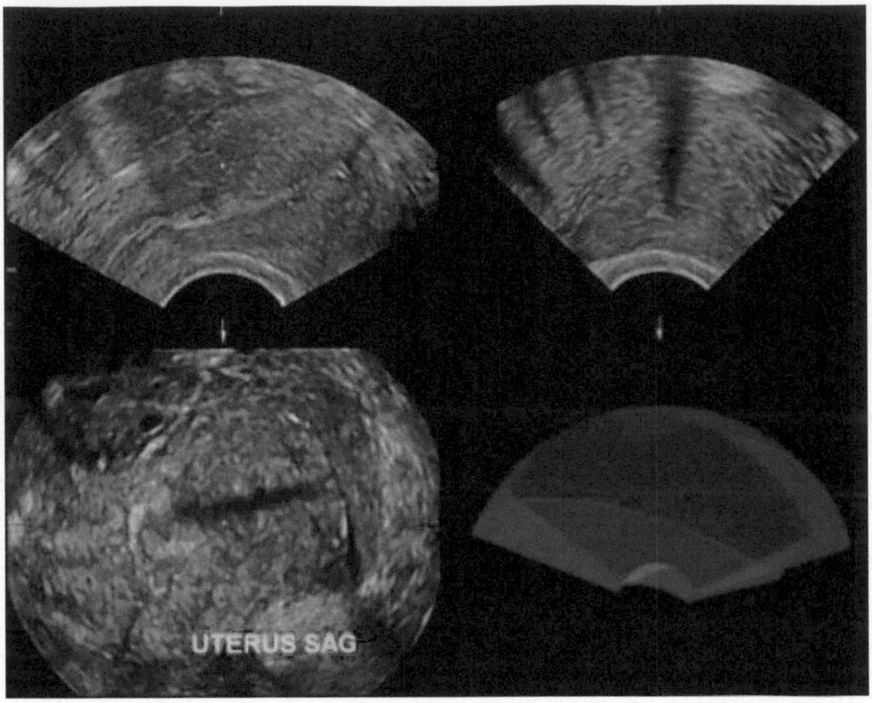

Fig. 12. IUD. 3D rendering of the IUD is made difficult because various components of the device lie in different planes.

number of follicles compared with 3D. In addition, volume calculations are known to be less accurate and reproducible with 2D compared with 3D ultrasound. The 2D ultrasound technique has traditionally calculated ovarian volume based on the formula for an ellipsoid structure (length × width × thickness × 0.5). The validity of this formula is lost in less ellipsoid ovaries. In 3D ultrasound, volume calculations are independent of the shape of the structure, and thus are much more accurate than 2D ultrasound for irregularly shaped structures. An initial study by Lam and colleagues[20] has shown that polycystic ovaries have more pronounced blood flow that is only apparent with 3D ultrasound and not seen with 2D ultrasound, which may be related to the fact that in 2D ultrasound, the examiner must arbitrarily select a single vessel instead of evaluating overall ovarian flow. The vessel selected in 2D ultrasound may not be representative of flow to the entire ovary. The 3D ultrasound technique allows for quantitative assessment of vascularization of a defined volume of tissue, which is not possible with 2D ultrasound.[19] Various studies have shown ovarian stromal echogenicity to be increased in patients with PCOS, but this criterion is still debatable. Because 3D ultrasound allows for quantitative evaluation of ovarian echogenicity, 3D ultrasound is more accurate and reproducible than subjective assessment of echogenicity performed in 2D ultrasound. Because of its decreased subjectivity compared with 2D ultrasound, increased use of 3D ultrasound may lead to new criteria regarding ovarian vascularity and echogenicity in patients with PCOS.

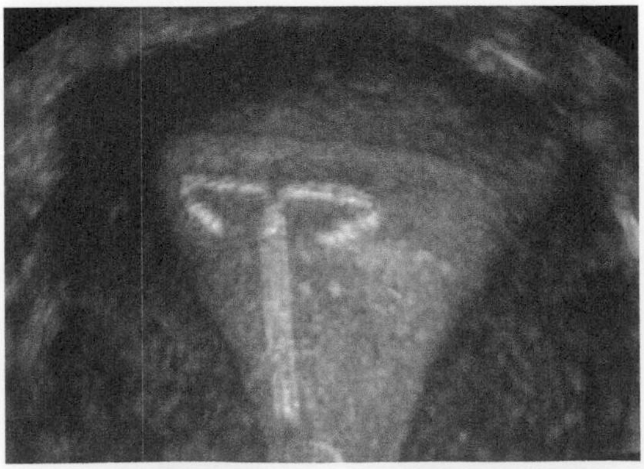

Fig. 13. IUD. 3D rendering shows the satisfactory position of the IUD in the endometrial cavity. (*Courtesy of* Beryl Benacerraf, MD, Boston, MA, USA.)

EVALUATION OF TUBAL PATENCY

Tubal patency is conventionally assessed using radiographic HSG to evaluate for free spill from the fallopian tubes. In addition, this technique shows the internal morphology of the tubes and

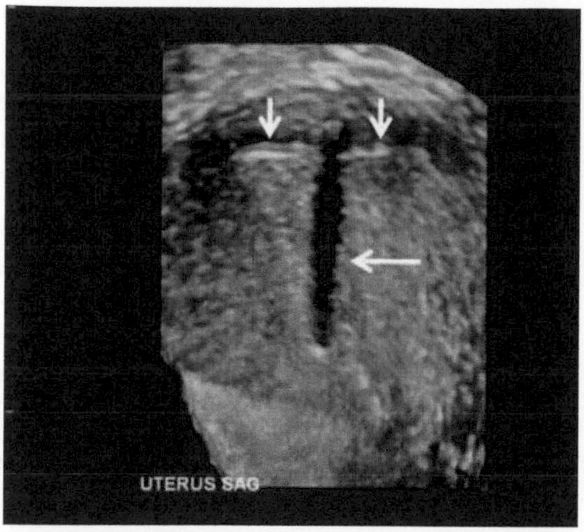

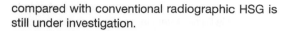

Fig. 14. IUD. When all the components of the IUD do not line up in the same plane, it is possible to show both the echogenic horizontal limbs (*short arrows*) and the negative shadow of the vertical limb of the device (*long arrow*).

can show the severity of narrowing and the location of the narrowest segments. There are studies, including those by Kiyokawa and colleagues[21] and Sladkevicius and colleagues,[22] showing the potential role for 3D ultrasound in evaluating tubal patency. Saline infusion or use of positive contrast agents was used with 3D sonography to evaluate for free spill. These results are encouraging and definitely need further investigation. However, the failure of ultrasound contrast agents to gain full Food and Drug Administration approval for routine use in the United States can slow down this initiative. As such, the role of 3D ultrasound is not yet clearly defined in this arena, as its accuracy compared with conventional radiographic HSG is still under investigation.

LIMITATIONS OF 3D ULTRASOUND

Larger Probes

Although 3D ultrasound is beneficial in several instances, it does have associated drawbacks. Probes used for 3D ultrasound are typically somewhat larger than 2D probes, especially for transabdominal applications. Theoretically this could result in increased discomfort in some patients, especially during a transvaginal examination. However, as the size is not significantly larger than conventional probes, this has not become a common problem in most clinics and can be significantly offset by the shorter time it takes to perform the examination. As probe design improves, this is not anticipated to be a disadvantage in the future.

Data Storage

Storage of the entire volume of ultrasound data is invaluable, allowing the entire examination to be reviewed at any time and in virtually any location. However, storage requirements are increased in 3D ultrasound because of the large size of the entire volume of data. Each volume set can require 3 to 18 MB of memory depending on the area of interest. This storage requirement may be further increased with added manipulation of data. Because of rapid advances in technology, media storage has become less expensive and more available than ever before. However, picture archiving and communication system capabilities must be kept in mind when evaluating the ability to store an increased amount of data.

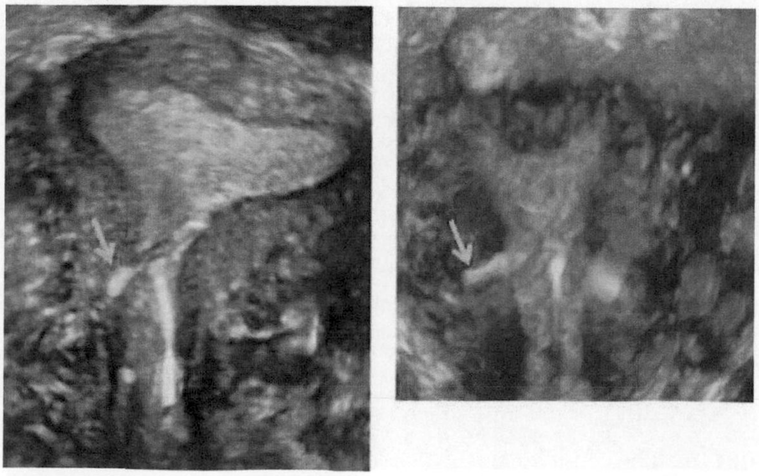

Fig. 15. Malpositioned IUD. 3D rendering shows horizontal limbs of the IUD (*arrows*) partially penetrating the myometrium that could complicate removal. (*Courtesy of* Beryl Benacerraf, MD, Boston, MA, USA.)

In 3D ultrasound, the size of the volume of data to be stored is finite. A very large structure may be difficult to acquire in one volume acquisition. For example, a significantly enlarged uterus may not be completely included in one volume. Evaluating the commonly encountered enlarged myomatous uterus can be problematic if the entire uterus cannot be captured in a single acquisition.[3] The increased spatial awareness gained with 3D ultrasound is lost if a structure, such as an enlarged myomatous uterus, cannot be included in one volume.

To circumvent the storage issues, some centers have saved volumetric data in off-line storage devices or storage media for later processing. Specific reconstructed images are then chosen for permanent storage in patient archives. This archiving also facilitates the ability to mail storage media to consultants in other institutions, who may be able to manipulate these volumetric data at different locations and render an opinion or diagnosis.

Operator Requirements

The acquired data software requires more user input, which incurs increased time and training of operators. Although the actual scan times are decreased, increased image manipulation by a specially trained sonographer or sonologist is required to obtain high-quality results.[1] In addition, the ability to view data in multiple planes may increase time of image interpretation. It is still not clear whether increased time spent in the processing phase is offset by the time savings during the scan.

The 3D ultrasound technique significantly increases spatial awareness; however, there is a possibility of orientation problems if the orientation is not recorded accurately during scan. Therefore, it is vital that the operator determines correct orientation of uterus at the time of scan because the correct orientation may not be apparent later (**Fig. 16**). False assumptions could easily be made based on incorrect orientation (**Fig. 17**).

Artifacts

The commonly encountered artifacts in 2D ultrasound are also present in 3D ultrasound (**Fig. 18**). Some of these artifacts are beneficial and frequently used for diagnosis in ultrasound. However, in 3D ultrasound there are additional artifacts related to 3D technique including those related to acquisition, volume rendering, and editing. For this reason, it is

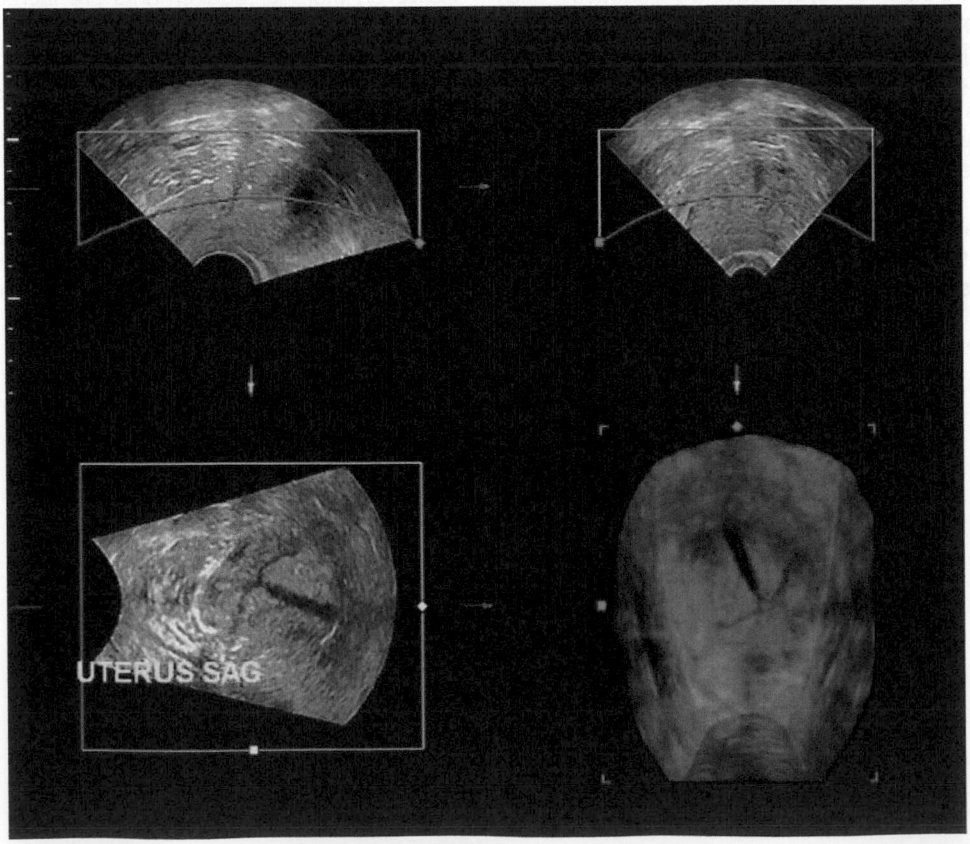

Fig. 16. Upside-down IUD. It is crucial to maintain meticulous orientation of the planes of display of the images to show the upside-down position of this IUD.

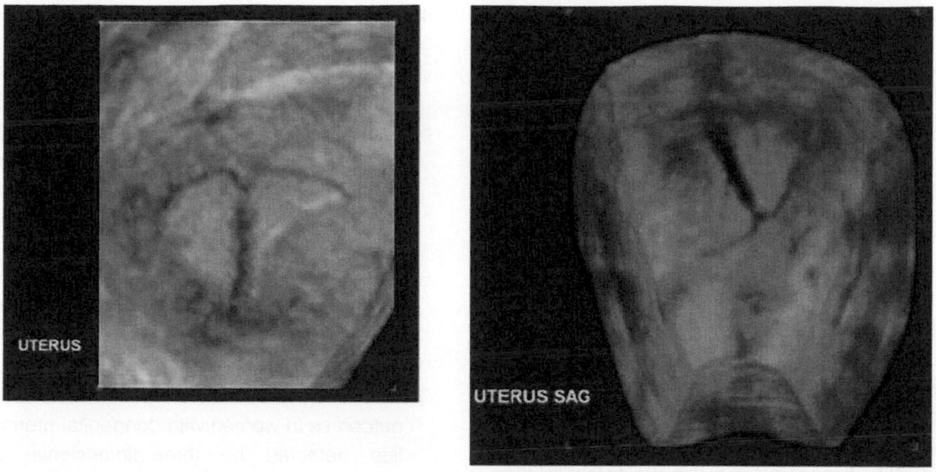

Fig. 17. Pitfall in image display. 3D-rendered images of **Fig. 16** initially erroneously rectified the position of the IUD in the endometrial cavity. Repeat processing with the proper orientation confirmed the upside-down position of the IUD.

vital that the sonographer or sonologist responsible for data manipulation be appropriately trained so as not to introduce additional artifacts that could be misinterpreted. Inappropriate settings may also lead to artifacts. A commonly described enhancement artifact of uterus occurs when the echogenic endometrium appears to spread beyond endometrium-myometrium interface.[3] In addition, motion artifacts may play a larger role in 3D ultrasound because of the need to obtain the entire volume

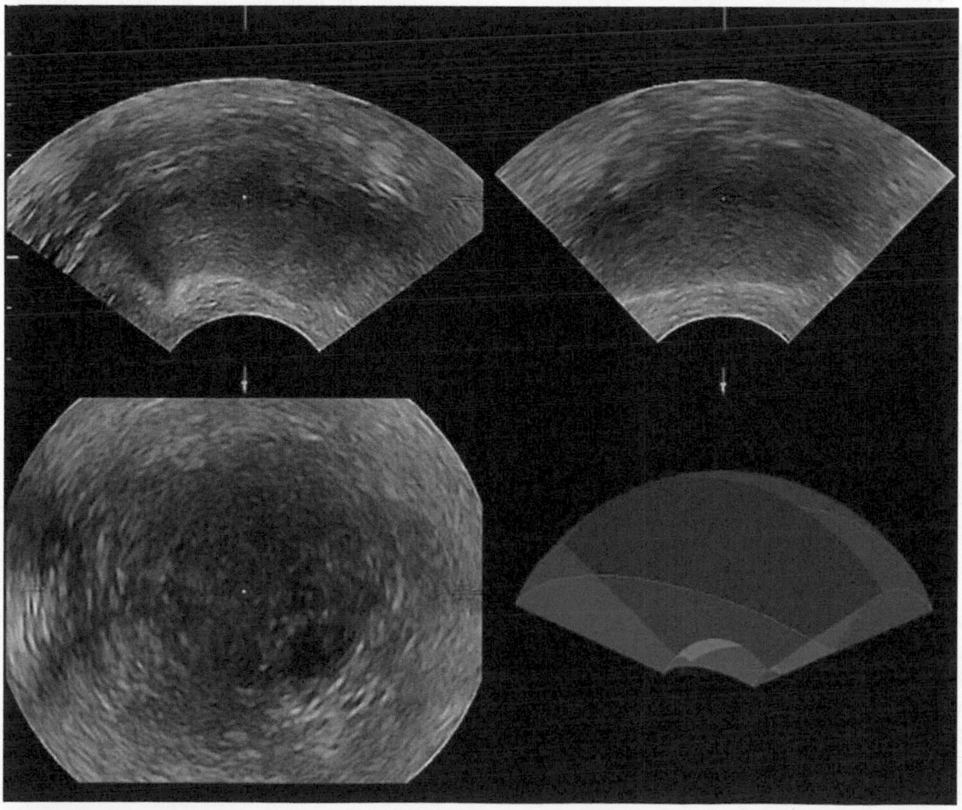

Fig. 18. Artifacts. Although 3D can be valuable as a supplement to 2D images, it can only be as good as the source images. The coronal plane on this study is rendered useless by the artifacts arising from adjacent bowel leading to suboptimal 2D images.

of data in a single acquisition. Suboptimal results may be seen in patients who are in pain or unable to hold their breath for a short period of time. It is in these circumstances that the 2D technique has a distinct advantage over 3D.

FUTURE CONSIDERATIONS

Telemedicine has an increasing role in medicine; however, ultrasound does not lend itself well to telemedicine applications because of the need of the physical presence of the interpreting physician in many instances. Oftentimes, the interpreting physician must be present at the examination to understand complex anatomy and pathology and to distinguish real from artifactual findings. However, 3D ultrasound may make telemedicine in ultrasound a more feasible possibility. The entire 3D volume of data can be completely reanalyzed at any time by any examiner without loss of any information. Data from a single examination may require less storage and in the future can be easily transferred wirelessly in a short time. Patient convenience can thus be increased, and discussion about cases between physicians may be more feasible. Tertiary consultation is also a more feasible possibility with 3D ultrasound.[23,24] With increasing use of telemedicine, remote consultations may be possible by mailing to a consultant volume data saved in storage media.

The growing interest in and use of 3D ultrasound in gynecology can only lead to more accurate diagnosis and more efficiency in the workplace. As technology improves, 3D ultrasound can be made more available and not remain limited to high-end equipment. The portability of ultrasound can bring this technology to the patient's bedside and optimize imaging in more critical patients who may not be able to come to the main ultrasound department for a standard examination. More operator-friendly, off-line work stations or processing software in ordinary personal computers can make this technique routine in all ultrasound departments, and change the way sonography is practiced.

REFERENCES

1. Downey D, Fenster A, Williams J. Clinical utility of three-dimensional US. Radiographics 2000;20:559–71.
2. Raine-Fenning N, Fleischer A. Clarifying the role of three-dimensional transvaginal sonography in reproductive medicine: an evidence-based appraisal. J Exp Clin Assist Reprod 2005;2:10.
3. Bega G, Lev-Toaff A, O'Kane P, et al. Three-dimensional ultrasonography in gynecology. J Ultrasound Med 2003;22:1249–69.
4. Pairleitner H, Steiner H, Hasenoehrl G, et al. Three-dimensional power Doppler sonography: imaging and quantifying blood flow and vascularization. Ultrasound Obstet Gynecol 1999;14(2):139–43.
5. Gruboeck K, Jurkovic D, Lawton F, et al. The diagnostic value of endometrial thickness and volume measurements by three-dimensional ultrasound in patients with postmenopausal bleeding. Ultrasound Obstet Gynecol 1996;8:272–6.
6. Kyei-Mensah A, Zaidi J, Pittrof R, et al. Transvaginal three-dimensional ultrasound: accuracy of follicular volume measurements. Fertil Steril 1996;65(2):371–6.
7. Woelfer B, Salim R, Banerjee S, et al. Reproductive outcomes in women with congenital uterine anomalies detected by three-dimensional ultrasound screening. Obstet Gynecol 2001;98(6):1099–103.
8. Homer HA, Li TC, Cooke ID. The septate uterus: a review of management and reproductive outcome. Fertil Steril 2000;73(1):1–14.
9. Lev-Toaff AS, Pinheiro LW, Bega G, et al. Three-dimensional multiplanar sonohysterography: comparison with conventional two-dimensional sonohysterography and x-ray hysterosalpingography. J Ultrasound Med 2001;20:295–306.
10. Sylvester C, Child TJ, Tulandi T, et al. A prospective study to evaluate the efficacy of two- and three-dimensional sonohysterography in women with intrauterine lesions. Fertil Steril 2003;79(5):1222–5.
11. Chang WC, Chang DY, Huang SC, et al. Use of three-dimensional ultrasonography in the evaluation of uterine perfusion and healing after laparoscopic myomectomy. Fertil Steril 2009;92(3):1110–5.
12. Fleischer A. Color Doppler sonography of uterine disorders. Ultrasound Q 2003;19(4):179–89.
13. Royo P, Alcazar JL. Three-dimensional power Doppler assessment of uterine vascularization in women with primary dysmenorrhea. J Ultrasound Med 2008;27(7):1003–10.
14. Alcazar JL, Galvan R. Three-dimensional power Doppler ultrasound scanning for the prediction of endometrial cancer in women with postmenopausal bleeding and thickened endometrium. Am J Obstet Gynecol 2009;200(1):44. e1–6.
15. La Torre R, De Felice C, De Angelis C, et al. Transvaginal sonographic evaluation of endometrial polyps: a comparison with two dimensional and three dimensional contrast sonography. Clin Exp Obstet Gynecol 1999;26(3–4):171–3.
16. Geomini P, Kluivers K, Moret E, et al. Evaluation of adnexal masses with three-dimensional ultrasonography. Obstet Gynecol 2006;108(5):1167–75.
17. Laban M, Metawee H, Elyan A, et al. Three-dimensional ultrasound and three-dimensional power Doppler in the assessment of ovarian tumors. Int J Gynaecol Obstet 2007;99(3):201–5.

18. Kalmantis K, Papgeorgiou T, Rodolakis A, et al. The role of three-dimensional (3D) sonography and 3D power Doppler in the preoperative assessment of borderline ovarian tumors. Eur J Gynaecol Oncol 2007;28(5):381–5.
19. Allemand MC, Tummon IS, Phy JL, et al. Diagnosis of polycystic ovaries by three-dimensional transvaginal ultrasound. Fertil Steril 2006;85:214–9.
20. Lam P, Johnson I, Raine-Fenning N. Three-dimensional ultrasound features of the polycystic ovary and the effect of different phenotypic expressions on these parameters. Hum Reprod 2007;22(12):3116–23.
21. Kiyokawa K, Masuda H, Fuyuki T, et al. Three-dimensional hysterosalpingo-contrast sonography (3D-HyCoSy) as an outpatient procedure to assess infertile women: a pilot study. Ultrasound Obstet Gynecol 2000;16:648–54.
22. Sladkevicius P, Ojha K, Campbell S, et al. Three-dimensional power Doppler imaging in the assessment of Fallopian tube patency. Ultrasound Obstet Gynecol 2000;16:644–7.
23. Heer IM, Strauss A, Muller-Egloff S, et al. Telemedicine in ultrasound: new solutions. Ultrasound Med Biol 2001;27(9):1239–43.
24. Alcazar J. Three-dimensional ultrasound in gynecology: current status and future perspectives. Curr Womens Health Rev 2005;1:1–14.

Pelvic Floor Imaging

Cecile A. Unger, MD[a], Milena M. Weinstein, MD[b,*], Dolores H. Pretorius, MD[c]

KEYWORDS

- Pelvic floor disorders • Pelvic floor imaging
- Pelvic floor ultrasound • Transperineal ultrasound

Pelvic floor disorders including urinary incontinence, pelvic organ prolapse, and anal incontinence have high prevalence in women of all ages,[1] can significantly decrease quality of life, and produce an economic effect. Proper evaluation of pelvic floor muscle function, strength, and integrity is an important component of diagnosis and treatment of pelvic floor disorders. In addition, the pelvic floor muscle training used to change the structural support and strength of muscle contraction requires clinicians to be able to conduct high-quality measurements of pelvic floor muscle function and strength. Studies have shown that up to one-third of women do not know how to contract their pelvic floor muscles correctly.[2] Therefore, it is also important to be able to assess pelvic muscle function and strength to document a patient's progress during interventions designed to improve their strength.[3] Approximately 1 in 10 women undergo surgery for pelvic organ prolapse by the time they reach the age of 70 years.[4] In addition, urinary incontinence often coexists with pelvic organ prolapse.[1] Urinary incontinence is defined by the International Continence Society as a complaint of any involuntary leakage of urine.[5] The most common type of incontinence is involuntary leaking in response to increased intra-abdominal pressures during exertion, cough, or sneeze. This type of incontinence is called stress urinary incontinence.[6] Urinary incontinence is more common in women than it is in men, and it affects women of all ages. The prevalence ranges from 9% to 72%, with an incidence that rises steeply with age.[7] Several studies have documented the effects that urinary incontinence have on quality of life; it is a debilitating disorder that affects women socially and physically.[6] The International Consultation on Incontinence defines anal incontinence as the involuntary loss of gas, liquid, or stool that causes a social or hygienic problem.[8] The prevalence of anal incontinence has been documented in several studies to range from 20% to 54%.[9,10] The underlying cause of this type of incontinence is often related to anal sphincter defects following vaginal deliveries.[11] Because these disorders are so prevalent and severely affect a woman's quality of life, it is important to understand normal pelvic anatomy and function to treat pelvic floor disorders appropriately.[12]

PELVIC FLOOR ANATOMY AND FUNCTION

The deep muscles of the pelvic floor are often referred to as the levator ani or the pelvic diaphragm. The muscles that comprise the levator ani include the pubococcygeus, puborectalis, and iliococcygeus. These muscles span the space between the obturator internus muscle laterally, the pubis symphysis anteriorly, and the coccyx posteriorly. The superficial muscles of the pelvic floor make up the urogenital diaphragm and include the ischiocavernosus, bulbospongiosus, and the transverses perinea superficialis (**Fig. 1**). These pelvic floor muscles are encased in fascia that is continuous with the endopelvic fascia, which surrounds the pelvic viscera and also contributes to pelvic support.[3] The levator hiatus is a funnel-shaped cleft in the muscles of the

Funding: None.
The authors have nothing to disclose.
[a] Department of Vincent Obstetrics and Gynecology, Massachusetts General Hospital, 55 Fruit Street, FND 5, Boston, MA 02114, USA
[b] Division of Urogynecology and Reconstructive Pelvic Medicine, Department of Vincent Obstetrics and Gynecology, Massachusetts General Hospital, 55 Fruit Street, FND 5, Boston, MA 02114, USA
[c] Department of Radiology, University of California San Diego, San Diego, CA, USA
* Corresponding author.
E-mail address: mweinstein2@partners.org

Ultrasound Clin 5 (2010) 313–330
doi:10.1016/j.cult.2010.04.002
1556-858X/10/$ – see front matter. Published by Elsevier Inc.

ultrasound.theclinics.com

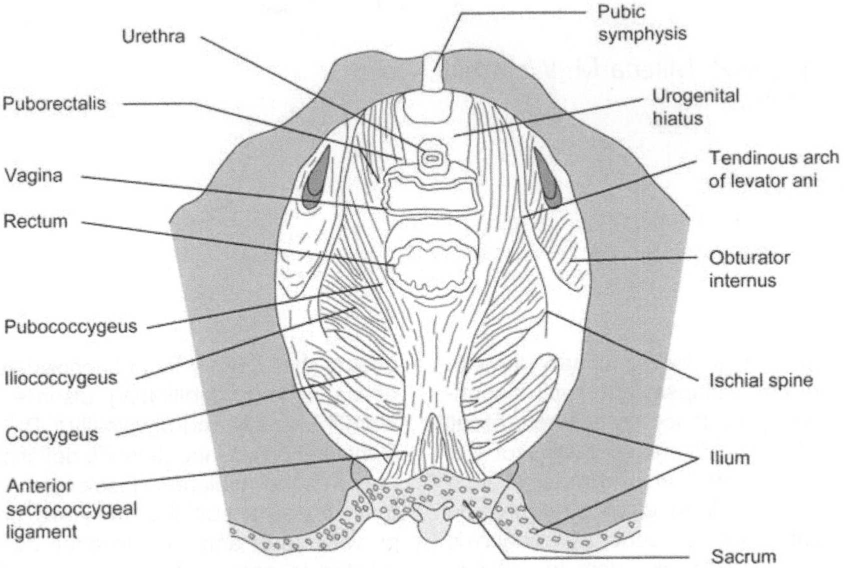

Fig. 1. Anatomy of the pelvic floor. Illustration: Rose Katz.

levator ani from which exit the urethra, vagina, and anal canal.[13] The puborectalis is the most inferior muscle of the pelvic floor and is composed of 2 limbs attached to the 2 pubic rami anteriorly; they merge posterior to the anal canal.[14] A normal anal canal is approximately 4 cm and represents the most distal portion of the gastrointestinal tract. The anal verge demarcates its most distal end. The structures surrounding the anal canal are responsible for maintaining fecal continence and include the involuntary internal anal sphincter (IAS), the voluntary external anal sphincter (EAS), and the puborectalis muscle (PRM). The IAS is responsible for approximately 80% of resting anal tone and where it terminates distally represents the junction of the subcutaneous and superficial components of the EAS, which is created from the downward extension of the PRM. The rectum, which is in communication with the anal canal, contains a longitudinal muscle layer that extends distally, separating the EAS and IAS, and anchors the sphincter complex to the fascia of the levator ani, as well as the pelvic side wall.[15] The perineal body separates the anus from the vagina. It is the central portion of the perineum that represents where the EAS, the bulbospongiosus, and the superficial and deep transverse perineal muscles meet. The presence of a thick perineal body is suggestive of a normal anal sphincter.[16]

The important role of the pelvic floor musculature is to perform voluntary contractions as well as involuntary, or reflex, contractions preceding or at the time of increased abdominal pressure. These types of contractions preserve fecal and urinary continence. In response to increased abdominal pressures, the superficial pelvic muscles, such as the anal and urethral sphincters, resist these pressures; and the levator ani muscles support the pelvic floor and counteract these pressures by contracting and creating a circular closing of the levator hiatus and an upward movement of the pelvic floor and perineum.[17–20] The PRM has an important role in pelvic floor support and conservation of continence. When this muscle contracts, the length of its 2 limbs is reduced, and this change lifts the anal canal anteriorly, compressing the structures within the levator hiatus against each other as well as the back of the pubic symphysis.[21] Because of their important role in urethral closure for urinary continence, these muscles are the target tissue in physical therapy for management of incontinence and other pelvic floor disorders.[22] In addition to the pelvic floor muscles, another important factor for urinary continence is the smooth and striated muscle contraction within the urethral wall, as well as the ligaments and the fascia that support the bladder and urethra in proper position during increased intra-abdominal pressure.[23] Fecal continence is maintained by the anorectal lift of the pelvic floor as well as the constricting of the anal canal. Urinary continence is preserved by the support applied to the bladder neck during pelvic floor contraction, as well as constriction of the urethral lumen.[17,18]

CONVENTIONAL IMAGING OF THE PELVIC FLOOR

Many imaging modalities have previously been used to evaluate the pelvic floor, including computed tomography, magnetic resonance (MR) imaging, and barium defecography.[24–26] These various forms of imaging have enhanced the diagnosis of many pelvic floor disorders, including pelvic organ prolapse.[12,27] Defecography uses fluoroscopy to evaluate the pelvic floor. It is an imaging modality that is appropriate for assessing pelvic organ prolapse because it uses contrast material to opacify the involved organs and it is used to evaluate their function in real time. The advantage of defecography is that it replicates the patient's symptoms, because it requires the patient to be upright during the evaluation. Organs of the anterior and posterior compartments of the pelvic floor can be examined, so that a patient can be evaluated for anterior and posterior prolapse.[25] Although defecography is useful to evaluate the interaction of rectal evacuation with the other pelvic organs and their relationship with the pelvic floor musculature, there is a significant disadvantage to defecography: it requires multiorgan opacification, which exposes patients to high-level radiation.[24,28] In addition, no studies have evaluated the reproducibility of the measurements obtained during defecography.

MR is used to evaluate the gross morphology of the pelvic floor anatomy and provides advanced soft-tissue differentiation because of its high spatial resolution. In addition, MR provides multiplanar imaging but avoids ionizing radiation and contrast material; it is also advantageous because it is not operator dependent.[25] T1-weighted images are usually taken in multiple planes. Coronal images show the structures from the anal verge to where the EAS meets the levator ani. Images can also be taken at the level of the puborectalis plane, which enables visualization of the IAS, EAS, and the levator ani, which makes this modality an excellent tool to evaluate for sphincter abnormalities and structural causes for incontinence.[25] The disadvantages of MR imaging are that it is the most expensive modality, it is time consuming, and it is not always readily available.[24,25,29] A significant disadvantage of using MR is its poor dynamic parameters in assessing pelvic organ descent during patient straining or squeezing and the need to place patients in nonphysiologic positions to look for prolapse.[25,29] Studies have shown that the prolapse parameters measured on MR correlate poorly with those seen on defecography[25] and therefore it is difficult to assess the degree of prolapse found in patients who undergo MR imaging.

ULTRASOUND IMAGING

Ultrasound has been widely used to explore pelvic floor abnormalities and dysfunction.[30–32] Real-time ultrasound can be used to look at the dynamic interaction involved in the pelvic floor as it relates to continence and pelvic organ prolapse. Studies have shown that ultrasound is superior as a clinical adjunct when compared with conventional methods, including anal manometry, electromyography, and defecography.[33] It is especially useful as a biofeedback tool for pelvic floor training.[19]

Endoanal Ultrasound

Endoanal ultrasound can be used to evaluate the anal sphincter complex to assist in the diagnosis of fecal incontinence. Many studies have shown that on ultrasound, fecal incontinence is strongly associated with anal sphincter defects; patients most often have a combined external and internal sphincter defect, or an EAS defect alone; isolated internal sphincter defects are rare.[16,34]

Endoanal ultrasound requires a high frequency transducer of 7 mHz or higher that can produce a 360° panoramic image to adequately visualize the anal sphincter complex.[35] Patients are usually placed in a prone or left lateral position because this facilitates the complete imaging of the anterior part of the sphincter complex as well as the perineum. Once the transducer is placed in the anal canal, it is rotated to the 12 o'clock position anteriorly. When the transducer is rotated in this direction, the images obtained are in the same orientation as those used for cross-sectional imaging of the entire body.[15] In this view, 4 anatomic layers can be visualized: the subepithelial layer, which is hyperechoic; the IAS, which is a hypoechoic ring with a thickness of approximately 1.35 to 2.67 mm; the longitudinal muscle, which is hyperechoic; and the EAS, which is hyperechoic and is the outermost layer, with a measured thickness of approximately 5.4 to 7.42 mm.[15,35] In the most cephalad region of the anal canal, the deep EAS is continuous with the PRM, which is a sling of mixed echogenicity that loops posteriorly around the anal canal (**Fig. 2**).[15]

Ultrasound allows for an easy visualization of the anal canal structures and thus is a perfect tool to assess the integrity of these structures.[25] Anal sphincter defects are seen as thickening and changes of echogenicity or asymmetry along the sphincter, described based on a clock face on which 12 o'clock is at the anterior position. Defects in the EAS appear hypoechoic, whereas defects in the IAS appear hyperechoic (**Fig. 3**).[15] Studies have shown good intraobserver and interobserver agreement on recognition of sphincter defects using endoanal ultrasound.[36] Results have also correlated with anorectal manometry findings in other studies; defects in the EAS are associated

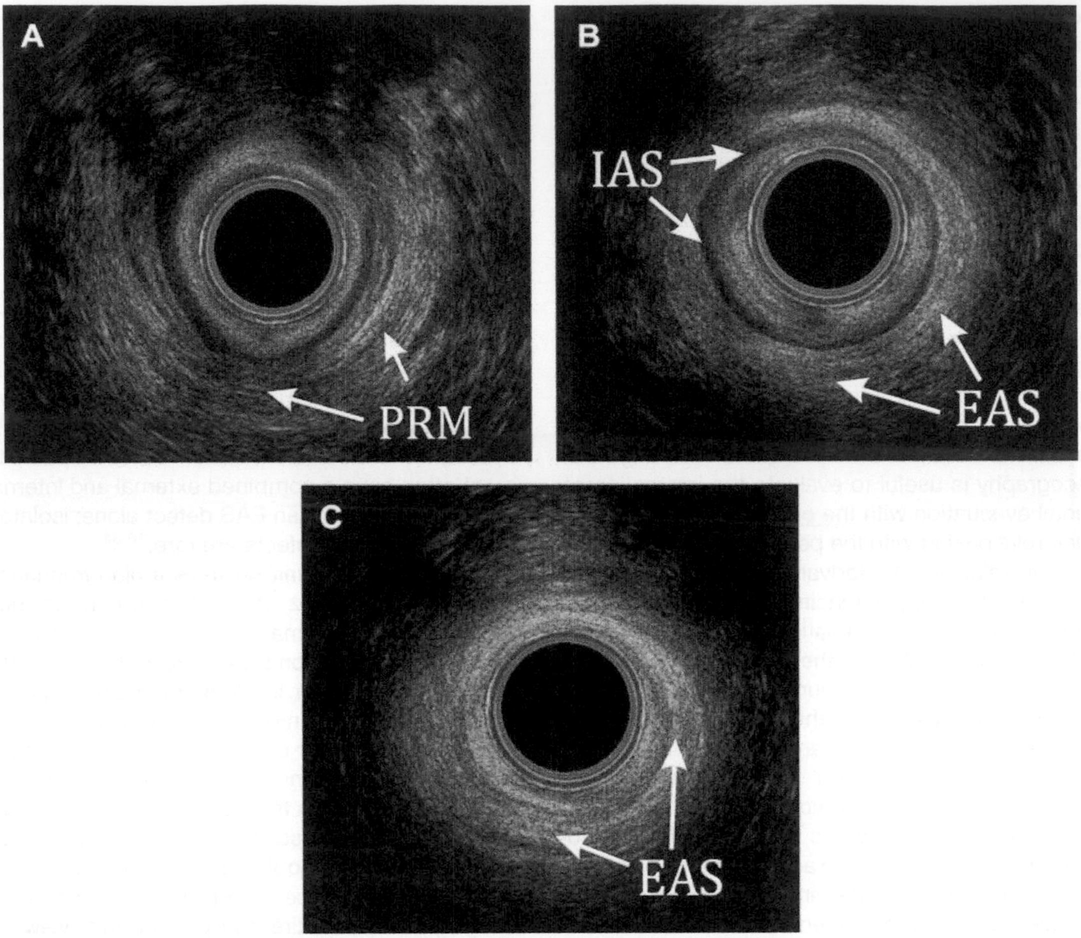

Fig. 2. Endoanal ultrasound with normal anal sphincter complex. (*A*) Proximal anal canal with puborectalis: endoanal ultrasound transducer is the round black circle in the middle, surrounded by echolucent anal mucosa and dark ring of the IAS. The IAS is surrounded posteriorly with the posterior portion of the PRM (*arrows*). (*Courtesy of* Dr Liliana Bordeianou.) (*B*) Midanal canal: the echolucent circle of the IAS (*arrows*), which is surrounded by an echogenic circle of the EAS (*arrows*). (*Courtesy of* Dr Liliana Bordeianou.) (*C*) Distal anal canal: the superficial portion of echogenic EAS (*arrows*) seen surrounding the transducer. This portion of EAS extends further distally than the IAS, which is normally not visible at the most distal extend of the anal canal. (*Courtesy of* Dr Liliana Bordeianou.)

with lower anal squeeze pressures, whereas defects in the IAS are associated with lower resting anal pressures.[37,38] Endoanal ultrasound is considered to be a sensitive study for anal sphincter defects; with sensitivity reaching 100% in some studies. This finding has been determined by comparing ultrasound findings with surgical findings at the time of anal sphincter repair for fecal incontinence, whereas other studies have compared ultrasound findings with sphincter defects confirmed histologically.[39–41] Furthermore, studies have shown that endoanal ultrasound can be used to show resolution of sphincter defects after sphincteroplasty, which has good correlation with patients' symptoms and resolution of incontinence.[42,43] Endoanal ultrasound can also be used as a means to detect sphincter defects early, before development of incontinence symptoms. Faltin and colleagues[44] showed that the use of ultrasound in addition to a standard clinical examination immediately post partum improved the detection of anal sphincter tears. The immediate repair of these tears significantly decreased the risk of severe fecal incontinence reported 3 months to 1 year after giving birth.

Perineal body measurement has been reported to enhance the evaluation of anal sphincter defects. This measurement can be obtained by positioning the patient in the left lateral position, placing the endoanal transducer inside the rectum, and slowly withdrawing the transducer so that the

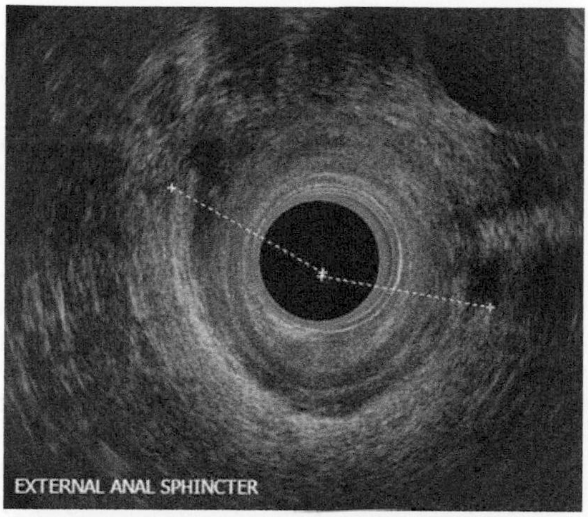

Fig. 3. Endoanal ultrasound of the midanal canal showing external and IAS defect (shown with calipers); the sphincter damage spans the area between 10 o'clock and 3 o'clock. (*Courtesy of* Dr Liliana Bordeianou.)

anal canal is visualized. A gloved finger is placed into the vagina and pressure is held against the posterior vaginal wall at the level of the midanal canal. The distance between the sonographic reflection of the fingertip and the inner border of the subepithelial layer is measured on a frozen ultrasound image.[16] Studies have found that thinning of the perineal body is a clinical finding among incontinent women who have anal sphincter defects. It has been shown that patients with a perineal body thickness of 10 mm or less are likely to have an anal sphincter defect 93% to 97% of the time.[16,45] Patients with a perineal body thickness of 10 to 12 mm are shown to have an indeterminate thickness of the perineal body, and anal sphincter defects can be found in approximately one-third of these patients. A perineal body thickness of greater than 12 mm was shown to be unlikely to be associated with a sphincter defect unless a patient had previously undergone reconstructive perineal surgery, at which point the risk of a defect was shown to be approximately 20%.[16]

Because the images obtained show the entire anal canal as it relates to the sphincter complex and the rest of the pelvic floor, endoanal ultrasound can be used to delineate fistulas, abscesses, and anal carcinomas.[25] Fistulas appear as hypoechoic tracts containing pockets of air that appear as focal hyperechoic areas.[15] The technique has also been used to evaluate patients with obstructed defecation, which is visualized as thickening of the sphincter muscle complex.[46] Patients with pelvic organ prolapse and urinary incontinence can also be evaluated with endoanal ultrasound. Patients with urinary incontinence have concomitant anal sphincter defects noted on endoanal ultrasound 52% of the time, and patients with other pelvic floor disorders have been shown to have additional anal sphincter defects 30% of the time.[34] These findings have been replicated in other studies as well, proving that there is a spectrum of pelvic floor disorders, with extensive overlap amongst the defects that can be seen on ultrasound.[47]

Endoanal ultrasound has also been used as biofeedback during pelvic floor exercises that are used to strengthen pelvic floor muscles for patients with prolapse and incontinence symptoms. No studies have shown that ultrasound using a transducer in the anal canal is better feedback than digital examination or anal manometry.[48] However, there is evidence that certain measurements can be obtained only with ultrasound and these measurements have better correlations with clinical outcomes than digital examination and manometry. The 2 measurements that have been studied are isotonic fatigue time and isometric fatigue contraction during pelvic floor squeezing. Pelvic floor training seems to improve these measures, which have been shown to correlate directly with a patient's improvement in quality of life and improvement in fecal continence symptoms. Endoanal ultrasound may not have any additional benefit during a physical therapy session in regards to biofeedback, compared with conventional methods of feedback; however, it seems that ultrasound may have an important role in determining physiologic measures, which correlate well with pelvic floor strength and improvement with training.[48]

Transperineal Ultrasound

Transperineal ultrasound was one of the first modes of ultrasound to be used to evaluate the soft tissues and viscera of the pelvic floor. An article written by Beer-Gabel and colleagues[24] describes the following technique for the use of transperineal ultrasound. The patient is positioned in the left lateral position, and acoustic gel is applied to the vagina and rectum. In other studies, patients have been placed in the dorsal supine lithotomy position.[49] The ultrasound transducer is then placed on the perineal body in the midsagittal plane to outline the pelvic floor muscles and organs. Images are obtained at rest, during maximal straining (Valsalva maneuver), and during pelvic squeeze so that real-time movement can be assessed. The transducer is then rotated 180° to visualize the anus and its surrounding structures, including the EAS and IAS. Sagittal evaluation of the anterior portion of the perineum shows the distal vagina, bladder, and urethra as well as the rectovaginal septum. These images are useful for the diagnosis of anterior vaginal wall prolapse (cystocele), posterior vaginal wall prolapse (rectocele), and for measuring the vaginal vault prolapse. Certain anatomic measurements can be taken in this view. These measurements include the perimeters of the PRM and the calculation of the anorectal angle as well as the posterior urethrovesical angle. The anorectal angle is measured where the longitudinal axis of the anal canal (designated with a line) meets the posterior border of the rectal wall. The urethrovesical angle or the urethrovesical junction is measured by creating a perpendicular line from the x-axis on the image, and following this line to the margin of the bladder base when the patient is at rest (**Fig. 4**).[50] The anorectal angle and the urethrovesical angle are measured at rest and at squeeze, which is helpful in the diagnosis of fecal incontinence, organ prolapse, and urinary incontinence.[24] In addition, this view allows for the dynamic function of the puborectalis to be measured. The puborectalis is visualized as a hyperechoic sling hugging the IAS in the transverse view and as a soft-tissue bundle in the sagittal view. The distance between the posterior margin of the symphysis pubis and posterior limit of the anorectal junction represents the perimeter of the puborectalis. The difference in length between the rest measurement and the squeeze measurement defines the dynamic activity of this muscle; the muscle usually shortens during a contraction

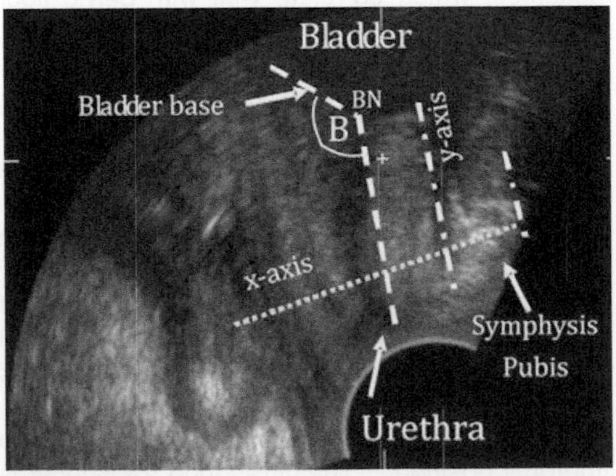

Fig. 4. The posterior urethrovesical angle measurement method with perineal ultrasound described by Schaer and colleagues.[50] The rectangular coordinate system was constructed with the y-axis at the inferior symphysis pubis and the x-axis perpendicular through the midsymphysis pubis. The posterior urethrovesical angle (B) was measured with a line through the urethral axis and the other line through the at least one-third of the bladder base.

(**Fig. 5**). When the transducer head is held in the transverse plane, oriented backward at 45°, at the level of the vaginal introitus, a different view of the anal sphincters can be captured as well. As in the longitudinal axis, the IAS appears hypoechoic, whereas the EAS appears hyperechoic.[24,49]

Transperineal ultrasound can be a useful tool. Investigators have described it as being applicable from a clinical perspective. It can be used to visualize the anal sphincter complex, which is useful in the grading of hemorrhoidal disease, evaluating the submucosal location of anal fistulas, and looking at sphincter defects. Studies have looked at the usefulness of conducting a physical examination alone after repair of a perineal injury from childbirth, versus using transperineal sonography as well to ensure proper sphincter repair. The digital examination is adequate to ensure proper restoration of the anatomy, which includes palpating for EAS thickness and perineal body length; however, ultrasound was determined to enhance evaluation by providing additional information on sphincter function.[51]

Endoanal ultrasound has been reported as one of the most reliable methods of identifying anal sphincter defects. However, images obtained by transperineal ultrasound have shown the same concentric layers and cross-sectional images as seen on endoanal ultrasound.[49] Many support the use of transperineal ultrasound for these reasons, as well as the other advantages, which include low cost, availability of equipment, and low degree of invasiveness for the patient.[49] It can also be used to visualize the contrast between the shapes of the pelvic organs at rest and during straining, which helps to diagnose posterior and anterior vaginal wall prolapse (rectocele and cystocele), enteroceles, and genital prolapse.[24] In addition, the urethrovesical junction during straining can be measured, which is useful for the diagnosis of stress urinary incontinence. Minardi and Parri[52] used transperineal ultrasound to assess the function and morphology of the urethral sphincter and detrusor muscle in the evaluation of dysfunctional voiding in patients with recurrent urinary tract infections. Via transperineal ultrasound, the urethrovesical angle, proximal pubourethral distance, and the urethral inclination were measured and calculated. The thickness of the bladder detrusor wall was measured at the bladder dome via a suprapubic ultrasound. The urethral sphincter volume was then measured with a transvaginal ultrasound transducer. They were able to show that patients who had recurrent urinary tract infections and dysfunctional voiding, shown on urodynamic testing, had higher urethral sphincter volumes and abnormal echogenicity of

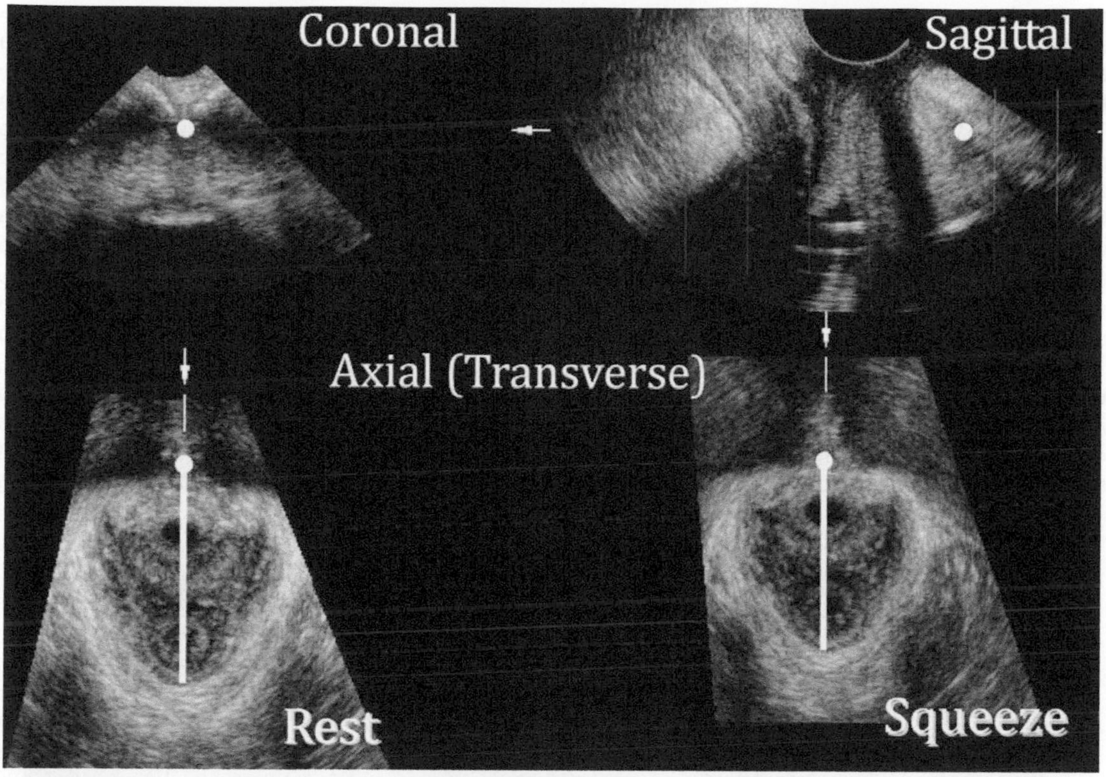

Fig. 5. Transperineal three-dimensional ultrasound of the pelvic floor hiatus: multiplanar image with coronal, sagittal, and axial (transverse) planes shown. The original volume was obtained at rest; the insert image of the axial pelvic floor hiatus is from a volume obtained during a sustained pelvic floor contraction (squeeze). Images show measures on the anterior-posterior (AP) hiatal length; the shortening of the AP length is a reflection of shortening as a result of the PRM shortening during pelvic floor contraction.

the urethral sphincters. In addition, they were able to use the calculated measurements of the posterior urethrovesical angle, proximal pubourethral distance, and the urethral inclination to diagnose urethral hypermobility, which was more common in patients with recurrent infections. Urodynamic testing on these patients significantly correlated with the calculated urethral sphincter volumes on ultrasound, showing the validity of these measurements. With all of this information, the investigators were able to create threshold ultrasound measurements for patients with dysfunctional voiding, and they propose that transperineal ultrasound be used as a first-line diagnostic test for evaluating patients with suspected urinary incontinence.[52]

Three-dimensional Ultrasound

Three-dimensional ultrasound has been used for the last 20 years and has been embraced by the obstetrics specialty in the last 5 years. Gynecologists are now starting to use this modality as an adjunct to study pelvic floor disorders.[53,54]

As mentioned earlier, MR imaging has been one of the modalities of choice for evaluation of the pelvic floor because it can identify the involved muscle groups, and has excellent spatial resolution. However, the major limitation of MR imaging is its failure to fully capture present-time pictures because spatial resolution is often spared as imaging time becomes faster. It is also expensive and time consuming and is less clinically convenient. As a result, the usefulness of three-dimensional ultrasound has been studied.[13,14,21,55]

Some studies have shown poor correlation between MR imaging and ultrasound, but some investigators believe that this is because previous studies did not use the same plane on ultrasound as was used on MR.[13] Another study showed that the 2 modalities correlate at rest, but there is no correlation during maximum Valsalva. This finding is likely because of the physical limitations of MR imaging. When using MR imaging, it is difficult to predict the end point during Valsalva and because MR is not performed under real time, the true plane needed to adequately evaluate pelvic floor function is not as available to the degree that it is in ultrasound.[13] In more recent studies, transperineal three-dimensional ultrasound has shown to be as effective, if not better, than MR imaging in imaging the pelvic floor.[13] This is because three-dimensional ultrasound contains cine loop capabilities, which allows for assessment of the functional anatomy of the pelvic floor with superior spatial and temporal resolution with multiple volumes of imaging obtained per second.[56] Three-dimensional ultrasound acquires volume datasets that can be used to produce single slices in any arbitrarily defined plane.[47]

The three-dimensional ultrasound technique used to evaluate the pelvic floor was described in a recent study conducted by Weinstein and colleagues.[14] The imaging is performed with subjects in the dorsal supine lithotomy position, using a transvaginal transducer placed on the midperineum, oriented in the midsagittal plane to obtain images of the anal sphincter complex. The ultrasound beam is directed in the cranial direction to visualize the pelvic floor hiatus as well as the PRM. The field of view is optimized by identifying the symphysis pubis on the left of the screen and the anal canal on the right side of the screen (**Fig. 6**A).[14] When the beam is directed in the posterior direction, the EAS and IAS are visualized. Images are captured at rest and during sustained anal sphincter and pelvic floor contraction. To visualize the anal sphincters three-dimensionally, the sagittal images of the anal canal are rotated in the horizontal direction and the axial images that are examined are the craniocaudal length of the IAS and EAS at 1-mm distances separating

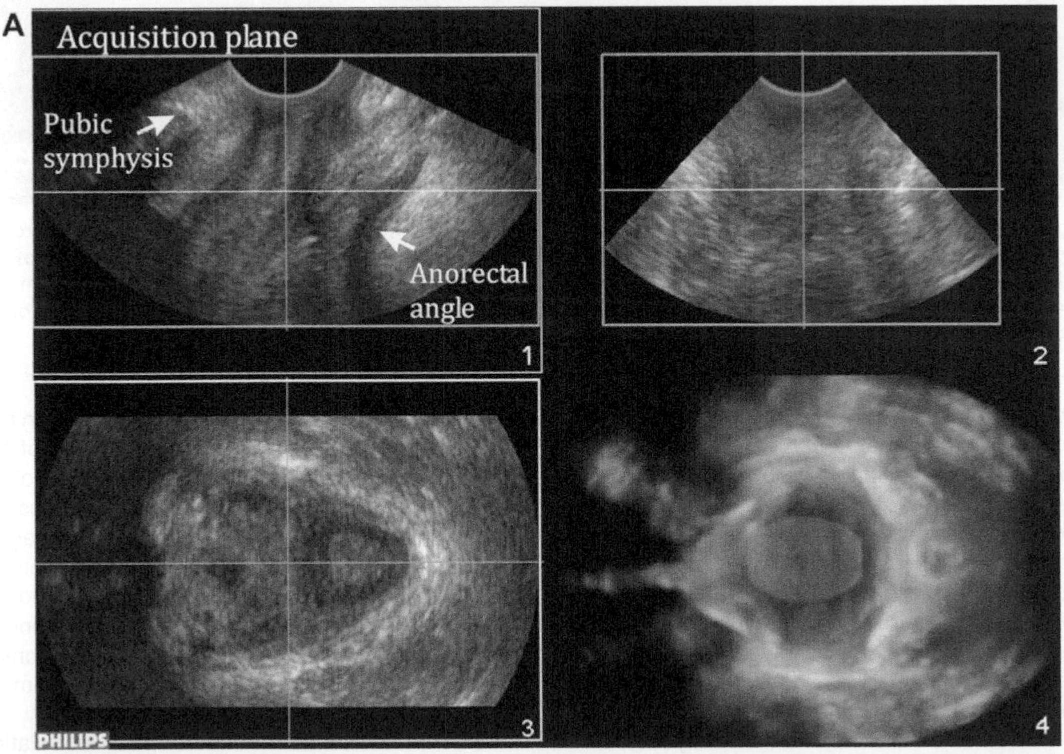

Fig. 6. (*A*) Transperineal ultrasound of the pelvic floor hiatus. Endovaginal ultrasound transducer positioned on the perineum and oriented cranially to obtain the three-dimensional volume. The acquisition plane-sagittal plane is optimized by visualizing the pubic symphysis and the anorectal angle. (*B*) Volume is rotated to orient the axial plane upright. The multiplanar of the three-dimensional transperineal volume is shown with coronal, sagittal, and axial (transverse) planes. (*C*) The dot marker is moved in the axial (transverse) plane in the area of the pubic symphysis. The pubic rami and pubic symphysis are visible in the coronal plane. The dot marker is positioned on the pubic symphysis. (*D*) In the sagittal plane the volume is rotated to align the pubic symphysis with the anorectal angle; this represents the PRM plane. The PRM is seen encircling the pelvic floor hiatus in the transverse image. (*E*) The transperineal view of the pelvic floor hiatus after completion of the volume rotation. The rendered thick slice (10 mm) allows for more detailed assessment of the hiatal structures. The pelvic floor hiatus anatomy includes a cross section of the urethra, vagina, and the anorectum. The hiatus is encircled by the PRM. The PRM can also be seen as a bundle abutting the anorectum at the anorectal angle in the sagittal plane.

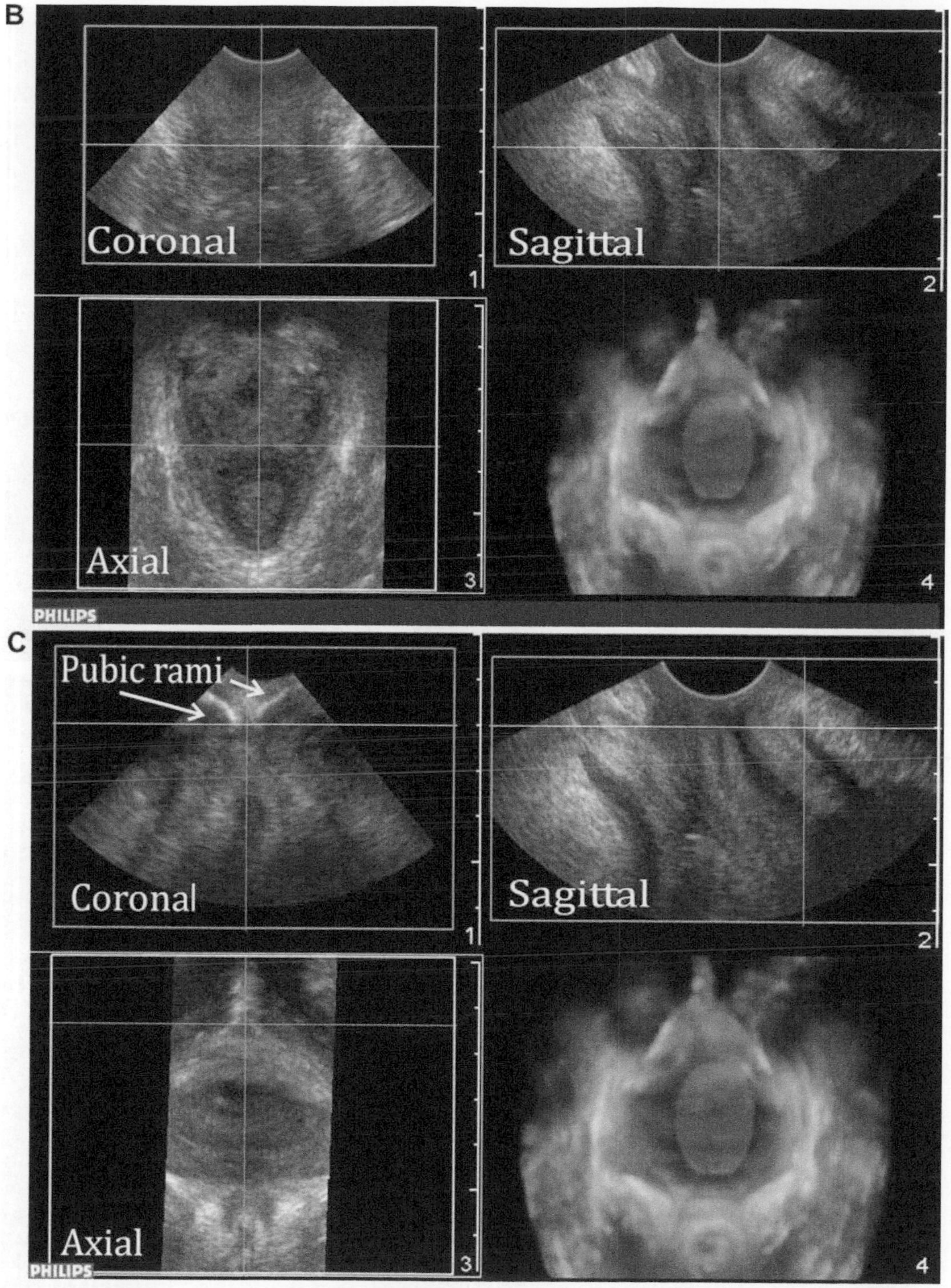

Fig. 6. (*continued*)

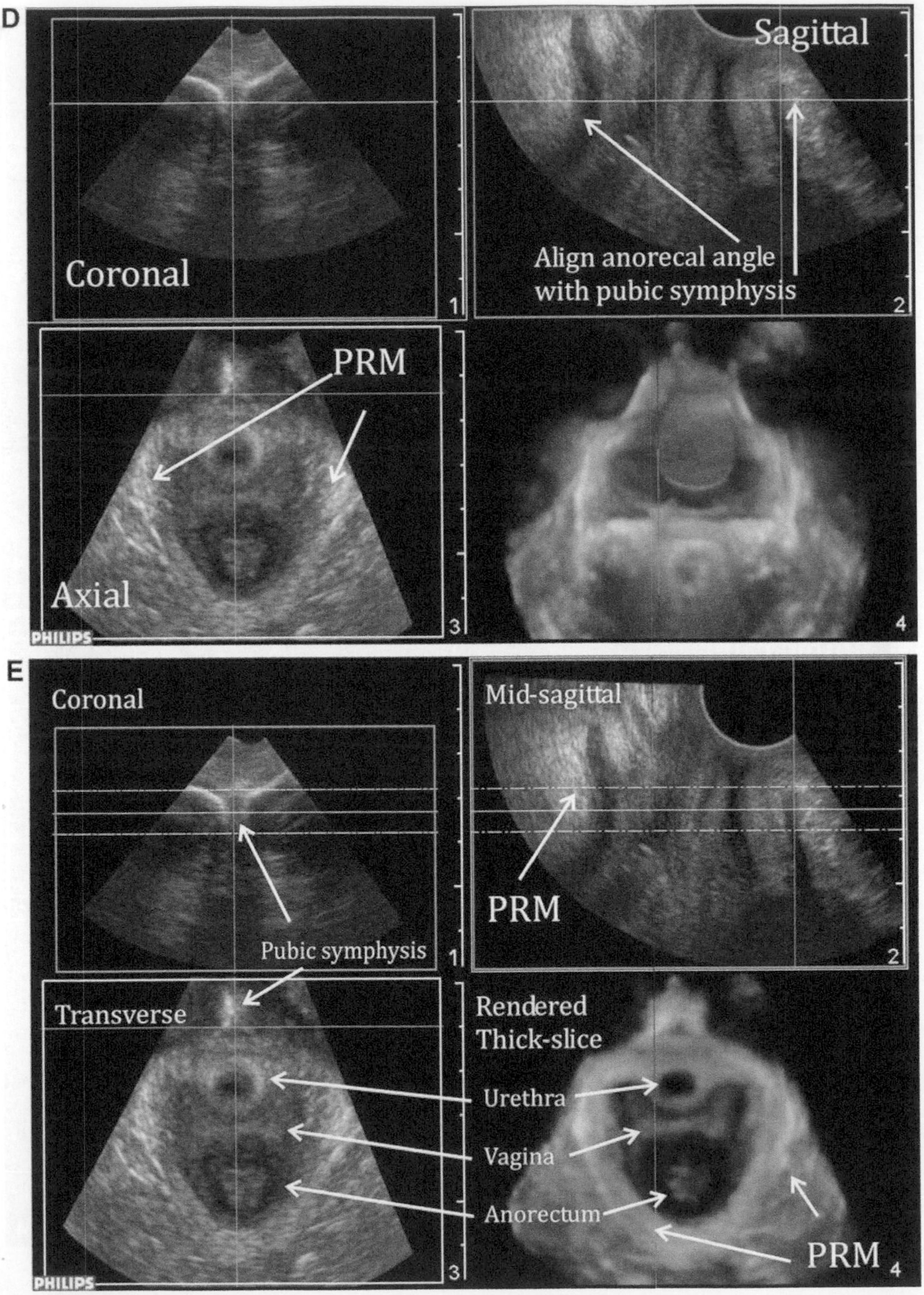

Fig. 6. (*continued*)

each image (**Fig. 7**). The lower edge of the pubic symphysis and anorectal angles are then identified and these landmarks are used to delineate the PRM. The puborectalis plane is defined by a straight line that connects these 2 landmarks (see **Fig. 6**A–D). The puborectalis inner perimeter is defined by a curvilinear measurement along the inner border of the PRM to its insertion site on the pubic ramus. The pelvic floor hiatus inner area is defined as the area within the PRM inner perimeter enclosed anteriorly by 2 straight lines, connecting the puborectalis insertion point on the pubic rami to the inferior edge of the symphysis pubis. The pelvic floor hiatus outer area is contained within the outer border of the puborectalis; it has the same borders as the pelvic floor hiatus inner area anteriorly. The puborectalis area is a calculated measurement obtained by subtracting the pelvic floor hiatus from the outer area. This measurement represents the cross-sectional area of the puborectalis.[14] Images are captured parallel to this plane, again, at 1-mm distances separating each image. In addition, a 10-mm-thick slice is captured, which integrates the volumes of data obtained (see **Fig. 6**E). This tool is used to assess the anatomic appearance of the muscles examined for any defects, to ensure that any defects noted on the two-dimensional images are real and not artifact. A shift from the midline in any of the pelvic floor hiatal structures is also measured, as any defect in the puborectalis may cause asymmetry in the pelvic floor hiatus. The anterior-posterior length of the pelvic floor hiatus is also calculated. This length is described as the distance between the pubic symphysis and an anorectal angle.[14]

Three-dimensional ultrasound has been shown to be a reliable method for detecting morphologic defects in the IAS, EAS, and puborectalis.[55] These defects have been identified in studies of women after childbirth, because this population has a high incidence of PRM and anal sphincter defects related to childbirth trauma.[57] Studies have shown that the most common injury related to childbirth is an avulsion injury of the insertion of the PRM on the pubic ramus (**Fig. 8**).[58] Detecting avulsions of the PRM has a potential clinical implication in women with fecal incontinence.[58,59] Contractions of the PRM are believed to decrease the anorectal angle and increase pressure in the proximal part of the anal canal, and when the EAS contracts, there is increased pressure in the distal part of the canal.[60] On three-dimensional ultrasound, these contractions and associated measurements are well captured.[61] Three-dimensional ultrasound can also visualize anatomic defects of the individual components of the anal sphincter (**Fig. 9**). For example, the anal canal may appear asymmetric when there is a defect, and this asymmetry is more pronounced during pelvic floor contraction or squeeze. Patients with fecal incontinence are shown to have sphincter complex and PRM defects compared with nulliparous patients with no symptoms of incontinence. Women who are parous and examined with ultrasound are shown to have more defects than nulliparous women, but fewer abnormalities when compared with women who have diagnosed fecal incontinence. In addition, women noted to have an anatomically defective puborectalis have longer anterior-posterior lengths of the pelvic floor hiatus compared with controls. Other measurements that can be obtained with three-dimensional ultrasound include the muscular component of the levator hiatus (the length of the suprapubic arch subtracted from the hiatal circumference) and the muscle strain on contraction (hiatal circumference subtracted from the hiatal circumference at rest). These measurements can raise suspicion for levator injuries or defects if they are abnormal. In addition, the images can be used to look for avulsion injuries, which appear as abnormal insertion of the PRM on the inferior pubic ramus. This image is best seen during maximal contraction of the pelvic floor (**Fig. 10**).[62]

Transperineal three-dimensional ultrasound has been compared with two-dimensional endoanal ultrasound and has been shown to be a better mode of imaging with many advantages. It allows better visualization of the entire puborectalis sling, which is not seen well on two-dimensional imaging.[21] In addition, using a cutaneous transducer is less invasive and is favored by patients, there is less operator-induced error in capturing adequate images, thin and thick slices of the ultrasound images are available, the entire pelvic hiatus can be visualized as well as any asymmetry in the hiatus or the vagina, and structures in the hiatus are well delineated compared with two-dimensional imaging. However, three-dimensional ultrasound is new technology and it is still at the preliminary stages of its clinical application in most clinical sites.

ULTRASOUND IN THE EVALUATION AND TREATMENT OF URINARY INCONTINENCE

Three-dimensional ultrasound has also been used in the assessment of patients with urinary incontinence by imaging the urethral morphology and measuring the urethra and its sphincter. Imaging has shown that women with stress urinary incontinence have urethral sphincters that are shorter, thinner, and smaller in volume.[63] There has been debate about the urinary continence mechanism, whether it is related to an extrinsic mechanism such as a sling that is located under the urethra that is pulled upward and compresses the urethra during pelvic floor contraction,[64] or whether it is related to an intrinsic mechanism such as striated sphincter that contracts down on the urethral lumen when the pelvic muscles contract.[65] With

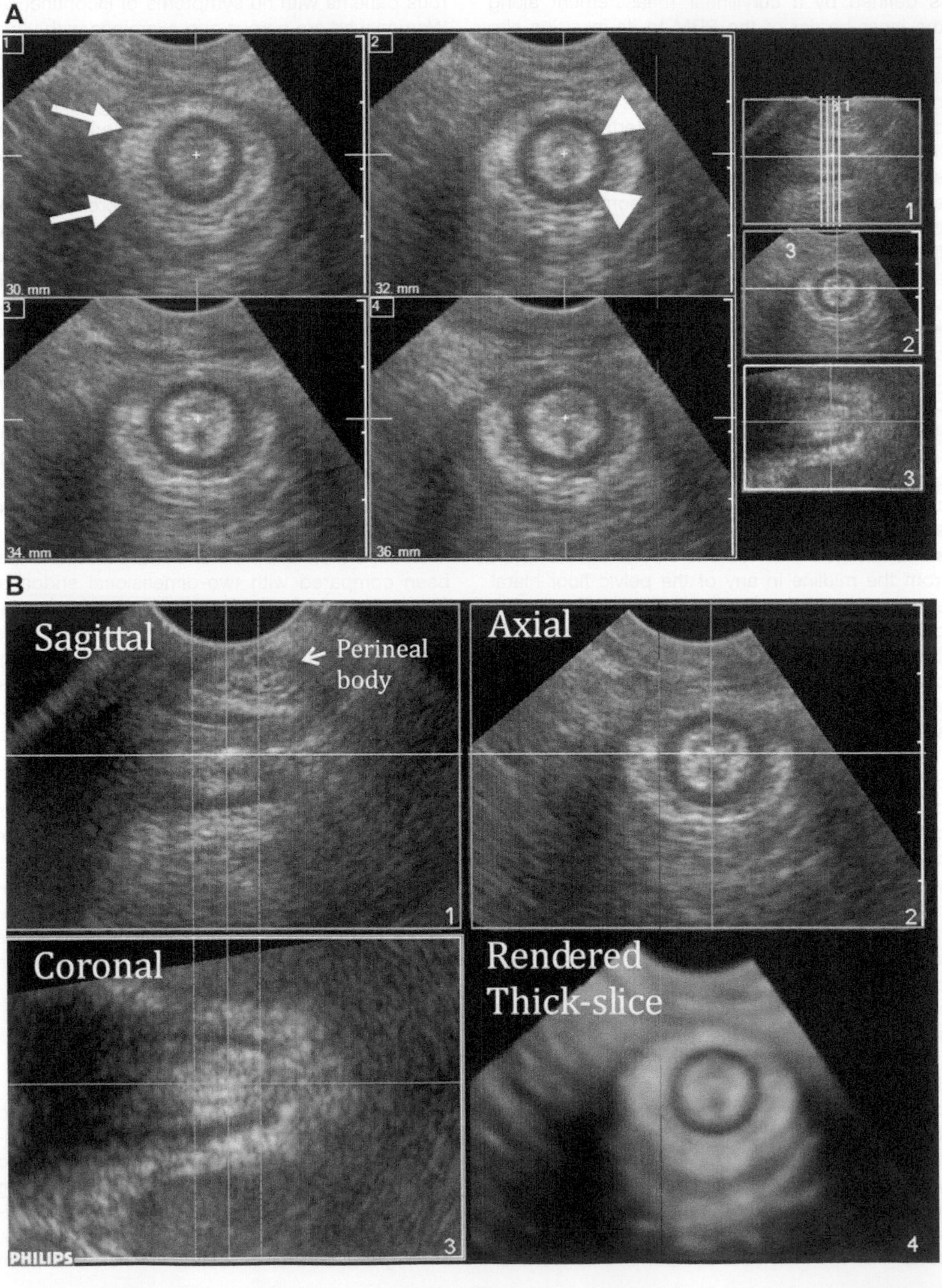

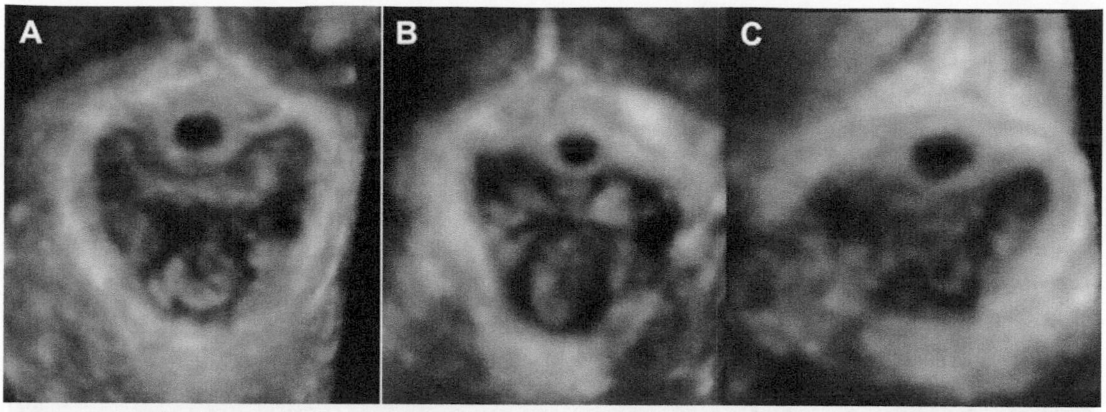

Fig. 8. An example of hiatal structure and the PRM without injury are shown (*A*). Examples of the PRM injury (*B, C*) on 10-mm-thick slice images of the PRM. The PRM injury is easily seen with asymmetry in hiatal structures. Note how urethra and vagina shift away from the midline to the side where the PRM injury is greater.

use of three-dimensional ultrasound Umek and colleagues[66] tried to elucidate the urethral continence mechanism. With use of a transrectal transducer, the morphology of the urethra was recorded and the urethral diameters, sphincter, and smooth muscle lengths as well as their thickness and volumes were measured. These investigators found that urethral diameters and sphincter thickness were smaller during pelvic floor contraction compared with pelvic floor relaxation. In addition, total urethral and sphincter volumes are smaller during contraction compared with relaxation. The smooth muscle complex of the urethra did not change in thickness or volume during contraction periods compared with relaxation periods. These investigators concluded that the urethral continence mechanism was extrinsic and occurs because of external compression by paraurethral tissues rather than intrinsic contraction of the urethral sphincter.[66]

Urethral bulking agents are used to improve continence by enhancing urethral coaptation. These agents are mostly used in urinary disorders that are attributed to intrinsic sphincter abnormalities or urethral hypermobility.[67] In 1993, Khuller and colleagues[68] imaged women using two-dimensional transperineal and transvaginal ultrasound after periurethral collagen injections. These investigators first correlated clinical symptoms of incontinence with urodynamic testing to test for improved sphincter function. They subsequently evaluated the collagen around the urethra with ultrasound and found that the parameter that was most correlated with improvement in continence was collagen intrusion into the bladder base, and not the cross-sectional area of the collagen. They concluded that increased collagen at the bladder neck improves clinical outcomes. This finding has also been replicated in other studies.[69] Studies have also reported an optimal periurethral location for bulking agents. This finding has been assessed using three-dimensional ultrasound, which is considered the best way to evaluate this parameter because it can measure the volumes of irregularly shaped structures; these measurements have been proved to be reproducible and reliable.[53] These studies have shown that the optimal periurethral location of the collagen is a circumferential or horseshoe distribution around the urethra. This type of

Fig. 7. (*A*) Cross-sectional (axial) multislice imaging of the normal anal canal in a nulliparous woman. The anal sphincter complex is shown at every 2-mm distance using the I-Slice function. The arrowheads mark the hypoechoic (*dark circle*) IAS; the arrows mark the hyperechoic (*white*) outer ring EAS; both sphincters are uniform and symmetric. The PRM is not seen here because the cross section is through the midportion of the sphincter complex and the PRM is a more caudal structure. (*B*) Transperineal three-dimensional ultrasound of the normal anal canal: the multiplanar of the ultrasound of the normal anal sphincter is shown with the corresponding planes: sagittal, coronal, and axial (cross-sectional). The rendered thick slice (10 mm) allows for integrated evaluation of the midanal sphincter portion. In the sagittal plane the perineal body is seen as an oval structure.

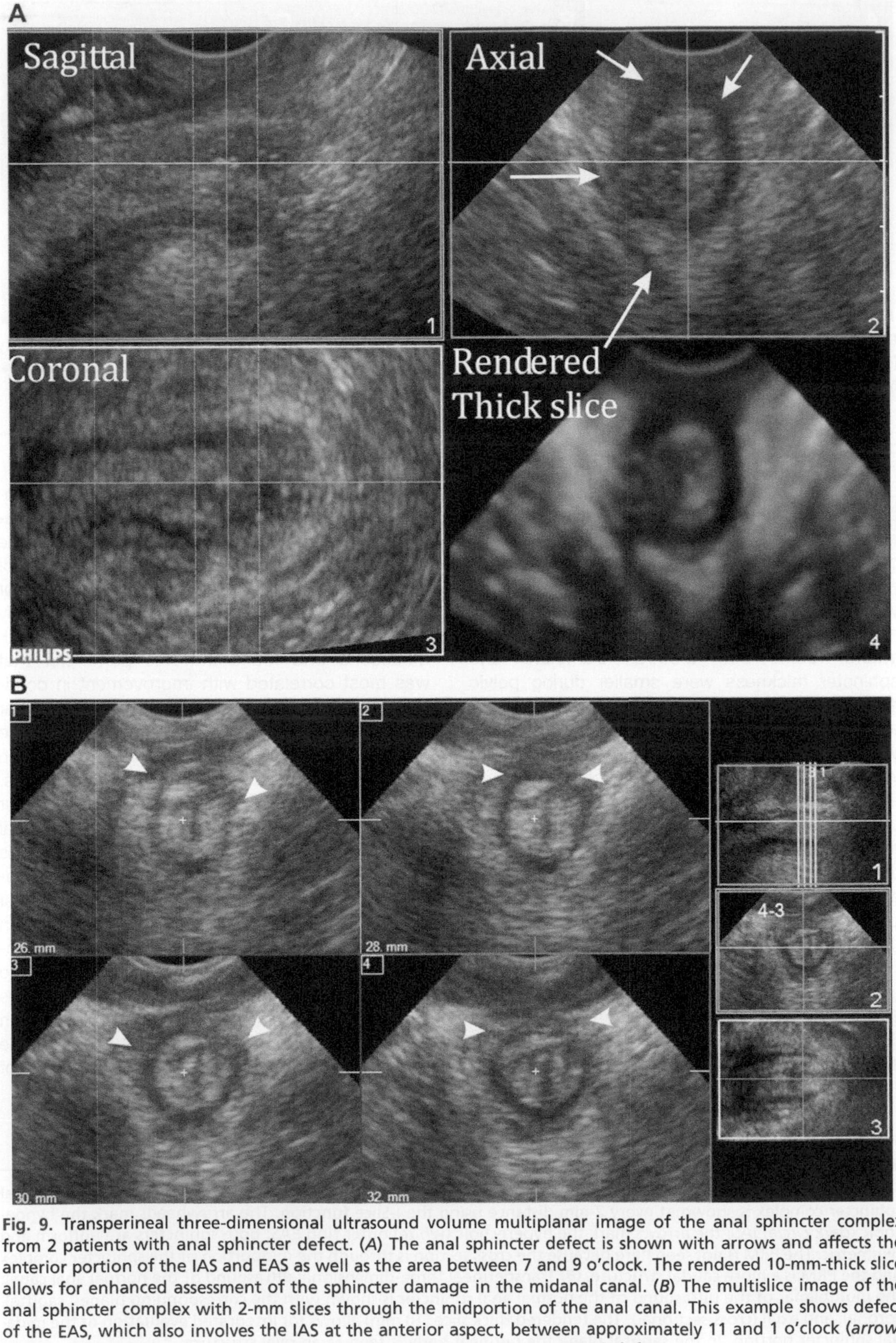

Fig. 9. Transperineal three-dimensional ultrasound volume multiplanar image of the anal sphincter complex from 2 patients with anal sphincter defect. (*A*) The anal sphincter defect is shown with arrows and affects the anterior portion of the IAS and EAS as well as the area between 7 and 9 o'clock. The rendered 10-mm-thick slice allows for enhanced assessment of the sphincter damage in the midanal canal. (*B*) The multislice image of the anal sphincter complex with 2-mm slices through the midportion of the anal canal. This example shows defect of the EAS, which also involves the IAS at the anterior aspect, between approximately 11 and 1 o'clock (*arrowheads*). The anal mucosa shows asymmetry toward the area of the EAS/IAS defect.

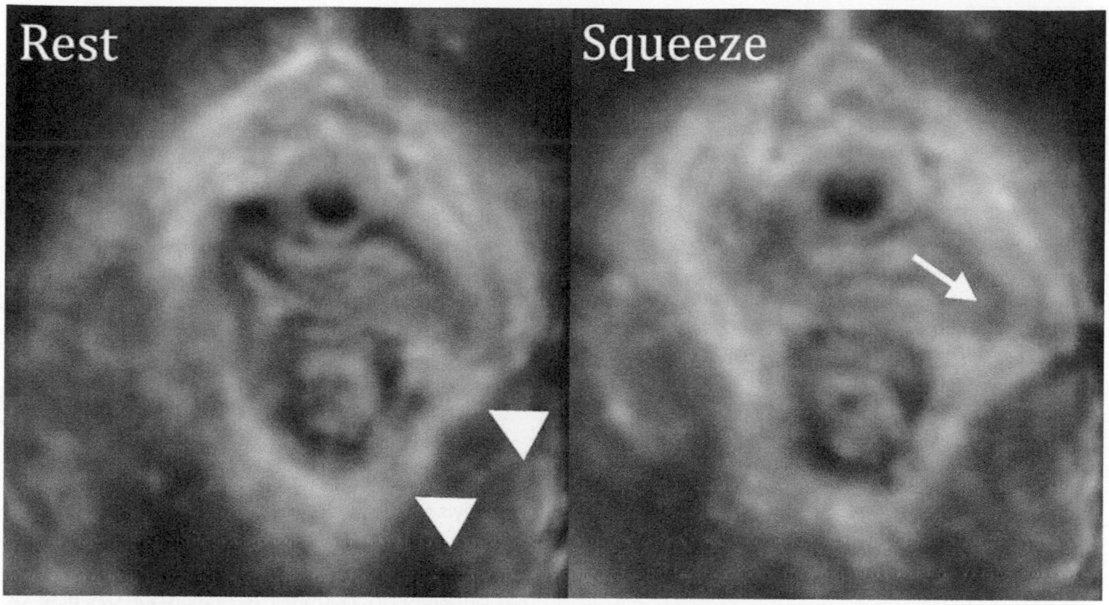

Fig. 10. Dynamic images of the pelvic floor hiatus at rest and during squeeze in the same parous woman. The injury of the PRM (*arrowheads*) is accentuated when during the pelvic floor contraction (squeeze) the pelvic floor hiatus bulges out toward the side of injury (*arrow*).

distribution contributes to a 60% to 80% improvement in continence, whereas an asymmetric distribution is associated with a significantly smaller improvement in continence symptoms.[53,70,71] Poon and Zimmern[53] describe the use of three-dimensional ultrasound as part of their standard algorithm in managing incontinence in patients who undergo periurethral collagen injection. If a patient has no or minimal improvement after collagen injection therapy and ultrasound shows low volume retention of collagen or an asymmetric distribution, the patient is offered a repeat injection in the area of deficiency. If there is no improvement but a circumferential pattern is seen on ultrasound, the injection is considered optimal and the patient is offered an alternative treatment.

Ultrasound can also show the spatial relationship between a suburethral sling, the urethra, and the symphysis pubis at rest and on Valsalva. Urethral slings are usually made out of mesh material, which is easily visualized on ultrasound because it is echogenic. It has been shown to move variably as an arc around the posterior symphysis pubis. Movement closes the gap between the mesh and the bony structure of the pelvic, thereby compressing the urethra during increases in intra-abdominal pressure. The ability to visualize the variability in the location and the movement of the sling allows clinicians to understand why there is variability in the efficacy of the sling and to help determine if the sling needs to be adjusted.[72]

SUMMARY

In summary, pelvic floor ultrasound is a valuable adjunct in elucidation of cause, diagnosis, and treatment of pelvic floor disorders. Three-dimensional ultrasound specifically has been shown to have many advantages over conventional imaging modalities. When using three-dimensional ultrasound, scanning times are short and the technique is noninvasive; there is less user dependency when compared with two-dimensional ultrasound, which contributes to the accuracy of measurements, there is no radiation exposure involved, and it allows for the capturing of images in real time.[53] In addition, three-dimensional ultrasound has proved to be especially useful in the imaging of pelvic organ prolapse as well as the evaluation and treatment of urinary and fecal incontinence, which are disorders that many women face. Proper evaluation of pelvic floor muscle function, strength, and integrity is an important component of diagnosis and treatment of pelvic floor disorders. In addition, the pelvic floor muscle training used to change the structural support and strength of muscle contraction requires clinicians to be able to conduct high-quality measurements of pelvic floor muscle function and strength. Ultrasound has proved to be an extremely useful modality to assess the pelvic floor and its function. As practitioners become more familiar with the advantages and capabilities of ultrasound, this tool should become part of routine clinical practice in evaluation and management of pelvic floor disorders.

REFERENCES

1. Lawrence JM, Lukacz ES, Nager CW, et al. Prevalence and co-occurrence of pelvic floor disorders in community-dwelling women. Obstet Gynecol 2008;111(3):678–85.
2. Bump RC, Hurt WG, Fantl JA, et al. Assessment of Kegel pelvic muscle exercise performance after brief verbal instruction. Am J Obstet Gynecol 1991;165(2):322–7 [discussion: 327–9].
3. Bo K, Sherburn M. Evaluation of female pelvic-floor muscle function and strength. Phys Ther 2005; 85(3):269–82.
4. Olsen AL, Smith VJ, Bergstrom JO, et al. Epidemiology of surgically managed pelvic organ prolapse and urinary incontinence. Obstet Gynecol 1997; 89(4):501–6.
5. Abrams P, Cardozo L, Fall M, et al. The standardisation of terminology of lower urinary tract function: report from the Standardisation Sub-committee of the International Continence Society. Am J Obstet Gynecol 2002;187(1):116–26.
6. Abrams P, Blaivas JG, Stanton SL, et al. Sixth report on the standardisation of terminology of lower urinary tract function. Procedures related to neurophysiological investigations: electromyography, nerve conduction studies, reflex latencies, evoked potentials and sensory testing. The International Continence Society. Br J Urol 1987;59(4): 300–4.
7. Hunskaar S, Burgio K, Diokno A, et al. Epidemiology and natural history of urinary incontinence in women. Urology 2003;62(4 Suppl 1):16–23.
8. Norton CCJ, Butler U, Harari D, et al. Incontinence management. In: Abrams P, Cardozo L, Khoury S, et al, editors. Incontinence. International Consultation on Incontinence, 2001, 2002. 2nd edition. Anal incontinence, vol. 2. Plymouth (UK): Health Publications; 2002. p. 987–1043.
9. Chen GD, Hu SW, Chen YC, et al. Prevalence and correlations of anal incontinence and constipation in Taiwanese women. Neurourol Urodyn 2003; 22(7):664–9.
10. Soligo M, Salvatore S, Milani R, et al. Double incontinence in urogynecologic practice: a new insight. Am J Obstet Gynecol 2003;189(2):438–43.
11. Nichols CM, Gill EJ, Nguyen T, et al. Anal sphincter injury in women with pelvic floor disorders. Obstet Gynecol 2004;104(4):690–6.
12. Shagam JY. Pelvic organ prolapse. Radiol Technol 2006;77(5):389–400 [quiz: 401–3].
13. Kruger JA, Heap SW, Murphy BA, et al. Pelvic floor function in nulliparous women using three-dimensional ultrasound and magnetic resonance imaging. Obstet Gynecol 2008;111(3):631–8.
14. Weinstein MM, Jung SA, Pretorius DH, et al. The reliability of puborectalis muscle measurements with 3-dimensional ultrasound imaging. Am J Obstet Gynecol 2007;197(1):68 e1–e6.
15. Chong AK, Hoffman B. Fecal incontinence related to pregnancy. Gastrointest Endosc Clin N Am 2006; 16(1):71–81.
16. Oberwalder M, Thaler K, Baig MK, et al. Anal ultrasound and endosonographic measurement of perineal body thickness: a new evaluation for fecal incontinence in females. Surg Endosc 2004;18(4): 650–4.
17. Deindl FM, Vodusek DB, Hesse U, et al. Activity patterns of pubococcygeal muscles in nulliparous continent women. Br J Urol 1993;72(1):46–51.
18. Peschers UM, Vodusek DB, Fanger G, et al. Pelvic muscle activity in nulliparous volunteers. Neurourol Urodyn 2001;20(3):269–75.
19. Yang JM, Yang SH, Huang WC. Biometry of the pubovisceral muscle and levator hiatus in nulliparous Chinese women. Ultrasound Obstet Gynecol 2006; 28(5):710–6.
20. Sapsford RR, Hodges PW, Richardson CA, et al. Coactivation of the abdominal and pelvic floor muscles during voluntary exercises. Neurourol Urodyn 2001; 20(1):31–42.
21. Jung SA, Pretorius DH, Padda BS, et al. Vaginal high-pressure zone assessed by dynamic 3-dimensional ultrasound images of the pelvic floor. Am J Obstet Gynecol 2007;197(1):52, e1–7.
22. Lose L. Simultaneous recording of pressure and cross-sectional area in the female urethra: a study of urethral closure function in healthy and stress incontinent women. Neurourol Urodyn 1992;11(2): 55–89.
23. Howard D, Miller JM, Delancey JO, et al. Differential effects of cough, Valsalva, and continence status on vesical neck movement. Obstet Gynecol 2000;95(4): 535–40.
24. Beer-Gabel M, Teshler M, Barzilai N, et al. Dynamic transperineal ultrasound in the diagnosis of pelvic floor disorders: pilot study. Dis Colon Rectum 2002;45(2):239–45 [discussion: 245–8].
25. Weidner AC, Low VH. Imaging studies of the pelvic floor. Obstet Gynecol Clin North Am 1998; 25(4):825–48, vii.
26. Healy JC, Halligan S, Reznek RH, et al. Patterns of prolapse in women with symptoms of pelvic floor weakness: assessment with MR imaging. Radiology 1997;203(1):77–81.
27. Altringer WE, Saclarides TJ, Dominguez JM, et al. Four-contrast defecography: pelvic "floor-oscopy". Dis Colon Rectum 1995;38(7):695–9.
28. Goei R, Kemerink G. Radiation dose in defecography. Radiology 1990;176(1):137–9.
29. Fielding JR, Griffiths DJ, Versi E, et al. MR imaging of pelvic floor continence mechanisms in the supine and sitting positions. AJR Am J Roentgenol 1998; 171(6):1607–10.

30. Falk PM, Blatchford GJ, Cali RL, et al. Transanal ultrasound and manometry in the evaluation of fecal incontinence. Dis Colon Rectum 1994;37(5):468–72.
31. Law PJ, Bartram CI. Anal endosonography: technique and normal anatomy. Gastrointest Radiol 1989;14(4):349–53.
32. Law PJ, Kamm MA, Bartram CI. Anal endosonography in the investigation of faecal incontinence. Br J Surg 1991;78(3):312–4.
33. Law PJ, Kamm MA, Bartram CI. A comparison between electromyography and anal endosonography in mapping external anal sphincter defects. Dis Colon Rectum 1990;33(5):370–3.
34. Nichols CM, Ramakrishnan V, Gill EJ, et al. Anal incontinence in women with and those without pelvic floor disorders. Obstet Gynecol 2005;106(6):1266–71.
35. Gantke B, Schafer A, Enck P, et al. Sonographic, manometric, and myographic evaluation of the anal sphincters morphology and function. Dis Colon Rectum 1993;36(11):1037–41.
36. Gold DM, Halligan S, Kmiot WA, et al. Intraobserver and interobserver agreement in anal endosonography. Br J Surg 1999;86(3):371–5.
37. Mimura T, Kaminishi M, Kamm MA. Diagnostic evaluation of patients with faecal incontinence at a specialist institution. Dig Surg 2004;21(3):235–41 [discussion: 241].
38. Saclarides TJ. Endorectal ultrasound. Surg Clin North Am 1998;78(2):237–49.
39. Sultan AH, Kamm MA, Talbot IC, et al. Anal endosonography for identifying external sphincter defects confirmed histologically. Br J Surg 1994;81(3):463–5.
40. Deen KI, Kumar D, Williams JG, et al. Anal sphincter defects. Correlation between endoanal ultrasound and surgery. Ann Surg 1993;218(2):201–5.
41. Farouk R, Bartolo DC. The use of endoluminal ultrasound in the assessment of patients with faecal incontinence. J R Coll Surg Edinb 1994;39(5):312–8.
42. Ternent CA, Shashidharan M, Blatchford GJ, et al. Transanal ultrasound and anorectal physiology findings affecting continence after sphincteroplasty. Dis Colon Rectum 1997;40(4):462–7.
43. Savoye-Collet C, Savoye G, Koning E, et al. Anal endosonography after sphincter repair: specific patterns related to clinical outcome. Abdom Imaging 1999;24(6):569–73.
44. Faltin DL, Boulvain M, Floris LA, et al. Diagnosis of anal sphincter tears to prevent fecal incontinence: a randomized controlled trial. Obstet Gynecol 2005;106(1):6–13.
45. Zetterstrom JP, Mellgren A, Madoff RD, et al. Perineal body measurement improves evaluation of anterior sphincter lesions during endoanal ultrasonography. Dis Colon Rectum 1998;41(6):705–13.
46. Nielsen MB, Rasmussen OO, Pedersen JF, et al. Anal endosonographic findings in patients with obstructed defecation. Acta Radiol 1993;34(1):35–8.
47. Jackson SL, Weber AM, Hull TL, et al. Fecal incontinence in women with urinary incontinence and pelvic organ prolapse. Obstet Gynecol 1997;89(3): 423–7.
48. Solomon MJ, Pager CK, Rex J, et al. Randomized, controlled trial of biofeedback with anal manometry, transanal ultrasound, or pelvic floor retraining with digital guidance alone in the treatment of mild to moderate fecal incontinence. Dis Colon Rectum 2003;46(6):703–10.
49. Kleinubing H Jr, Jannini JF, Malafaia O, et al. Transperineal ultrasonography: new method to image the anorectal region. Dis Colon Rectum 2000;43(11): 1572–4.
50. Schaer GN, Koechli OR, Schuessler B, et al. Perineal ultrasound for evaluating the bladder neck in urinary stress incontinence. Obstet Gynecol 1995; 85(2):220–4.
51. Shobeiri SA, Nolan TE, Yordan-Jovel R, et al. Digital examination compared to trans-perineal ultrasound for the evaluation of anal sphincter repair. Int J Gynaecol Obstet 2002;78(1):31–6.
52. Minardi D, Parri G, d'Anzeo G. Perineal ultrasound evaluation of dysfunctional voiding in women with recurrent urinary tract infections. J Urol 2008; 179(3):947–51.
53. Poon CI, Zimmern PE. Role of three-dimensional ultrasound in assessment of women undergoing urethral bulking agent therapy. Curr Opin Obstet Gynecol 2004;16(5):411–7.
54. Timor-Tritsch IE, Platt LD. Three-dimensional ultrasound experience in obstetrics. Curr Opin Obstet Gynecol 2002;14(6):569–75.
55. Weinstein MM, Pretorius DH, Jung SA, et al. Transperineal three-dimensional ultrasound imaging for detection of anatomic defects in the anal sphincter complex muscles. Clin Gastroenterol Hepatol 2009;7(2):205–11.
56. Dietz HP, Shek C, Clarke B. Biometry of the pubovisceral muscle and levator hiatus by three-dimensional pelvic floor ultrasound. Ultrasound Obstet Gynecol 2005;25(6):580–5.
57. Sultan AH, Kamm MA, Hudson CN, et al. Anal-sphincter disruption during vaginal delivery. N Engl J Med 1993;329(26):1905–11.
58. DeLancey JO, Kearney R, Chou Q, et al. The appearance of levator ani muscle abnormalities in magnetic resonance images after vaginal delivery. Obstet Gynecol 2003;101(1):46–53.
59. Dietz HP, Lanzarone V. Levator trauma after vaginal delivery. Obstet Gynecol 2005;106(4):707–12.
60. Choi JS, Wexner SD, Nam YS, et al. Intraobserver and interobserver measurements of the anorectal angle and perineal descent in defecography. Dis Colon Rectum 2000;43(8):1121–6.
61. Padda BS, Jung SA, Pretorius D, et al. Effects of pelvic floor muscle contraction on anal canal

pressure. Am J Physiol Gastrointest Liver Physiol 2007;292(2):G565–71.
62. Abdool Z, Shek KL, Dietz HP. The effect of levator avulsion on hiatal dimension and function. Am J Obstet Gynecol 2009;201(1):89 e1–5.
63. Athanasiou S, Khullar V, Boos K, et al. Imaging the urethral sphincter with three-dimensional ultrasound. Obstet Gynecol 1999;94(2):295–301.
64. DeLancey JO. Structural aspects of the extrinsic continence mechanism. Obstet Gynecol 1988;72(3 Pt 1):296–301.
65. Bø K, Stien R. Needle EMG registration of striated urethral wall and pelvic floor muscle activity patterns during cough, Valsalva, abdominal, hip adductor, and gluteal muscle contractions in nulliparous healthy females. Neurourol Urodyn 1994;13(1):35–41.
66. Umek WH, Laml T, Stutterecker D, et al. The urethra during pelvic floor contraction: observations on three-dimensional ultrasound. Obstet Gynecol 2002;100(4):796–800.
67. Monga AK, Robinson D, Stanton SL. Periurethral collagen injections for genuine stress incontinence: a 2-year follow-up. Br J Urol 1995;76(2):156–60.
68. Khullar V, Cardozo LD, Abbott D, et al. GAX collagen in the treatment of urinary incontinence in elderly women: a two year follow up. Br J Obstet Gynaecol 1997;104(1):96–9.
69. Elia G, Bergman A. Periurethral collagen implant: ultrasound assessment and prediction of outcome. Int Urogynecol J Pelvic Floor Dysfunct 1996;7(6):335–8.
70. Defreitas GA, Wilson TS, Zimmern PE, et al. Three-dimensional ultrasonography: an objective outcome tool to assess collagen distribution in women with stress urinary incontinence. Urology 2003;62(2):232–6.
71. Radley SC, Chapple CR, Mitsogiannis IC, et al. Transurethral implantation of macroplastique for the treatment of female stress urinary incontinence secondary to urethral sphincter deficiency. Eur Urol 2001;39(4):383–9.
72. Dietz HP, Wilson PD. The 'iris effect': how two-dimensional and three-dimensional ultrasound can help us understand anti-incontinence procedures. Ultrasound Obstet Gynecol 2004;23(3):267–71.

Index

Note: Page numbers of article titles are in **boldface** type.

Ultrasound Clin 5 (2010) 331–336
doi:10.1016/S1556-858X(10)00119-2
1556-858X/10/$ – see front matter

G

H

I

L

M

N

O

Printed and bound by CPI Group (UK) Ltd, Croydon, CR0 4YY
03/10/2024
01040359-0012